EARLY MANAGEMENT
OF HEARING LOSS

PROCEEDINGS OF THE WINNIPEG CONFERENCE ON EARLY MANAGEMENT OF HEARING LOSS

Winnipeg, Manitoba, April 26–29, 1980

This conference, like its predecessors, was made possible by a grant from the Elks Purple Cross Deaf Detection and Development Program, a philanthropic effort maintained, operated, and funded through the generosity of the Benevolent and Protective Order of Elks of Canada and their auxiliary, The Order of the Royal Purple. The editors and all the conference participants wish to thank the members of those organizations for their contribution in time, money, and personal effort. Without them, it could not be done!!

Grune & Stratton Rapid Manuscript Reproduction

EARLY MANAGEMENT OF HEARING LOSS

Edited by

GEORGE T. MENCHER, Ph.D.

Nova Scotia Hearing and Speech Clinic and
Dalhousie University
Halifax, Nova Scotia, Canada

SANFORD E. GERBER, Ph.D.

Speech and Hearing Center
University of California
Santa Barbara, California

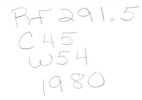

GRUNE & STRATTON

A Subsidiary of Harcourt Brace Jovanovich, Publishers
NEW YORK   LONDON   TORONTO   SYDNEY   SAN FRANCISCO

Library of Congress Cataloging in Publication Data

Winnipeg Conference on Early Management of Hearing
  Loss, 1980.
  Early management of hearing loss.

  "Proceedings of the Winnipeg Conference on Early
Management of Hearing Loss, Winnipeg, Manitoba,
April 26–29, 1980."
  Bibliography
  Includes index.
  1. Hearing disorders in children—Congresses.
2. Children, Deaf—Rehabilitation—Congresses.
I. Mencher, George T.   II. Gerber, Sanford E.
III. Title. [DNLM: 1. Hearing disorders—In infancy
and childhood—Congresses.   2. Hearing disorders—
Therapy—Congresses.   WV 271 E12]
RF291.5.C45W54 1980   618.92'0978   80–25992
ISBN 0–8089–1346–8

Grune & Stratton, Inc.
111 Fifth Avenue
New York, New York 10003

Distributed in the United Kingdom by
Academic Press Inc. (London) Ltd.
24/28 Oval Road, London NW 1

Library of Congress Catalog Number 80-25992
International Standard Book Number 0-8089-1346-8

Printed in the United States of America

TO THE CHILDREN
who make it possible for us to enjoy our work.

TABLE OF CONTENTS

viii   Contents

Contents   ix

LIST OF CONTRIBUTORS

PATRICK ALEXANDER, Ph.D.
Consultant, Division of Speech
 and Hearing
British Columbia Ministry of Health
Victoria, British Columbia, Canada

GYLFI BALDURSSON
Supervisor of Audiology
Nova Scotia Hearing and Speech
 Clinic
Halifax, Nova Scotia, Canada

OLE BENTZEN, M.D.
Professor of Audiology
The State Hearing Institute
Århus, Denmark

DENZIL N. BROOKS, Ph.D.
Principal Physicist
Manchester Area Health Authority,
 South District
Regional Audiology Unit
Withington Hospital
Manchester, England

DAVID J. BYRNE, M.Ed.
Director, Niagara Research Unit
Mary Sheridan Unit
Borocourt Hospital
Reading, Berkshire, England

ROBERT K. COULLING
Executive Director and Chairman
 of the Board
Elks Purple Cross Deaf Detection
 and Development Program
Regina, Saskatchewan, Canada

VICTOR deC. MAGIAN, M.D.
ENT Consultant
Office of Hearing Conservation
Department of Health and Social
 Development
Winnipeg, Manitoba, Canada

MARION P. DOWNS, M.A.
Professor of Audiology
Division of Audiology
University of Colorado
Health Sciences Center
Denver, Colorado

MOSHE FEINMESSER, M.D.
Professor and Head
Department of Otolaryngology
Hadassah University Hospital
Jerusalem, Israel

GARY FISHMAN, M.D.
Rose F. Kennedy Center for
  Research in Human
  Development and Mental
  Retardation
Yeshiva University
New York, New York

SANFORD E. GERBER, Ph.D.
Professor and Chairman
Department of Speech
University of California
Santa Barbara, California

GRACE M. HARRIS, M.A.
Supervisor, Society for Crippled
  Children and Adults of
  Manitoba
Winnipeg, Manitoba, Canada

JOHN T. JACOBSON, Ph.D.
Associate Professor of Audiology
Dalhousie University
School of Human Communication
  Disorders
Halifax, Nova Scotia, Canada

JANNE HARTVIG JENSEN, M.D.
Division of Audiology
The State Hearing Institute
Århus, Denmark

CHAYA LEVI, M.A.
Division of Audiology
Department of Otolaryngology
Hadassah University Hospital
Jerusalem, Israel

DANIEL LING, Ph.D.
Professor, School of Human
  Communication Disorders
McGill University
Montreal, Quebec, Canada

EDGAR J. LOWELL, Ph.D.
Director, John Tracy Clinic
Los Angeles, California

ENELDA LUTTMAN, B.A.
Director, Orientacion Infanitil Par
  Rehabilitation
Protasic Table 103
Mexico City, Mexico

GEORGE T. MENCHER, Ph.D.
Director, Nova Scotia Hearing and
  Speech Clinic
Professor of Audiology
School of Human Communication
  Disorders
Dalhousie University
Halifax, Nova Scotia, Canada

LENORE MENCHER, M.A.
Co-ordinator, Hearing Screening
  Program
Nova Scotia Hearing and Speech
  Clinic
Halifax, Nova Scotia, Canada

KENNETH L. MOSES, Ph.D.
Clinical Psychologist
930 Maple Avenue
Evanston, Illinois

KEVIN P. MURPHY, Ph.D.
Audiology Unit
Royal Berkshire Hospital
Reading, Berkshire, England

LINDA W. NOBER, Ed.D.
Assistant Professor of Special
  Education
Westfield State College
Westfield, Massachusetts

JERRY L. NORTHERN, Ph.D.
Professor of Otolaryngology
Head, Division of Audiology
University of Colorado
Health Sciences Center
Denver, Colorado

VALERIE PARROTT, M.Sc.
Clinical Audiologist
Janeway Child Health Centre
St. John's, Newfoundland, Canada

AGNES H. LING PHILLIPS, Ph.D.
Associate Professor of Audiology
School of Human Communication
   Disorders
Dalhousie University
Halifax, Nova Scotia, Canada

DOREEN POLLACK, L.C.S.T., B.A.
Director, Speech and Hearing
   Services
Porter Memorial Hospital
Denver, Colorado

CAROL A. PRUTTING, Ph.D.
Associate Professor of Speech
   Pathology
Speech and Hearing Center
University of California
Santa Barbara, California

ROBERT J. RUBEN, M.D.
Chairman and Professor
Department of Otolaryngology
Albert Einstein College of
   Medicine
Yeshiva University
Bronx, New York

MARTHA RUBIN, Ph.D.
Director, Lexington Hearing and
   Speech Centre
Lexington School for the Deaf
Jackson Heights, New York

MICHAEL R. SEITZ, Ph.D.
Associate Professor
Department of Biocommunications
University of Alabama at
   Birmingham
Children's Hospital
Birmingham, Alabama

D. ROBERT SHEA, M.D.
Consultant Pediatrician
Department of Pediatrics
Glenrose Hospital
Edmonton, Alberta, Canada

ANDREE SMITH, Ph.D.
Director, Audiology Department
Children's Hospital of Eastern
   Ontario
Ottawa, Ontario, Canada

LILLY TELL, M.A.
Division of Audiology
Department of Otolaryngology
Hadassah University Hospital
Jerusalem, Israel

**MADELEINE VAN
   HECK-WULATIN, Ph.D.**
Assistant Professor
Department of Psychology
North Central College
Naperville, Illinois

PREFACE

The Third Elks International Conference was held in Winnipeg, Manitoba, April 26–29, 1980. Entitled "Early Management of Hearing Loss," it was a natural extension of the previous two meetings, "Early Identification of Hearing Loss" and "Early Diagnosis of Hearing Loss," held in Halifax, Nova Scotia (1974), and in Saskatoon, Saskatchewan (1978), respectively. Once again, our outlook was international, there being representatives from six different countries, each reporting a variety of experiences and points of view.

We sought specific management techniques and proposals we could offer the reader. Unfortunately, management recommendations are not as easily quantified, or so clearly defined, as those for identification and diagnosis. Although there is uniformity both in some of the habilitative procedures and in the extent to which they succeed, unfortunately it was difficult for us to isolate which specific procedures help achieve which specific successes. That is to say, while we seemed to know when there had been success in management, we had difficulty defining what it is that successful programs have in common. Some of the participants drafted a statement on early language development. The fact that we could not unanimously agree on its acceptance and universality (see Editors' Comment on pages 1–5) reminds us that we do not know when and how to make some of the most critical decisions in early management. As the conference progressed, it became more and more obvious there was a lack of quantitative and prognostic data on management. Thus, a principle outcome of the conference is an appeal for quantitative, if descriptive, research in the area of methods of achieving language development for the severely hearing-impaired baby.

A major portion of the conference dealt with medical management, and in its formal papers presented the pediatric, otologic, and multi-disciplinary perspectives. They stressed, as did all the others, the growth, gaps, and obligations outlined in the keynote address of Grace M. Harris. In response, we wrote recommendations and passed resolutions dealing with medical management.

The conference attendees also considered family—child management. Of major concern was the problem of counselling the family who learns they have a child with a hearing impairment; and just as important, starting the family on a constructive road with an auditory habilitative program. We, therefore, wrote recommendations on family counselling.

As one might expect, the issues of audiological management appear to be even more easily defined than those of family—child management. Yet, even there, we had to deal with the elusive. One issue concerned the potential of acoustic trauma associated with over-fitting a hearing aid on a baby. Discussion included such issues as, "What should be recommended? How much amplification is 'too much?' Is there an absolute limit for any child? Can children with mild conductive hearing losses benefit from amplification?"

The acoustic impedance battery was also reviewed. Those procedures continue to have applicability, not only in diagnosis, but in the ongoing evaluation of the hearing impaired child. Children with sensory—neural hearing impairment are not exempt from middle ear disease, and we recommend they should be screened with impedance on a regular basis. Furthermore, since reflex testing procedures appear to have applicability in evaluating the effectiveness of amplification, we recommend consideration of this procedure as well.

Conferences and their proceedings do not arise spontaneously from the soil of Manitoba. Like hearing-impaired infants, they are conceived, developed, born, raised, and sometimes, habilitated. We may take credit for conception, and some of the labour pains involved in preparing the conference and editing the proceedings, but delivery of the particular infant has rested with several persons very important to us. As always, Robert K. Coulling is "the Grandfather" of the Elks Conference, if we are the fathers. It is entirely through the generosity and concerned efforts of the BPO Elks and their auxiliary, The Order of the Royal Purple, under the firm, guiding, and often sweaty palm (from good old-fashioned hard work) of Bob Coulling that these conferences are possible. We must repeatedly express gratitude to the Elks and, especially thank and praise

Bob, on behalf of the hearing-impaired infants who benefit from their endeavors.

If Bob is the grandfather of the Elks Conferences, certainly Ms. Marion Neild is the mother of this one. Ms. Neild made all of our local arrangements in Winnipeg and stayed with us from early in the morning until late at night doing all the nasty, little chores which needed to be done. It seemed that she was always quietly and efficiently in the background, and all the little details that needed attention got it. We are grateful to her for making the Winnipeg Conference fun.

The Manitoba Speech and Hearing Association was of great benefit to us from early on. The public meetings on the first day and one-half were within their purview and came off admirably. As our leprechaun in residence, Kevin Murphy, was heard to say, "A tip o' me hat ta ya!!"

What can we say about Debbie Jorgenson? She stayed up late at night to type our papers, got up early in the morning to type our papers, went upstairs to type our papers, and through it all had the brightest smile around. To Debbie we owe whatever organization we maintained throughout the entire conference.

Other people and groups also deserve special thanks. The Audio-Visual Department at the Izaak Walton Killam Hospital for Children in Halifax came through again. Horst Peppel recorded all the sessions and made the transcription of the questions-answers possible. The Board of Directors and staff of the Nova Scotia Hearing and Speech Clinic tolerated George Mencher's absence and allowed him time to prepare the text, as the University of California at Santa Barbara staff did for Sandy Gerber.

The seventeen conferees from six countries who joined the two of us in Winnipeg are the ones who obviously made the conference occur. Each of them worked hard, diligently, intelligently, and with great concern for the other's point of view. We told them at the beginning of the conference that we would fight, argue, scream, and yell; but when we went home, we would love each other again. We hope that is true. Certainly, we love them for their brilliance and their devotion to the hearing-impaired child. We offer the following resolution to them:

WHEREAS, we invited only Superstars to this Conference;

AND WHEREAS, those invited exceeded expectations, proved that they were better than ordinary superstars, and have contributed so much toward improving the quality of life of their fellow man;

RESOLVED: Henceforth they shall be known as Super-Duper-Stars

AND WE MEAN IT!!

Above all, our gratitude goes to those very children to whom this volume is dedicated. They make it worthwhile.

And last but never least, the most tolerant ladies in the world, Lenore and Louise, let us do it again. We only hope it justifies your sacrifices.

George T. Mencher, Ph.D.
Sanford E. Gerber, Ph.D.

EARLY MANAGEMENT
OF HEARING LOSS

RECOMMENDATIONS FROM THE WINNIPEG CONFERENCE ON THE EARLY MANAGEMENT OF HEARING LOSS

Preamble

The primary focus of this conference is <u>early</u> management with the ultimate goal of maximizing the quality of life of the child who has a hearing loss. This conference, as the previous two conferences, emphasizes the care of the infant up to the age of six months, but not to the exclusion of the older baby. Help for the infant who has a hearing loss, and his family, begins at the time of identification, irrespective of age, and continues through and beyond infancy.

All of us who take responsibility for management, recognize individual differences, but must also attend to general principles of child and family psychosocial development. These principles are best employed through systematic and well-organized delivery of services by a team of professionals. We are concerned about the deleterious effects upon the infant with hearing impairment of inaction or inadequate support at each development stage. Thus, as advocates for the child who has a hearing impairment, we urge the implementation of the following resolutions.

We resolve to assure -- and, where possible, to provide -- all means which accrue to the benefit of the hearing impaired infant. These means include early identification, early diagnosis, and early management -- procedures which are both sequential and simultaneous. We recognize the difference between the ideal and the reality. Here we resolve the ideal in the wish that in so doing, the reality will come closer to it. The reality is that there is diversity across habilitative practices, but there are commonalities. For the benefit of the infant, we stress the commonalities.

I. Editor's Comment

Management of hearing loss has, to this point, been less of a quantitative science than either identification or diagnosis. Consequently, some of the recommendations which follow tend to be more in the form of what habilitationists and researchers might do, than in the form of what diagnosticians and clinicians should do.

The recommendations follow the arbitrary sequence of medical management, audiological management, family-child management, and general habilitative management. Those for medical management are, undoubtedly, more tangible than those concerned with general habilitative management. However, we believe that all are truly far-reaching and, we hope, will have a significant impact on the treatment of hearing impaired children all over the world.

These recommendations were drafted only after detailed discussion and concern. The participants at the conference met and discussed each of the issues, divided into sub-committees for the purpose of drafting proposed resolutions, and then met as a committee of the whole to review, consider, debate, and adopt or reject the work presented by each sub-committee. Each recommendation has received extensive review and is bound to a detailed research base or the combined experience of a group of the world's foremost experts in early management of hearing loss.

The recommendations we offer were adopted unanimously by all those in attendance, and thus represent commonalities which may be found amongst the divergent philosophies of early management of hearing loss.

Noticeably absent is a specific recommendation as to the best method to develop language in the severely impaired infant. The reader should not assume that this is an over-sight. On the contrary, that topic occupied a great deal of our time; indeed, more so than any other topic. After much discussion, a sub-committee was formed to draft a statement with respect to a common procedure we could all recommend. After long hours of debate and discussion, the statement was brought to the entire group for review, modification, and, if possible, adoption. We could not agree to unanimously accept the statement as written and, thus, there is no recommenda-tion for a specific procedure for the development of language in hearing impaired infants. It is not our purpose to side with any of the groups which sought to pass or reject the statement, but merely to reflect arguments so that the reader may follow our discussion and, we hope, have a better under-standing of all the issues. The statement which was rejected may be seen as Figure 1.

FIGURE 1:   Statement of Speech and Language Development

NOT ADOPTED

Because the use of spoken language offers the widest
range of opportunity for personal, social, linguistic, educational and economic development, hearing-impaired infants
should be given optimal opportunity to develop spoken language communication from early infancy.   Thus, we recommend
whenever and wherever possible, to begin training with a
spoken language communication approach.

To suggest that speech development is best fostered by
early and exclusive interaction through spoken language is
not to claim that all children can, or should be expected to
develop high level speech communication skills through the
use of residual hearing.   It would be appropriate to support
the use of a visual-oral system (e.g., Cued Speech) with that
minority of children who have little or no useful audition,
or who fail to develop verbal skills adequately through an
early auditory-oral approach.   It would be equally appropriate to support the use of manual codes, sign systems, sign
language (such as American Sign Language), and/or fingerspelling as a supplement or alternative to auditory-oral
training, or their use in the context of total communication
with those whose parents wish it; with those who cannot learn
to communicate by speech; with those whose spoken language,
given exemplary teaching, cannot be developed sufficiently to
realize their potential both pre-academically and personally;
and those, who, at a later stage, having acquired high levels
of oral skills, wish to become bilingual in speech and sign
and, thus, be able to communicate with their non-oral peers.
One of the most profound problems we face as professionals
is knowing when and how to make these decisions.

Ongoing monitoring in the form of objective evaluation
may indicate necessary modifications of the program.   A high
priority should be given to the improvement of evaluation
measures.   If a change to another type of program is deemed
necessary, it should be on the recommendation of the management team, which will include the teacher-clinician working
with the child.

Some of the attendees at the conference believe that, for the majority of hearing impaired infants, spoken language alone should be utilized during the early training period. They believe that if spoken language does not prove to be optimal as the prime communicative system for the child, then at some later point an alternative approach or approaches should be utilized. They believe that the early and exclusive use of oral language will, for the majority of hearing impaired children, enhance the development of speech and, thus, lead to normal psychosocial development and function within the hearing world. They also believe that simultaneous use of a manual and oral system will inhibit development of spoken language and, thus, restrict achievement of full potential. They argue that because you cannot predict the success of language and speech development, it is essential to give the child every opportunity to develop an oral language before inhibiting it with a manual system.

The other group of participants believe that the child should be submerged in a total communication environment utilizing both spoken language and the sign language of the country, a bilingual approach. They believe that early use of all modes of communication encourages language development, thereby enhancing early psycho-social and cognitive development. They also believe that a true total communication approach will not restrict or limit normal speech development, nor restrict achievement of full potential within the hearing world. They argue that because you cannot predict the success of language and speech development, it is essential to give the child every opportunity to develop language and that a total (auditory-oral-manual) approach will provide that opportunity without inhibiting the development of oral language.

The issue, therefore, is whether you begin with an oral language and, if deemed necessary, offer an alternative at a later date; or, begin by offering a total or parallel language environment consisting of both spoken and sign languages. At present, there are conflicting research findings with respect to both of these positions and the associated issues. We are in need of further research to be able to differentiate the effects of deafness from those of methodological management and, additionally, to develop tools for predicting which children will learn and function best under which management system. One of the recommendations of this conference (Recommendation Number 20) speaks specifically to that point.

One of the most profound issues facing professionals at this time is learning how and when to make the intervention decision. Even so, the single most significant issue to which we all unanimously agreed was, no matter which methodology or philosophy to which we subscribe, we are all profoundly committed to working toward the welfare of those with hearing impairment.

George T. Mencher, Ph.D.

Sanford E. Gerber, Ph.D.

II.   Position Statement

The conference attendees unanimously agreed to two
philosophic concepts which, while certainly part of the
recommendations of the meeting, lend themselves to a slightly
different format for their presentations. They are offered
here as Position Statements.

A.   POSITION STATEMENT: FAMILY/CHILD MANAGEMENT

   1.   Our approach to management begins with the primacy
        of the family:

        a)   Therapy should not abrogate the rights and
             responsibilities of the family,

        b)   The family cannot discharge this responsibility
             without proper information,

        c)   The family cannot absorb information without
             appropriate emotional support for their personal
             growth,

        d)   The family is to be regarded by professionals
             as valuable team members who will contribute to
             the corpus of information upon which long-term
             and continuing diagnostic therapy will be based.

   2.   Information for the parents, to be given over time
        as part of the ongoing, individualized diagnostic
        therapy program, is identified under the following
        headings:

        a)   Knowledge of hearing, hearing loss and amplifi-
             cation,

        b)   Knowledge of care, maintenance, and function of
             hearing aids,

        c)   The creation of a normal living, learning and
             linguistic environment, which includes:

             (1)   normal child development and behaviour
                   management,
             (2)   speech and language development,
             (3)   addressing problems in addition to hearing
                   loss,
             (4)   alternate methods of communication,
             (5)   relationship of child to society,

    d)   Genetics,

    e)   How to evaluate an educational system,

    f)   Problems when deafness is not the major
        disability,

    g)   Availability and utilization of community
        services,

    h)   Legal rights.

3. Parents should be given emotional support to cope with the hearing loss with the fact that, at the present state of knowledge, with the exception of conductive problems, the loss is not likely to respond to medical treatment. This support should be directed to individual needs, but groups provide a potent method of support. Parent-to-parent support is to be encouraged, particularly in rural or dispersed communities. Professionals must not, and should not, abrogate the rights and responsibilities of the parents, and particularly, should not intervene in such a manner as to interfere with the family's opportunities to learn and grow with experience. Professional over-zealousness can be counter-productive to the parents' development of independence.

B. POSITION STATEMENT: MODEL FOR DEVELOPING COMMUNICATION

Habilitation in infancy must be based on a normal developmental model. Within such a model communication is viewed as synergistic behaviour,* thus, no part of the system can be regarded separately, and all must be considered in guiding management.

The communicative system involves the interaction of two persons, as illustrated in the following model:

----

* "Synergy means behaviour of whole systems unpredicted by the behaviour of their parts taken separately." -

R. Buckminster Fuller, <u>Synergetics</u> (New York: MacMillan Co.), 1975.

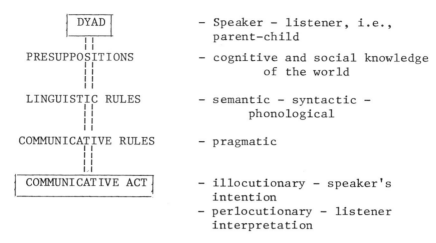

DYAD	– Speaker – listener, i.e., parent-child
PRESUPPOSITIONS	– cognitive and social knowledge of the world
LINGUISTIC RULES	– semantic – syntactic – phonological
COMMUNICATIVE RULES	– pragmatic
COMMUNICATIVE ACT	– illocutionary – speaker's intention – perlocutionary – listener interpretation

It is essential that there be common terminology as broad guidelines are developed within a developmental model for serving the infant who is hearing impaired. These guidelines provide information for the content and sequencing of communicative behaviour.

Broad Guidelines

The communicative system is viewed as having the following integral parts which should be viewed as synergistic in nature and should be addressed in early management:

    1. Social and emotional

    2. Cognitive

    3. Pragmatic

    4. Semantics

    5. Syntax

    6. Phonology

Within the framework of these six components of the communicative system are outlined broad guidelines for habilitative planning along developmental lines. It is felt that these guidelines apply, regardless of methodology, and can, therefore, be utilized in the early intervention

COMMUNICATIVE DEVELOPMENTAL GUIDELINES FOR FIRST TWO YEARS

0 - 12 Months

Cognitive and Social: Behaviours prerequisite to the establishment of the first word: symbolic play, tool use, imitation, communicative intentions (showing, pointing and giving).

Phonological: Stimulation and development of babbling.

12 - 18 Months

Establishment of a first lexicon: Pragmatic - Semantic

Pragmatic	Semantic	
describe	agent	action
request	location	negation
response	object	possession
label	event	recurrence

18 - 24 Months

Establishment of beginning syntax: Semantic - Syntactic and Pragmatic

Semantic - Syntactic:	
agent - action	recurrence
agent - object	adjectival
action - object	description
negation (denial,	possession
rejection, non-	
existence)	

Pragmatic:
child can use language in expanded contexts and for a variety of reasons.

NOTE: These guidelines should be used within a + or - 6 mo. range to account for individual rates of development.

9

of verbal, vocal, and/or non-verbal behaviour.

REFERENCES

Included is a list of references which will be helpful
in the early management of the young, deaf child.

Bradford, L.W. and Hardy, W.G. (eds.) Hearing and Hearing
    Impairment (New York: Grune and Stratton), 1979.

Bates, E., et al. The Emergence of Symbols (New York:
    Academic Press), 1979.

Bloom, L. and Lahey, M. Language Development and Language
    Disorders (New York: John Wiley and Sons), 1978.

Brown, R. A First Language (Cambridge: Harvard University
    Press), 1973.

Calvert, D.R. and Silverman, S.R. Speech and Deafness
    (Washington, D.C.: Alexander Graham Bell Association
    for the Deaf, Inc.), 1975.

Conrad, R. "Let the Children Choose", International Journal
    of Pediatric Otorhinolaryngology 1:317 - 329, 1980.

Erickson, E. Childhood and Society (New York: Norton), 1950.

Harris, G.M. Language for the Preschool Deaf Child (New York:
    Grune and Stratton), 3rd edition, 1971.

Jaffe, B.F. (ed.) Hearing Loss in Children (Baltimore,
    Maryland: University Park Press), 1971.

Ling, D. and Ling, A.H. Aural Habilitation (Washington, D.C.:
    Alexander Graham Bell Association for the Deaf, Inc.),
    1978.

Northcott, W.H. Hearing-Impaired Children, Birth to Three
    Years, and Their Parents, Curriculum Guide ·(Washington,
    D.C.: Alexander Graham Bell Association for the Deaf,
    Inc.), 1975.

Piaget, J. The Language and Thought of the Child (Cleveland:
    World Publishing), 1928. (or any other text on Piaget's
    developmental stage theory of development).

Pollack, D. Educational Audiology for the Limited Hearing
    Infant (Springfield, Illinois: Charles C. Thomas), 1970.

Prutting, C.A. and Skarakis, E.A. "Communication Develop-
    ment", in Audiometry in Infancy, S.E. Gerber (ed.) (New
    York: Grune and Stratton), 1977.

Schlesinger, H. and Meadow, K. Sound and Sign: Childhood
    Deafness and Mental Health (Berkeley, California: Univer-
    sity of California Press), 1972.

Schlesinger, I.M. and Manir, L. Sign Language of the Deaf:
    Psychological, Linguistic and Sociological Perspectives
    (New York: Academic Press), 1978.

Simmons-Martin, A. and Calvert, D.R. Parent-Infant Inter-
    vention - Communication Disorders (New York: Grune and
    Stratton), 1979.

III. Recommendations Unanimously Adopted

    1. WHEREAS, the resolutions and recommendations of
        both the Halifax, Nova Scotia, (1974), and Saskatoon,
        Saskatchewan, (1978), conferences are still applic-
        able and germane to the early identification and
        diagnosis of hearing loss;

        AND WHEREAS, in the intervening years the recommen-
        dations of those conferences have been widely
        adopted and successfully applied.

        BE IT RESOLVED
        We re-affirm the resolutions and recommendations of
        the Nova Scotia Conference on the Early Identifica-
        tion of Hearing Loss and the Saskatoon Conference on
        the Early Diagnosis of Hearing Loss (see Appendices
        1 and 2).

2. WHEREAS, the infant is a complex organism with many
    interrelated systems;

    AND WHEREAS, hearing loss exists in such a complex
    organism;

    AND WHEREAS, infants with hearing impairment may have
    other organ systems affected, and the onset of other
    defects may occur at the time of the hearing impair-
    ment, or at a later time;

    AND WHEREAS, a hearing impaired infant will benefit
    from the consultation of many specialists.

    BE IT RESOLVED
    A team of consulting specialists should be involved
    in the diagnosis and ongoing monitoring of the hear-
    ing impaired child and that, ideally and whenever
    possible, the following expertise should be avail-
    able: audiologist, developmentalist, educator of
    the deaf, geneticist, otolaryngologist, pediatrician,
    psychiatrist, psychologist, social worker, speech-
    language pathologist, and visiting nurse, as well
    as the availability of other specialists, where
    relevant; and

    BE IT FURTHER RESOLVED
    The team should be responsible for:

    1) initial diagnosis of hearing loss and assessment
        of pediatric, psychosocial and speech-language
        status;*

    2) ongoing review of achievement in educational pro-
        gram and audiological, medical**, psychosocial
        and speech-language status;

---

*   All infants identified as hearing impaired should have
    ophthalmological, neurological, developmental, vestibular
    and otological evaluations at the time of diagnosis; and
    all families that have known genetic factors or in which
    genetic factors cannot be ruled out, should be given
    appropriate genetic counselling.

** Including the "second look" described by Downs in this
    volume, in The Team Approach to Congenital Deafness.

3. WHEREAS, it is not common knowledge in the medical
    community that the hearing ability of an infant may
    be assessed immediately after birth;

    AND WHEREAS, it is not common knowledge in the
    medical community that there are efficacious pro-
    cedures for the care of hearing impairment in
    infants which are available at any age;

    AND WHEREAS, this lack of information is deleterious
    to the case finding and referral of infants for
    diagnosis and care;

    AND WHEREAS, physicians must be able to make appro-
    priate referrals.

    BE IT RESOLVED
    1) A course in communicative disorders and a demon-
        stration of competence should be required of all
        medical students before they receive the degree
        of medicine;

    2) All physicians in training in the area of primary
        practice, pediatrics, neurology, ophthalmology,
        and otolaryngology should be required to study
        and demonstrate competence in communicative dis-
        orders, and this should be part of the criteria
        for specialty certification in these areas; and

    3) Continuing education in communicative disorders
        should be required of all physicians who
        practice primary care, pediatrics, neurology
        and otolaryngology.

4. WHEREAS, the delayed identification of additional
    disorders and disabilities creates problems for the
    effective management of children with hearing
    impairment;

    AND WHEREAS, the growth of information concerning
    deafness and its complications is increasing
    rapidly;

AND WHEREAS, the presence of hearing impairment in children who have other disabilities may be a serious barrier to both diagnosis and management.

BE IT RESOLVED
1) Those responsible for providing health care services be alerted to the significance of multiple disability, its identification and management;

2) Preparation and training of health care providers should take into account the most recent developments in information available concerning multiple disabilities;

3) Those providing services to the hearing impaired and/or multiply handicapped children should have easily available access to various types of continuing education.

5. WHEREAS, hearing impaired infants can, and frequently do, acquire other otological diseases;

AND WHEREAS, hearing disorders of hearing impaired infants can be progressive.

BE IT RESOLVED
1) Hearing impaired children less than three years of age should have at least three examinations each year by an otologist and an audiologist; and

2) The frequency of otological evaluation should be increased to more than three per year if conditions in the child indicate a change or changes in the disease process(es).

6. WHEREAS, treatment of the hearing impaired infant with hearing aids is a critical component in the development of optimal spoken language;

AND WHEREAS, following suspicion of hearing loss and estimate of hearing sensitivity, there is a need to use amplification as soon as possible after birth in order to avoid the deleterious effects of delay;

AND WHEREAS, appropriate amplification should be provided within a five to six week period after identification of hearing loss.

BE IT RESOLVED
1) Hearing impaired infants, regardless of age, should be provided with amplification as soon as possible after an estimate of diminished hearing sensitivity is made;

2) Intervention should be of the same quality of care for all children, regardless of other handicaps;

3) There should be ready availability of hearing aids for immediate use; and

4) Consideration should be given to limiting the SSPL 90 (See ANSI S3.22 - standard for specification of hearing aid characteristics, 1976), of hearing aids to 120 dB SPL for pure sensory-neural losses, and appropriately higher SPLs for mixed or conductive losses or other cases, according to the clinician's judgment.

7. WHEREAS, post auricular aids have the advantage of improved signal-to-noise ratio, and localization in space;

AND WHEREAS, ear level aids produce electro-acoustical characteristics in an infant's ear comparable to body-worn aids.

BE IT RESOLVED
Post-auricular aids should be the fitting of choice for infants whenever possible, but that body-worn aids are still an acceptable alternative.

8. WHEREAS, ventilating tubes have been successfully
    placed in the tympanic membranes of infants who also
    have sensory-neural hearing loss;

    AND WHEREAS, this form of treatment has resulted in
    an improved hearing level;

    AND WHEREAS, this form of treatment is compatible
    with the use of a hearing aid.

    BE IT RESOLVED
    1) Ventilating tubes, when indicated, may be placed
        in the tympanic membranes of infants who use
        hearing aids; and

    2) Hearing aids can be worn effectively when
        ventilating tubes are in place.

9. WHEREAS, the complete battery of impedance tests,
    when performed by knowledgeable and skilled profess-
    ionals, has been shown to correlate highly with
    pneumatic otoscopy;

    AND WHEREAS, middle ear disease may have a substan-
    tial bearing on the effectiveness of hearing aid
    amplification;

    BE IT RESOLVED
    1) Skilled and knowledgeable professionals should
        be the operators for the infant impedance
        program;

    2) The impedance battery (tympanometry and acoustic
        reflex measurement) should be used:
        a. as a prerequisite for hearing aid evaluation;
            and
        b. routinely, to monitor the middle ear status
            of those wearing hearing aids.

    3) Every center or professional dealing with hear-
        ing impaired children should have access to the
        impedance battery; and

4) The frequency of testing should be at least that
    recommended for otologic/audiologic examination
    (Resolution # 5). Especially should it be more
    frequent in infants wearing hearing aids who are
    in the at-risk groups for middle ear effusion
    (Resolution # 11).

10. WHEREAS, studies have shown a high incidence of
    middle ear effusion in otherwise normal infants;

    AND WHEREAS, children with constant or fluctuating
    middle ear effusion are at risk for short or long
    term auditory language learning problems and
    emotional problems.

    BE IT RESOLVED
    1) No infant should be allowed to have more than
        three months of recurrent or constant middle
        ear effusion without medical intervention, and
        if this is not efficacious, educational inter-
        vention should be immediately instituted; and

    2) Educational intervention can be concomitant
        with an ongoing medical intervention.

11. WHEREAS, there are populations who are at particu-
    lar risk for middle ear effusion, and that these
    include:

    Cleft Palate and Cranio-facila anomalies
    Down's Syndrome
    Other relevant syndromes*
    Post-natal viral infections
    Premature infants, particularly those who have
      experienced naso-tracheal intubation
    Rubella or other prenatal viral diseases.

---

* cf. Saskatoon proceedings, Early Diagnosis of Hearing
        Loss, Appendices C and E.

BE IT RESOLVED
1) Systematic pneumatic otoscopy and impedance
   testing (tympanometry and acoustic reflex tests)
   should be done on those populations known to be
   at risk for middle ear effusion during the first
   year of life; and

2) Those responsible for pediatric management
   should also be aware of evidence suggesting
   a higher incidence of middle ear effusion in
   infants who are not breast fed.

12. WHEREAS, the early habilitation of hearing impaired
    children is currently being carried out by a variety
    of professionals including speech-language patholo-
    gists, audiologists, and/or teachers of the hearing
    impaired;

    AND WHEREAS, the training for any one of these pro-
    fessional fields provides certain sets of competen-
    cies required for this work, and these may differ
    from one of these groups to another;

    AND WHEREAS, in no case can such competencies, how-
    ever essential, be considered sufficient;

    AND WHEREAS, each of these types of professionals
    lack skills that have generally been developed by
    the remaining two;

    AND WHEREAS, adequate habilitative education of
    hearing impaired children depends upon the knowledge
    and skills of individuals responsible for direct and
    indirect intervention; and that such skills are of
    a multi-disciplinary nature;

    BE IT RESOLVED
    1) A new type of professional should be trained
       with appropriate and sufficient competencies
       in speech-language pathology, audiology, coun-
       selling, child development and education of the
       hearing impaired to be the providers of habili-
       tative education. For the purpose of this con-
       ference, such professionals are termed
       habilitationists.

2) Agencies, institutions and organizations responsible for credentialing, certification and
licensing should address their procedures
accordingly.

13. WHEREAS, not all children are capable of developing
adequate spoken skills.

BE IT RESOLVED
Those professionals responsible for habilitative
educational management of children who require
alternative communication methods should obtain
those additionally required competencies.

14. WHEREAS, early habilitative education of hearing
impaired children is a multi-faceted process;

AND WHEREAS, each facet should be evaluated as
objectively as possible;

AND WHEREAS, the critical habilitative treatment and
educational placement of each individual child must
be based on objective assessment.

BE IT RESOLVED
Habilitationists should examine each facet of the
treatment program and the results of criterion
referenced tests and observations at least twice
yearly, filing a report as part of the child's
permanent record.

15. WHEREAS, it is imperative that each child progress
at his or her optimal rate;

AND WHEREAS, the habilitationist is responsible for
maintaining high standards of work in all relevant
areas;

AND WHEREAS, skills and experience differ from one habilitationist to another.

BE IT RESOLVED
Habilitationists engaged in this work should be regularly assisted, supported, supervised and evaluated by senior habilitative personnel.

16. WHEREAS, a good understanding of all information is essential to the engagement of parents in the habilitation process.

BE IT RESOLVED
The sharing of information, the interpretation of the results of evaluations, and the demonstrations of techniques essential to habilitation be done in such a fashion as to take into account the psycho-social impact of the hearing impairment on the family.

17. WHEREAS, the establishment of attachment and trust is a reciprocal process between parents and infants;

AND WHEREAS, parent-infant interaction forms the basis for the development of a broad range of communication skills;

AND WHEREAS, a diagnosis of hearing impairment may precipitate a grief reaction which may be disruptive to parent-infant interaction.

BE IT RESOLVED
1) Family counselling* should be a primary aspect of habilitation;

---

* Family counselling is defined as a process that focuses on affect to facilitate psychosocial growth, and to minimize the negative, emotional effects of crises on the child and family.

2) Family counselling should be aimed at fostering
    the development and use of both new and exist-
    ing supportive networks; that is, the extended
    family, parent groups, parent organizations,
    and the habilitative team; and

3) Counselling and guidance should be initiated
    immediately upon informing the parents of sus-
    pected or confirmed hearing impairment.

18. WHEREAS, each partner has his/her own unique
     approach toward managing stress;

     AND WHEREAS, professionals must know how to recog-
     nize and how to interact with parents and refrain
     from judgment or condescension;

     AND WHEREAS, there is a unique body of knowledge
     and skills required for counselling.

     BE IT RESOLVED
     The following elements should be included in the
     curricula of members of the habilitative team:

     (1) the dynamics of grieving;

     (2) the dynamics of coping;

     (3) basic techniques of counselling;

     (4) participating in group processes which focus
          on the clinician's personal experiences and
          attitudes toward the affective states of
          grieving.

19. WHEREAS, relating affectively to families in crises
     is emotionally stressful.

     BE IT RESOLVED
     1) Professionals should receive periodic inservice
         training and support in the psychosocial aspects
         of habilitation, including ongoing professional-
         centered consultation with a mental health

specialist; and

2) Professionals should seek to develop supportive
    networks for themselves, including such mechan-
    isms as in-house staff meetings to encourage
    interaction on psychosocial issues, and group
    experiences at regional and national professional
    associations designed to enhance personal insight
    into psychosocial issues.

20. WHEREAS, little is known about the most effective
    methods or procedures required for the training of
    individual hearing impaired children in infancy;

    AND WHEREAS, most of the persons in parent/child
    programs are not equipped by training or experience,
    to develop program evaluation systems;

    AND WHEREAS, methods presently in use may, or may
    not be, adequate.

    BE IT RESOLVED
    1) Research pertaining to the various proposed
        early habilitative educational procedures should
        be encouraged and supported;

    2) High priority should be given to the provision
        of support for research into methods of program
        assessment; and

    3) High priority should be given to the provision
        of support for research into methods of evaluat-
        ing the progress of a child with a hearing
        impairment.

21. WHEREAS, there are many other areas of research
    necessary to improve early management procedures.

BE IT RESOLVED
We encourage the following:

1) Continued research into the use of both electric
    response audiometry and impedance audiometry;

2) Development of a paradigm for hearing aid
    selection and fitting for infants;

3) Development of specially designed hearing aids
    and ear molds to meet infants' needs;

4) Further studies to clarify the use of impedance
    batteries on infants under 7 months of age;

5) Further investigation into the effects of middle
    ear effusion early in life, and into various
    interventions including hearing aid use;

6) Continued research into immunology and middle
    ear diseases regarding infecting agents and
    allergenic factors;

7) Development of a communication profile including:
    a. ability to perceive difference limens for
        intensity, frequency and duration (DLI, DLF,
        DLT);
    b. developing listening skills;

8) Evaluation of current tests (e.g., BOEL) and
    development of other tests that might help in
    public health screening.

APPENDIX A

EDITED RECOMMENDATIONS FROM THE NOVA SCOTIA CONFERENCE ON THE
EARLY IDENTIFICATION OF HEARING LOSS*

We are biologically programmed to develop certain skills
in response to certain inputs. Language learning is one such
skill which must be gained very early in life. Hearing is
the most expedient basis for normal language acquisition and
language is the keystone of modern society. Hearing loss must
be identified as early as possible in the first 2 years of
life so that its effects may be diminished to a point where
the hearing impaired child may mature to a full role in
society.

The subtleties of hearing impairment require esoteric
and intensive assessment. This Conference was convened to
evaluate the methods of assessment and to make recommendations for their realization and implementation by making
guidelines which lead to practical results. To those purposes the Conference adopts the following resolutions.

1) RESOLVED: A high risk register or file should be univer-
    sally implemented on the basis of the five points of the
    1973 supplementary statement of the Joint Committee on
    Infant Hearing Screening (Appendix 1): and the follow-up
    procedures of that statement should also be universally
    implemented.

    This conference also recognizes that children who fall
    into the designated high risk categories delineated by
    the Joint Committee on Infant Hearing Screening often
    suffer from other communication disorders.

2) RESOLVED: As a supplement to the high risk register an
    agency may employ behavioural screening tests as in the
    appended model. (See Appendix 2).

    Any tests recommended in the future must also satisfy

---

*   Mencher, G.T. (ed.) Early Identification of Hearing Loss
        (Basel: Karger), 1976.

    Gerber, S.E. and Mencher, G.T. Early Diagnosis of Hearing
    Loss (New York: Grune and Stratton), 1978.

the requirements contained in the 1970 statement of the
Joint Committee on Infant Hearing Screening with respect
to stimuli, response patterns, environmental factors,
status at the time of testing, and behavior of observers.
(See Appendix on page 15 of Gerber and Mencher, Early
Diagnosis of Hearing Loss.)

We believe the reasons for the intensive studies of these
variables are:

a) Different stimuli may activate different components
    of the auditory system;

b) Different response criteria may be selectively sensi-
    tive to different aspects of hearing disturbances;

c) Different observers bring special sensitivities to
    the test procedures; and

d) Different infants in different psycho-physiolological
    states offer varying types of responses, each with
    different clinical meaning.

We believe that to control these variables the acoustic
stimulus must be carefully specified as to its intensity
and frequency (energy content), duration, rise and fall
time (shape), interstimulus interval (pattern of presentation), and informational content. Criteria must
specify changes of behavior accepted as response differ-
entiated from behavioral changes during control periods.
The psycho-physiological states of the infant must be
operationally defined and determined in relation to the
test procedure. Finally, the physical and physiological
factors of the infants environment must be described, and
where possible, stabilized.

In light of the resolutions made here, and in view of the
guidelines that we have and will recommend, we encourage
field trials of automated techniques, such as the crib-
o-gram, since it meets the criteria set down previously.

3) RESOLVED: Because the high risk register or other
    screening program cannot be expected to detect all
    hearing impairment, a provision within the health care
    system should be made for hearing testing later in infancy
    as part of any public health - well baby care program.
    In order to identify both ear disease and hearing loss,
    the following procedures are recommended:

a)   In order to determine if ear disease is present some
     examination of the status of the middle ear should be
     employed at every health visit.

b)   A system should be designed in each country to dis-
     tribute and evaluate a questionnaire provided to the
     parents to ascertain the child's reaction to sound,
     at least twice in each of the first two years of life.

c)   At approximately seven months of age behavioral hear-
     ing tests should be employed universally. The kinds
     of tests that are recommended should employ stimuli
     that have been measured on appropriate instrumentation
     for frequency and intensity content. Signals con-
     sisting of no greater than 45 dB (C scale) measured
     at the ear canal, and at least one stimulus centered
     at high frequencies (2000 - 4000 Hz), and one at low
     frequencies (500 - 1000 Hz) should be employed.

d)   We recognize the impracticality, at the present time,
     of implementing the specifications presented above
     in all testing situations involving the seven month
     old child, and therefore suggest as interim procedures
     which are also acceptable, the documented protocols
     attached.*

e)   At the time of regular health visits close to the
     age of twelve and eighteen months, additional screen-
     ing tests are desirable.

4)   RESOLVED: At two years of age a child should be evaluated
     for hearing, speech and language function. Delivery
     systems must be designed by each country.

5)   RESOLVED: In view of the fact that hearing loss may
     develop at older ages, and although we are dealing with
     the child 0 - 2 years, we urge that periodic screening
     for hearing should be mandated beyond the age of two and
     that complete assessment of communication skills be
     required for entrance to school.

---

*   See Gerber, S.E. and Mencher, G.T. Early Diagnosis of
     Hearing Loss (pages 15 - 20) for copies of those documents.

6) RESOLVED: Persons who implement the recommendations of
    this conference should be given special training in the
    procedures that have been specified, and the World Health
    Organization and other health agencies offer interdisci-
    plinary training courses to this effect. These courses
    should be designed and outlined by responsible interna-
    tional groups such as represented by this conference.

7) RESOLVED: Continued research into the causes, prevention,
    and early detection of hearing loss is essential.

    We specifically recommend continued research in the
    following areas:

    a) Comprehensive studies of genetic and other kinds of
        hearing impairment, with special emphasis on longi-
        tudinal audiologic studies concerning the natural
        history and time of onset;

    b) Continued exploration of procedures for the early
        differential diagnosis of all forms of auditory
        disorders in children;

    c) Automated hearing testing units be studied with age
        levels beyond the newborn period;

    d) The relationships between prenatal environment and
        hearing loss be studied.

APPENDIX 1

Supplementary Statement of Joint Committee on Infant Screening
(July, 1972)

    In light of the urgent need to detect hearing impairment
as early as possible, a 1970 statement of the Joint Committee
urged further investigation of screening methods but discouraged routine hearing screening which is not research
oriented. In consonance with that statement, and in view
of the information that application of high risk data can
increase the detectability of congenital hearing impairment
perhaps as much as tenfold, the Committee considers it appropriate to make additions to the 1970 statement.

The Committee recommends that, since no satisfactory
technique is yet established that will permit hearing screening of all newborns, infants AT RISK for hearing impairment
should be identified by means of history and physical examination. These children should be tested and follow-up as
hereafter described.

I.   The criterion for identifying a newborn as AT RISK for
     hearing impairment is the presence of one or more of
     the following:

     A. History of hereditary childhood hearing impairment.
     B. Rubella or other nonbacterial intrauterine fetal
         infection (e.g., cytomegalovirus infections, Herpes
         infection).
     C. Defects of ear, nose, or throat. Malformed, low-
         set or absent pinnae; cleft lip or palate (including
         submucous cleft); any residual abnormality of the
         otorhinolaryngeal system.
     D. Birthweight less than 1500 grams.
     E. Bilirubin level greater than 20 mg/100 ml serum.

II. Infants falling in this category should be referred for
     an indepth audiological evaluation of hearing during
     their first two months of life and, even if hearing
     appears to be normal, should receive regular hearing
     evaluations thereafter at office or well-baby clinics.
     Regular evaluation is important since familial hearing
     impairment is not necessarily present at birth but may
     develop at an uncertain period of time later.

APPENDIX 2

Suggested Protocol for a Behavioral Hearing Screening Test

1.   TEST STIMULUS: A random noise having a low frequency
     attenuation of 30 dB or more per octave below 750 Hz; a
     maximum of 90 dB sound pressure level at the pinna; a
     rise-decay time of five (5) milliseconds or more; a
     duration of 0.5 to two (2) seconds; an interest interval
     minimum of fifteen (15) seconds.

2. INFANT RESPONSE: Any generalized body movement which
    involves more than one limb and which is accompanied by
    some form of eye movement.

3. SCORING CRITERIA: Controlled by one of two methods:
    a) Scorer does not know when a stimulus is actually
        present, or,
    b) Two observers score an infant's reponses independent
        of one another.

    Furthermore, two (of eight maximum) stimulus responses
    should be positive to score as a "pass" and a "failure"
    should be retested at least once (with a cumulative
    positive response score of more than 20%) before being
    considered a true test "failure".

4. PRETEST STATE: The pre-test behavioural state of an
    infant is an important determinant in governing the
    initiation of a response and must be controlled or
    described in specific terms. This protocol calls for
    a sleeping infant (eyes closed, no observable body
    movement for at least fifteen (15) seconds prior to
    stimulation).

5. TEST ENVIRONMENT: The ambient noise level at the time
    of the typical test should be measured and reported.

APPENDIX B

EDITED RECOMMENDATIONS OF THE SASKATOON CONFERENCE ON THE EARLY DIAGNOSIS OF HEARING LOSS*

Hearing is essential for the normal development of speech
and language. Therefore, impairment of hearing loss poses a
serious handicap to the child's entire psychosocial

---

* Gerber, S.E. and Mencher, G.T. (eds.) Early Diagnosis of
  Hearing Loss (New York: Grune and Stratton), 1978.

development. The objective, as presented in the First
Canadian Conference on Hearing Loss (held in Toronto in 1964)
was alleviation of the handicap to auditory communication
which is imposed by an early and severe auditory impairment.
That objective is still valid today. Alleviation of the
handicap is best begun at the earliest possible age; this
requires identification, diagnosis, and habilitation.

The Nova Scotia Conference (held in Halifax in 1974)
emphasized the early identification of hearing loss, advocating specific screening techniques. The success of an early
identification program depends, however, not only on screening, but on appropriate and adequate follow-up procedures for
diagnosis. The resolutions of the present conference deal
with the methods for the confirmation of the presence and
degree of hearing loss within the first six (6) months of
life as accurately, as rapidly and as economically as possible.

1) WHEREAS, the general principles and recommendations
    advocated at the Nova Scotia Conference on Early Identi-
    fication of Hearing Loss (1974) are still applicable
    and valid;

    RESOLVED: this conference endorses and reaffirms the
    principles and recommendations of the Nova Scotia
    Conference (See Appendix A).

2) WHEREAS, the high risk register has proven effective for
    the early identification of hearing loss; and

    WHEREAS, anoxia at birth has also been associated with a
    significant number of hearing losses;

    RESOLVED: A category is to be added to the high risk
    register as follows "Significant asphyxia associated
    with acidosis" (See Appendix 1).

3) WHEREAS, uncertainty about a possible hearing impairment
    in an infant is disruptive of normal family function;

    RESOLVED: In cases of parental concern about hearing
    impairment, it is recommended that a child of any age
    be immediately referred for audiologic evaluation.

4) WHEREAS, the parent is often the earliest identifier of a hearing loss;

RESOLVED: In cases of parental concern about hearing impairment, it is recommended that a child of any age be immediately referred for audiologic evaluation.

5) WHEREAS, physical examination in the diagnosis of hearing loss in infants adds greatly to the total information about the child and to the understanding of the etiology of the hearing loss;

RESOLVED: A comprehensive assessment of any child suspect for hearing loss should include these procedures:
A. Essential to the Assessment

    1. Standard pediatric examination
    2. Pneumatic otoscopy and/or oto-microscopy
    3. Fundoscopic examination
    4. Appropriate observations for specific physical abnormalities (See Appendix on pages 21 - 29, Gerber, S.E., and Mencher, G.T. (eds.) Early Diagnosis of Hearing Loss).

B. Strongly Recommended in the Assessment

    1. General laboratory examinations
    2. Appropriate serology examination for toxoplasmosis, rubella, cytomegalovirus and Herpes
    3. Urinalysis
    4. Family audiograms

C. Include When Indicated

    1. Thyroid function
    2. Polytomography of middle and inner ear (Except in established cases of antenatal infections)
    3. Electrocardiogram
    4. Chromosomal study
    5. Flourescent trepanemal antibody (FTA) - absorption test for syphilis
    6. Appropriate testing for Mucupolysaccharidosis

6) WHEREAS, correct diagnosis and appropriate treatment require as much information as possible about the auditory function of a suspect infant;

RESOLVED: A comprehensive auditory assessment of a suspect infant should include:

A. An extensive behavioral history by parental report
B. Observations of behavioral responses to appropriate
   auditory stimuli
C. Visual Reinforcement Audiometry (where age appropriate)
D. Acoustic immitance measurements (includes tympano-
   metry, acoustic reflex, and static compliance)
E. Electric response audiometry as indicated (See
   Appendix 2 and Resolution 7).

7) WHEREAS, electric response audiometry (such as described
   in Appendix 2) has been demonstrated to be a useful and
   appropriately sensitive tool in the recognition and
   diagnosis of hearing loss in newborn children as well as
   other difficult to test infants;

   RESOLVED: Diagnostic centers in which qualified administration of the test is available should include electric
   response audiometry (ERA) in their battery of tests for
   the evaluation of children who are suspected of hearing
   impairment.

8) WHEREAS, there is clear evidence that a significant proportion of children in the neonatal intensive care unit
   will have a hearing loss; and

   WHEREAS, preliminary evidence suggests auditory brainstem
   response (ABR) audiometry may be a useful screening-
   diagnostic tool in the earliest possible evaluation of
   those children;

   RESOLVED: Further research focusing on the use of
   auditory brainstem response audiometry (ABR) in the
   newborn intensive care unit is encouraged.

9) WHEREAS, the high risk register does not permit the
   identification of all infants with hearing impairment,
   nor those with a delayed onset of hearing impairment; and

   WHEREAS, observations of behavioral responses to acoustic
   stimuli can be made by trained and well supervised
   personnel and are appropriate for screening infants from
   approximately five (5) to seven (7) months of age;

   RESOLVED: Screening should be conducted routinely on all
   infants attending well-baby clinics and other health
   facilities; and, further, infants suspected of hearing
   loss through such a screening should be referred for

more detailed audiological investigation.

10) WHEREAS, significant hearing impairment can occur early in life through postnatal causes;

RESOLVED: Children having had meningitis, encephalitis, skull fracture or ototoxic medication should be closely investigated for possible hearing impairment.

11) WHEREAS, middle ear effusion can occur in the newborn and in infants; and

WHEREAS, middle ear effusion may persist chronically for months or years producing a mild, bilateral hearing loss; and

WHEREAS, prolonged mild hearing loss may produce speech, language, educational, and behavioral problems;

RESOLVED: Particular attention should be paid to those newborns likely to have sustained middle ear effusion (see Appendix D , pages 31 - 32, Gerber, S.E., and Mencher, G.T. (eds.) Early Diagnosis of Hearing Loss (Grune and Stratton), 1978.) As with all children, these newborns should be closely followed, and the effusion be considered a problem if it is sustained (more than three months) or is recurrent (over 50% of the time for six months). Diagnosis should be based upon pneumatic otoscopy, tympanometry, and audiometry. Further, if a sustained or recurrent problem is diagnosed, educational intervention should be applied in the form of language stimulation programs and/or low level amplification in addition to ongoing medical or surgical treatment.

12) WHEREAS, parent-infant bonding is of critical psycho-social importance; and

WHEREAS, the parent is the advocate for the child; and

WHEREAS, parents are often ignored in the course of the evaluation and treatment of their child;

RESOLVED: In order to understand the implications of the diagnostic findings and habilitative plans, parents should be extensively involved in the diagnostic and habilitative process.

13) WHEREAS, the medical, paramedical, and educational professions are too little aware of the practicality of early identification and diagnosis of hearing loss;

RESOLVED: This conference encourages active educational programs and dissemination of information within all concerned professions regarding the availability of methods to assess auditory function in infants and neonates; and, further, this conference advocates that this information be included in the curricula of medical schools and speciality training programs.

14) WHEREAS, having provided several resolutions concerning the early diagnosis of hearing impairment, this conference has offered to the remedial professions an opportunity whereby counselling and early remedial programs may be instituted;

RESOLVED: This conference encourages the institution of early guidance, counselling, and intervention programs aimed at the alleviation of the handicap to auditory communication which is imposed by an early and severe auditory impairment, provided always that such programs are conducted by trained personnel who, where appropriate, are under proper supervision.

APPENDIX 1

Statement Re Significant Asphyxia

In the past many neonates with fetal distress and low Apgar scores have been examined with a low incidence of hearing loss. However, as regional neonatal intensive care units expand and greater numbers of ill infants are transferred for special care, those term infants requiring neonatal intensive care because of antenatal and/or birth anoxia or birth trauma are now more readily identified. Those infants with hypoxic encephalopathy with persisting abnormal neurological signs* or neonatal convulsions secondary to anoxia have

* For clinical signs see: Sarnat HB: Neonatal encephalopathy following fetal distress. Arch Neurol 33:696, 1976.

a high incidence of neurosensory hearing loss as well as
other developmental disabilities.

A specific level of acidosis (arterial pH) is not given
here as an indicator of subsequent handicap as in some areas
it may not be measured or vigorous treatment may alter the
pH level prior to measurement. A pH level of < 7.3 associated with asphyxia has been associated with hearing loss.

APPENDIX 2

Statement Re Electric Response Audiometry (ERA)

1. Auditory brainstem response

Two forms of the auditory brainstem response test are
recognized; both of them test only the peripheral auditory
mechanism. The simpler test uses unfiltered clicks as
stimuli and tests primarily the sensitivity of the ear to
frequencies above 1500 Hz. It is particularly applicable
as an early follow-up test of babies at six (6) weeks of age.
A more elaborate test, still under development, uses filtered
clicks and yields a four frequency (500, 1000, 2000 and 4000
Hz) audiogram. The test is applicable to all ages; for both
of these tests, sedation is not usually required for infants
below three months of age.

The auditory brainstem response test should not be used
alone, but only as part of a battery of tests that also
includes impedance audiometry and behavioral tests. Furthermore, an audiogram may be generated from middle component
evoked potentials using tone burst stimuli (see below).

The auditory brainstem response test, which is relatively
expensive and time-consuming, need be used only if behavioral
testing is not feasible or yields equivocal results. The
auditory brainstem response test must be administered by
adequately trained personnel.

The simpler auditory brainstem response test has the
demonstrated capability of producing diagnostic data equal
to or exceeding that described in monographs by Davis (1976)
and by Picton et al (1977). The report of such a test should
include, for each ear:

1. Latency of Wave V response as a function of the
   clicks;
2. Threshold estimate;
3. Statement of the type of hearing loss found, if any;
4. Measurement of the I-to-V interval of the brainstem
   responses.

The procedures and capabilities of the auditory brainstem response test are still under development. Diagnostic
centers which make use of it must remain aware of developments
in the state of their art.

If the auditory brainstem response test yields negative
or equivocal results, electrocochleography may be considered
to assess the physiological state of the cochlea.

2. Middle component evoked potentials

Another technique for eliciting frequency specific information is the use of the middle components. Equipment used
for the auditory brainstem response test may also be used
for the middle components; only the filter settings and
length of the recording epoch need be changed. Likewise,
adequately trained personnel should administer the test.

While the middle components have been shown to yield
frequency specific information (Thornton et al., 1977;
McFarland, et al., 1977), these potentials have not been
used in extensive clinical trials. The exact origin of the
response is also unknown. However, it is felt that information may be obtained from the entire auditory pathway with
these potentials.

TEMPUS FUGIT!! HOW TIME FLIES BY!!

Robert K. Coulling

Elks Purple Cross Deaf Detection and Development, Regina, Saskatchewan

It seems like only yesterday that I was given the opportunity and privilege on behalf of 51,000 members of the B.P.O. Elks of Canada, and the 17,000 dedicated Ladies of their auxiliary, The Order of the Royal Purple, who make it all possible through their national charity, The Elks Purple Cross Fund, to welcome the contributors and participants to the second International Conference sponsored by the Elks Purple Cross Deaf Detection and Development Program to study the Early Diagnosis of Hearing Loss to Saskatoon.

Again, it seems such a short time ago since Doctor Mencher and I discussed the possibility of the first conference to be held in Halifax in 1974.

So -- here we are in Winnipeg in April of 1980, and again, major events in the interest of the hearing impaired child will unfold; and new techniques and new plans for further study of the welfare and rehabilitation of those so impaired will take place.

You are the participants. The children and their families are the benefactors, and the Elks and their ladies have reached another goal in their objective to help others.

On behalf of my Organization, I bid you all a most warm and sincere welcome.

PROLOGUE: THE WAY WE WERE

George T. Mencher
Gylfi Baldursson
Lenore Mencher
Nova Scotia Hearing and Speech Clinic, Halifax, Nova Scotia

There are certain words common to sister professions in
most situations. Usually, terminology is well understood by
all. This, however, is one of those circumstances whose
nature requires a very specific definition so that we all, as
audiologists, speech pathologists, teachers of the deaf,
psychologists, physicians, or whatever we represent, understand and agree to what we mean when we say "early identification, early diagnosis and early management". I am sure
that some believe the discussion will concern 2 and 3 year
olds, while others may expect a focus on younger age groups,
but just how much so will vary from one individual to the
next. By definition, then, when we say early identification,
we mean at birth; when we say early diagnosis, we mean within
the first few weeks; and when we say early management, we
mean as early as possible in life, even beginning within the
first month. In fact, the by-word for this conference is:
"If he is over 3 months of age -- he is a geriatric!"

Case E.L. is just one of several which illustrate the
situation (Figure 1). This child was 2 days of age when she
failed the identification procedure. She was less than 1
month when she failed in the audiology centre, and she
reached the ripe old age of 6 weeks before we had a confirmed
diagnosis of a sensory-neural hearing loss. Audiological
counselling was, of course, ongoing. At 2 3/4 months of age,
this deaf baby and her family were enrolled in a formal early
management program. Even at that, it took too long because
we were delayed 3 weeks while the family was away. We had a
confirmed diagnosis at 6 weeks and we could have, and should
have, started detailed management at that age. In point of
fact, it took longer to get the ear molds back from the
factory and to obtain the hearing aid then it did to confirm
deafness in what, at birth, appeared to be a normal baby.

All of the procedures implemented by our center which
led to this baby's program are the direct results of the Nova
Scotia Conference on Early Identification of Hearing Loss and

the Saskatoon Conference on the Early Diagnosis of Hearing
Loss, the two international predecessors to this conference,
also sponsored by the Elks Purple Cross Deaf Detection and
Development Fund. Those two meetings brought forth, between
them, some 21 recommendations (see Recommendations of this
Conference – Appendices 1 and 2) which were, to this day, the
state of the art in early identification and diagnosis: The
Way We Were.

FIGURE 1: PROGRESS OF E.L.

History:	Asphyxia, acidosis, negative family history, – "depressed", lathargic, incubator 3 days.
Sept 16/79	D.O.B.; BW – 3000 g; Gestation period 40 weeks.
Sept 18/79	Failed newborn screening; scheduled for follow-up.
Oct 11/79	Failed behavioural audiological testing at NSHSC.
Nov 1/79	Failed behavioural audiological testing at NSHSC.
Nov 2/79	Failed ABR (confirmed as a hearing loss).
Nov 9/79	Failed retest ABR and behavioural examination; Seen by ENT, results essentially negative; Referred for further medical examinations – sent for earmolds. Family away 3 weeks.
Dec 2/79	Counselling for use of hearing aid(s). Early management program set up with Dr. Phillips.
Dec 13/79	Given loaner aid (body type) – parents asked to alternate between ears and observe.
Dec 17/79	Gets new aid (Post-auricular).

There is no point in reviewing each specific recommendation,
as I am sure most of you are familiar with them. Consider,
however, what they look like as a group – a composite – in
application, and as part of an ongoing, screening-
diagnostic-management program.

FIGURE 2:   PROTOCOL FOR INFANT HIGH RISK AND BEHAVIOURAL
            HEARING SCREENING

Screening

1. List of daily admissions are collected.
2. Babies' charts are checked for Hi-Risk factors (@
    Joint Committee recommendations).
3. All mothers are requested to complete questionnaire
    "For Mothers of Newborn Infants".
4. All mothers are briefly interviewed to clarify or
    expand on answers at time of questionnaire collec-
    tion, for further screening on hi-risk factors.

Testing

1. Babies tested behaviourally include:
    a. those suggesting any hi-risk factor
    b. any baby whose mother requests a hearing test
    c. all babies in the Special Nursery Care or
        Intensive Care Units
    d. all babies going for adoption.

2. Babies are tested in a quiet location while sleeping.
3. Stimulus as per the Nova Scotia Conference (either
    Sandon or Apriton).
4. Two positive responses are needed to pass the test.
    A positive response = eye blink and generalized
    limb and/or body movement.
5. The testor alternates two trials each at 90 dB and
    100 dB or a maximum of eight trials.
6. Responses are recorded on Test Sheet after agreement
    by two observers.
7. If baby does not pass on initial test, it is
    retested. If it fails again, it is referred to
    the Hearing and Speech Clinic for audiological
    assessment.

Recording
1. Data entered on the record includes:

FIGURE 2 (continued)
       a. baby's name
       b. mother's room number
       c. date of birth
       d. date of test
       e. gestation (in weeks)
       f. birth weight
       g. days in incubator
       h. high risk category or non-risk
       i. remarks (why baby is being tested)
       j. pass/fail

2. An additional separate record is kept on all babies in Special Nursery Care Unit.

Reporting

1. A report is sent to the physician attending every high-risk baby, alerting them to the specific high risk factor, and requesting their cooperation in administering regular hearing tests for the first few months. The same is true for non-risk infants who failed the behavioural testing procedure.

2. A monthly list is kept and sent to the Provincial Department of Public Health Nurses of all high-risk babies, and non-risk babies who failed the testing procedure.

3. A monthly report is provided for the Director of the Hearing and Speech Clinic, the Supervisor of Audiology of the Clinic, and the Hearing Screening Coordinator which includes:
       a. the number of live births and mothers interviewed.
       b. the number of babies on the high risk register and their category breakdown.
       c. the number of babies tested behaviourally and their category breakdown.
       d. the number of failures and their category breakdown.
       e. a list of babies who failed.

4. Referrals on Downs Syndrome, Cleft Palate, and Cerebral Palsy children to speech pathology division for enrollment in special parent programs.

At the Nova Scotia Conference, the emphasis was on identification; that is, screening. Our program at the Grace Maternity Hospital in Halifax mirrors the methods outlined at that Conference (Figure 2). January 1 through December 31, 1979, represents a typical year. There were 4,910 babies born in the Grace during that period of time. Of those, (Figure 3), 669 were on the high risk register, which included the addition of asphyxia as a result of the recommendations in Saskatoon. Those babies constitute 13.6% of the newborn population. In addition, because of research underway at our center, we isolated 373 children not at risk for hearing loss who had spent time in the intensive care unit, 119 children up for adoption, and 535 babies meeting the other special requirements of our project. All of those sub-groups were behaviourally screened utilizing the arousal response and procedures outlined in Nova Scotia in 1974 (Figure 4). After the initial screening, those who failed were rescreened. Eventually, 101 infants were referred to our clinic for detailed evaluation.

FIGURE 3:   HIGH RISK INFANTS REQUIRING BEHAVIOURAL SCREENING
(N = 669/13.6% of population of 4910)

January 1, 1979 - December 31, 1979

Category	Number	%
A. Affected Family	319	47.7
B. Breathing Difficulty (asphyxia)	189	28.3
C. Congenital Rubella	3	.1
D. Defect of ENT	111	16.6
E. Elevated Bilirubin	2	.1
S. Small at Birth	45	6.7

Utilizing the recommendations of the Saskatoon conference, our audiology division undertook the very difficult task of differential diagnosis of hearing loss with babies

FIGURE 4:   SCHEMATIC DIAGRAM OF NEWBORN HEARING SCREENING AND DEAFNESS DETECTION PROGRAM

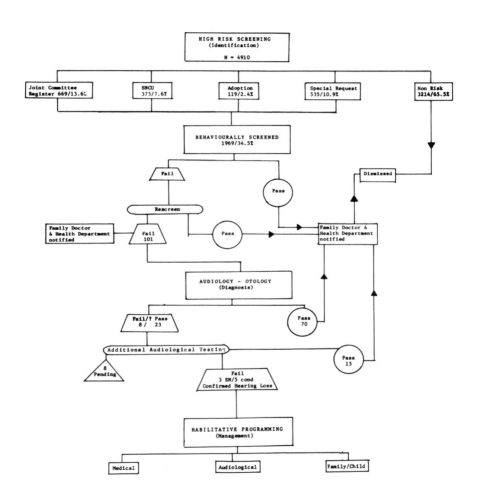

NOVA SCOTIA HEARING & SPEECH CLINIC   DEAF DETECTION & DEVELOPMENT PROGRAM

(January 1, 1979 - December 31, 1979)

as young as 2 days of age. Remember, for the most part,
these were infants on the high risk register for hearing loss
and who had twice failed a behavioural screening. One of the
initial major tasks was to develop a behavioural protocol and
scoring system which would be fairly rigid, but flexible
enough to be used with tiny babies (Figure 5). After the
initial visit to our clinic, 70 of the 101 babies were

FIGURE 5:   PROTOCOL FOR TESTING INFANTS FROM GRACE MATERNITY
            HOSPITAL OR FROM CRIB-O-GRAM PROGRAM

Stimuli/Pass Levels

Age	NB 3K	NB 4K	NB 1K	PN	Voice
0 - 6 weeks	80 dB	80 dB	85 dB	70	65 dB

Expected Response: eye widening, APR, startle, ½ startle,
                    limb movement, aroused from sleep.

If responses to standard stimuli are inconclusive or absent,
consider other testing with noisemakers, warble tones, bone
conducted stimuli + impedance.

1. If a child gives a definite response to all five stimuli
    within pass range, score as PASS. No retest is necessary.

2. If responses are present but vague and inconsistent,
    score as inconclusive. Send test results to mother
    immediately, marked as "inconclusive." Set up ABR
    appointment and re-evaluate within one month.

3. If responses are consistently absent to one or more
    stimuli, score as FAIL. Send results to mother immedi-
    ately, marked "inconclusive". Set up ABR and
    re-evaluation appointment within 2 weeks.

4. For older children, follow Downs' Auditory Behaviour
    Index (D).

---

cleared and dismissed. Of the remaining 31, 8 were definite
failures according to our protocols, while 23 were still
questionable. Subsequently, we have retested and cleared 15

of those 23, 8 are still pending, and we have confirmed at
least 8 hearing losses (3 sensory-neural and 5 conductive).
It should be noted that all 3 of the confirmed sensory-
neural hearing losses were on the high risk register; one
being a case of severe asphyxia and two being of low birth
weight (Figure 6). It does seem, however, that low birth
weight for gestational age may be a better guideline than
the recommended and arbitrary   < 1500 grams.

FIGURE 6:   SUMMARY OF NEWBORN SCREENING PROGRAM, GRACE
                MATERNITY HOSPITAL

January 1, 1979 - December 31, 1979

Live Births: 4910

Behaviourally Screened: 1969 (34.5%)

Failed - Referred to Audiology: 101 (6% of those screened,
                                        or 2% of the entire
                                        population)

Confirmed Hearing Loss: (a)   3 sensory-neural
                          (b)   5 conductive

Thus far, I have refrained from comment about the 5
children with confirmed conductive hearing loss and/or middle
ear problems. First of all, we really don't know if any of
them has a sensory-neural component as well. Further, we are
also interested in the possibility that one or more of these
children may develop a sensory-neural hearing loss of latent
onset, something which has been reported to occur with
rubella and other viral diseases. Further still, it is our
opinion that these children also require early management
programs. Granted, the primary emphasis may be medical, but
audiological and family-child management seem just as critical
for these babies at this early stage of their development.
Undoubtedly, we here will need to address ourselves to that
question.

The identification program I have described thus far, centers in a maternity hospital with, what are primarily normal children. We also operate a program through the neonatal intensive care unit at the Izaak Walton Killam Hospital for Children. That ICU serves 4 Maritime provinces. The Nova Scotia Hearing and Speech Clinic operates a crib-o-gram in that nursery. In fact, we have had 3 different prototypes of that system in operation in the hospital over the last 5 years. We are currently evaluating the new microprocessor unit in parallel with the earlier mechanical strip chart model. While there appear to be some problems in test-retest reliability and consistency, both systems seem to work. Of the 152 babies evaluated last year, 28 failed (18.4%). Of those, 4 - while still less than 3 months of age - were confirmed as having a sensory-neural hearing loss. An additional 3 are still under investigation. We do not consider the high risk register or any other factors in the neonatal ICU, we simply test every baby just prior to discharge. It is interesting to note, however, that all 4 crib-o-gram babies with confirmed hearing loss were on the high risk register. That means that all 7 babies identified in Halifax last year were on the high risk register.

Some of you may be aware of the new Telephone Pioneers Auditory Brainstem Response Screening program developed by Doctor Philip Peltzman in California. We were the first center in Canada to obtain one of those units (Figure 7). We are using it alongside the crib-o-gram in the ICU at the Killam Hospital in a check and balance program. Although there are some minor mechanical problems which slow things down a bit, I am pleased to report that the instrument works extremely well. The difficulties center on electrode placement (we use 2 ear clips and a forehead attachment) and over-sensitivity to artifact (Figure 8). It is too early to report data, as we have only recently initiated the use of the instrument on a regular basis.

One question which always lingers is "How much did this whole identification and diagnosis program cost?" Considering only the high risk and behavioural protocol, and including all salaries and equipment and all audiology visits for failures, billed at $35.00 per hour, the 1979 year cost $2.12 per child. That is, $2.12 for each of the 4,910 babies born in Halifax. Another way of looking at it is that it cost $1,301.15 to identify and diagnose each of the hearing impaired children, including all of the audiology appointments.

FIGURE 7:   SYNAP II AUDITORY BRAINSTEM RESPONSE INSTRUMENT
            DESIGNED BY THE TELEPHONE PIONEERS OF AMERICA
            (PHOTO COURTESY OF DR. PHILLIP PELTZMAN).

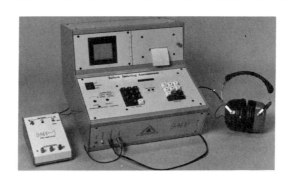

At the same time, the crib-o-gram project cost $41.44 per baby tested, or $1,575.00 per hearing-impaired child. I hasten to add, however, that that figure is quite distorted in that the price of the instrument is included in toto in the one year. That figure would be considerably less if the cost of the instrument were to be amortized over three or five years. If we project over a four year life expectancy for the instrument, and the number of deaf children identified is approximately the same each year (3 or 4), we would project a cost of $18.20 per baby tested, including all audiology visits. Remember also, however, that we are not utilizing the machine to its fullest capacity, and if we increase the number of babies tested, the cost will go down even further, proportionately.

Another frequent question concerns the amount of audiology time required to evaluate all the children on the high risk register or, as is the situation with our program, only those who fail the behavioural screening. If we consider the high risk register only, without behavioural screening, 669 children (13.6% of 4,910) would have been seen for, at most, 15 minute initial audiology appointments. That constitutes a total of 335 hours, less than 5 weeks of an audiologist's time per year. Even better yet, if the register and behavioural screening are set together, time committments are even less. Only 50 high risk babies failed the behavioural screening in Halifax and were referred to audiology. At 15 minutes per initial appointment, that constitutes less than 13 hours per year, or less than ½ of 1 week's work for the audiologist

FIGURE 8: TYPICAL TRACING FROM SYNAP II AUDITORY BRAINSTEM RESPONSE SYSTEM PRODUCED BY THE TELEPHONE PIONEERS FOR THE INFANT HEARING ASSESSMENT PROJECT. SHOWN ARE WAVES I, III, AND V AS RECORDED FROM A 45 DAY OLD F BABY WHILE STILL IN A NEONATAL INTENSIVE CARE UNIT

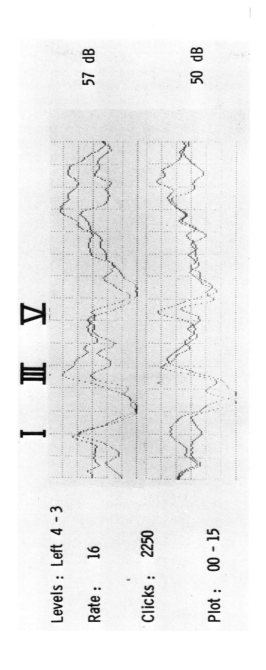

49

responsible for evaluating babies at the initial visit and,
of course, clearing most of them. I would suggest that
those children requiring a second visit or more have problems –
hearing or otherwise – which require care; and cost and time
commitment by an audiologist become secondary in those situations. Clearly, for those cases the problem is no longer a
function of the false positives and false negatives of the
screening procedure, but rather one of the children themselves.
In Figure 9, I have illustrated my projection for time commitments in some major regions in North America. I have chosen
California, as it is the most populous area; British Columbia
as it is probably average in population for both United States
and Canada; and Nova Scotia as it is typical of the less
populous regions in both countries. Further, I have utilized
30 minutes for the appointments, rather than 15 minutes as I
did earlier. In point of fact, the initial visits for the
101 nursery failures averaged 15 minutes each, but by using
30 minutes here, any errors in estimates will be on the con-
servative side. As can be seen, even in California the
amount of time required is quite small.

FIGURE 9:   PROJECTED AUDIOLOGY WORKLOADS FOR FOLLOW-UP TO
                    HEARING SCREENING PROGRAM

Audiologist's clinical work load: 25 patient contact hours
                x 48 weeks = 1200 work hours per year

Hours required for newborn failures at 30 minutes per child
(a very high estimate)

Area	High Risk Only (13.6%)	Behavioural Failures (7% of High Risk)
Nova Scotia	920	65
British Columbia	2,591	182
California	22,930	1,605

One last comment about our screening program. We are
proud of the fact that our program has been in existence for
2½ years, has identified 7 babies with sensory-neural hearing

loss, and that we have yet to see in our clinic a child born
in one of our hospitals who has been screened and who has a
hearing loss which we missed. Because we are the largest
and best equipped audiology center in the Maritimes, it is
likely that we would have seen such a child. We are currently
in contact with all the centers around us and searching for
additional cases.

What is the bottom line of all this? We have had babies
enrolled in an early management program as young as 75 to 85
days of age. In other words, the Nova Scotia and Saskatoon
conference recommendations and the system we evolved from
them works! When we say early management of sensory-neural
hearing loss, we mean babies of just weeks, or a few months
of age. Even so, nothing is perfect, perhaps least of all
clinical procedure. It is important, then, in spite of our
successes, to review some of the problems we see, both in
theory and method.

First of all, early identification itself is an issue.
I am not sure if the problem is one of complacency or confusion. We know that the high risk register/behavioural screening program is a good system, but advocacy by audiologists
and/or medical personnel, coupled with action, is inadequate
in both Canada and the United States. Unfortunately, unless
screening procedures are universally applied within a region,
the programs that do exist will fail because they will not
detect a sufficient number of infants with hearing impairment
to keep interest and quality and, thus, of course, the programs themselves sustained. Further, we cannot deny that the
system has flaws. Children with moderate hearing losses will
not be detected, nor will that supposed 20% with latent onset
of profound hearing loss. Unfortunately, those complications
(low numbers and limited population) lead to confusion about
what to expect from a program and/or complacency about starting one. Often the value of the entire program is lost, in
spite of successes in the only stated goal of these programs;
that being, the early identification of deaf or severely
hearing-impaired babies.

Next we come to the crib-o-gram; in principle, an excellent system. Although basically the same as the arousal procedure, it is automated and, therefore, I suppose, better.
But it costs too much. Further, because of some procedural
problems, it has had to undergo periodic review. It appears
as though the manufacturer did not properly field test the
microprocessor unit until they had clearly demonstrated it

has good reliability and validity before they put it on the
market. The crib-o-gram is currently undergoing standardization and, although it has promise for the future, that will
not be realized until standardization is complete and the
price is reduced.

Finally we come to ABR screening. I can tell you from
direct hands-on clinical experience that the Synap II unit of
the Infant Hearing Assessment Program of the Telephone Pioneers
does everything it purports to do. The problem is, it takes
too long. ABR is not, at the present state of the art, a
screening procedure. You cannot spend 30 minutes or more per
baby in a routine screening, especially when you can use a
behavioural test that lasts for 1 minute or less as a preliminary screen. The Telephone Pioneers Program is excellent for
a first follow-up of behavioural failures, but until the
entire procedure, including electrode placement, can be
accomplished in 5 minutes or less, it seems unrealistic to
consider it a screening device. The use of volunteers does
not really make any difference in that situation.

It is true, of course, that we do have many audiologists
and physicians urging early identification. We have some high
risk programs. We have the crib-o-gram in use in some centers
but still undergoing scientific review. We have ABR programs
touted as the ultimate in early identification. Yet, the
instruments are in very short supply or very expensive, and
the procedure is so time consuming that it is really not a
screening tool. The end result has got to be mass confusion
on the part of the general public. Doctor X in community Y
does not know which way to turn and/or which program to implement. The only saving grace is that there is the knowledge
that a program is necessary and he wants one. I suppose in
spite of the problems, even that is progress.

Now we come to diagnostic procedures. The confusion is
even greater in that realm. Consider the medical recommendations of the Saskatoon Conference (Figure 10). There is no
question they are all valid recommendations. The question is,
at what point should, or can, they be applied and for what
purpose. For example, most of the time the TORCH battery of
tests is administered after confirmation of hearing loss in
an attempt to determine the etiology and not as a diagnostic
battery for hearing loss per se. Family audiograms are rarely
done during the diagnostic period and polytomography is certainly not done on babies. In short, most of the procedures
can be applied but most also have very severe limitations.

FIGURE 10:   MEDICAL RECOMMENDATIONS FROM SASKATOON CONFERENCE
ON EARLY IDENTIFICATION OF HEARING LOSS

A. Essential to the Assessment

1. Standard pediatric examination
2. Pneumatic otoscopy and/or otomicroscopy
3. Fundoscopic examination
4. Appropriate observations for specific physical
    abnormalities.

B. Strongly Recommended in the Assessment

1. General laboratory examinations
2. Appropriate serology examination for toxoplasmosis,
    rubella, cytomegalovirus and herpes
3. Urinalysis
4. Family audiograms.

C. Include When Indicated

1. Thyroid Function
2. Polytomography of middle and inner ear
3. Electrocardiogram
4. Chromosomal study
5. Flourescent trepanemal antibody (FTA) - absorption
    test for syphilis
6. Appropriate testing for mucopolysaccharidosis.

Another critical problem in the area of diagnosis is with
audiology itself. Look at the track record of the Nova Scotia
Hearing and Speech Clinic - and I like to think of it as one
of the best in Canada. We have trouble deciding if a baby has
"passed", is "probably o.k.", or has a hearing loss. True, we
have criteria and guidelines for each of these categories, but
the truth is, those are almost pro forma. The clinicians
still do a tremendous amount of "seat of the pants" testing
which is based on experience and good clinical intuition.
Although it most often works, that is not always the case.
Thus, firm diagnosis may be delayed and, if so, then so will
early management. What benefit is screening and failing a
baby at 2 days of age, only to have diagnosis and management
delayed?

ABR offers, on the surface, what appears to be the
ultimate solution -- diagnosis by machine. But is it a
panacea? How many times have clinicians said, "Well, I see
an appropriate pattern here, but not there," or, "I think
this is a response." The procedure is, without a doubt, an
excellent tool but still just that, a tool, and one which
requires what is, in the end, a subjective interpretation of
procedures, but subjective nevertheless.

Finally, Case K.M. (Figure 11) illustrates an obvious
weakness typical of most early identification programs: the
unfortunate and, perhaps unnecessary, lag between the time a
hearing loss is suspected by audiology and the time of
institution of formal habilitative family/child management
programming. It also clearly illustrates the complexities
and intricacies of early diagnosis. Consider a high risk
infant with a sensory-neural hearing loss compounded by middle
ear problems and yet, through behavioural audiometry, ERA
testing of early and late components, and medical-otological
examination, the child is identified and firmly diagnosed by
3 months of age as having a mixed, moderate to severe, slop-
ing hearing loss. And further, the infant was inaccessible
for testing for one of those three months while it was still
in an incubator.

Certainly there is complacency in the development of
identification programs and confusion as to which one to
use. Perhaps even worse, there is complexity, indecision,
and even greater confusion during diagnosis. Even so, in
spite of all those difficulties, the system works. We know
that we are seeing more and more children under 2 months of
age with confirmed hearing loss. We have recommendations and
procedures designed to help us identify and diagnose hearing-
impaired babies and to bring them to management. But then
what are we going to do with them? What are we going to do
for them? How will we treat them and their families during
those first few months, during that first year of life?
Clearly, those questions carry with them certain connotations;
for example, we are not dealing with children per se, but
rather with methods - methods of helping handicapped children
and their families bond to each other and adjust to the
presence of a hearing loss; methods of initiating language
and speech skills; methods designed to assist children to
develop to their fullest potential.

FIGURE 11:   PROGRESS OF K.M.M.

History:	Small at birth, premature; Twin "B", adoption
Dec 3/79	D.O.B.; BW - 1470 g; gestation period - 34 weeks (in incubator 24 days)
Dec 28/79	Failed screening, left hospital before behavioral testing could be done at NSHSC
Feb 5/80	Failed behavioural audiology testing at NSHSC
Feb 6/80	Failed ABR (confirmed as hearing loss)
Feb 19/80	Failed again at clinic; tests seem to suggest moderate to severe loss, better responses to lower frequencies.
Feb 26/80	Failed again in clinic; ENT reports possible serous otitis bilaterally. Family/child management program instituted
Mar 11/80	Cortical evoked potential results suggest sloping hearing loss (moderate to severe)
Apr 16/80	Loaner hearing aid fit re appointment with ENT, Counselling

---

During the next few days we will complete our presentations here and adjourn to closed sessions where we will labour over many important issues. After all our discussions we will bring forth a series of recommendations which will offer a solid base for the early management of hearing loss no matter where it is found and to what extent it exists. No doubt there will be disagreement before the recommendations are offered and again before they are adopted. There will be compromise. No doubt we will spend many hours considering oral vs. total, and monaural vs. binaural, and directive vs. reflective, and individual vs. group, and so on and so on and so on. We are 19 people from 6 countries, but we all have one goal in mind: delineation of the most effective procedure for the early management of a baby with a hearing loss.

It has been said that "The education of all children
begins from the moment of birth." Why should the deaf
child's education be delayed? An early and good start in
life is his right. It has also been said that, "... intelligently and wisely applied knowledge garnered over the months,
leaves mothers and fathers little time to dwell upon themselves and their deaf child in self-pity. Far more time and
energy are being directed towards finding out what to do and
doing it." Our job, ladies and gentlemen, is to develop
that knowledge so that the parents may develop the children.
The challenge is before us here and now. We have been
brought a baby, a tiny infant, diagnosed as hearing impaired.
What will we do with him? What will we do for him? What
will we do to him?

GROWTHS, GAPS, AND FUTURE OBLIGATIONS: KEYNOTE ADDRESS

Grace M. Harris
The Society for Crippled Children and Adults of Manitoba, Winnipeg, Manitoba

Personnel in various fields of human endeavour, who have been seriously involved through the years in the positive advancement of civilization, are always aware of the importance of keeping up with the past. They do so in order to avoid repetition of derogatory actions, no matter how impressively they are re-articulated or semantically manipulated. To properly view the past is to selectively maintain, without indiscriminate experimentation, that which could be successfully applicable at any time in the world's ever-changing societies. It is also to act responsibly when spanning the voids which restrict the potential value of developments, now and in the future. Thus, they are in a position to recognize the growth and change which can effectively contribute to the improvement of human functioning.

Available information suggests there has been extensive improvement in the earlier, and thus more successful, management of hearing loss. Public action regarding hearing impaired children has moved from early disposal of a majority through death, through isolated institutionalization, to more and better residential day-school and clinical settings. Earlier identification of hearing loss followed by immediate intervention has resulted in more children who function normally earlier in life; more successful integration into our communication-controlled world; and, indeed, in far less cost to society as a whole.

The increase over the last 30 to 40 years in the number of disciplines providing services pertinent to hearing loss has contributed greatly to better management. Whereas, until the rather recent past, it was family doctors and teachers who had primary responsibility for attention to children with limited hearing, there now are many more personnel involved/available. Included among those making provisions or offering services might be: general practitioners, pediatricians, otolaryngologists, neurologists, geneticists, psychiatrists, psychologists, family counsellors, parents/guardians, and families, audiologists at research, clinical and educational levels, technologists, hearing aid dispensers, developmental

and child study personnel, public awareness support personnel
such as service clubs, community groups, and public relations
officers, speech-language pathologists, educators of the
hearing and hearing impaired from the earliest years and
ongoingly, administrative and governmental leaders, and others
whose attention would be required by hearing impaired children
with one or more other disabilities.

Under conditions of well-organized and well-coordinated
interdiscriplinary action, the findings of each discipline can
be best evaluated in conjunction with those of the other disciplines, resulting in decision making which will accrue to
the benefit of each hearing impaired child. "Team-work", so
crucially important, exists in actuality only where all members work together diligently, guiding each individual child
toward reaching his/her full potential. Each person within
each discipline does indeed have ongoing responsibility to
monitor his/her own knowledge and his/her own delivery of
services to young individuals having limited hearing. When
that responsibility is met, along with continuing education
and affiliation and participation through one's professional
associations - regional and national - the result can only be
a promotion of higher functioning for all hearing impaired
children. Knowledgeable and co-operative interdisciplinary
action has prevented, and indeed has an ongoing obligation to
continue to prevent, application of such derogatory and dark-
age tactics as:

1) generalizing and categorizing on the basis of the
   characteristics of the hearing loss, apart from all other
   individual human factors;

2) unnecessary segregation;

3) bad integration, which is often more debilitating than
   segretation;

4) toleration of administrative and governmental refusal to
   make further services possible which are validly needed;

5) many others which merely pay homage to failure, which no
   human being can afford, and do nothing for the child.

Obviously the "real" team is mandatory to successful management of hearing loss.

Medical developments and services so very important to the health of mankind continue to grow in depth and in number. Years of research and competent application have brought forth many successes, as in medical management of outer and middle ear problems. Progress being made toward successful use of the inner ear implant is encouraging, a worthy process which should be broadly supported. Medical progress in the areas of RH and blood factors, rubella immunization, management of drugs from prenatal through early childhood periods, viral diseases and ear infections, genetic counselling of parents and potential parents, has resulted in prevention of all forms of hearing loss. Highly aware and knowledgeable medical personnel, particularly among family physicians and pediatricians, do act immediately in response to high risk factors and/or a parent's suspicion of hearing loss. Referral directly to the appropriate specialist(s) makes possible the early identification of an existing hearing loss, and subsequent early intervention.

It remains a fact, however, that a major gap in management of hearing loss is created by a lack of early identification, at birth or very early life, for the majority of impaired children. Inappropriate advice to suspecting parents and/or misdiagnosis, primarily by family doctors and pediatricians, continue to be rampant. Whereas most children with a more severe hearing loss can be identified within the first year of life, a majority are not yet, nor are they appropriately referred. Many, even in larger metropolitan areas where pertinent services do exist, are not identified until well past 2 years of age. The most crucial age-range for learning and successful functioning by even the most "normal" of children in any society is 8 months to 2 years. There is no way that any hearing impaired child identified at a later age can, even with the best of follow-up services, compensate for that from which they have been unnecessarily deprived. It is indeed the responsibility of medical educators and physicians to activate programs for the early identification of hearing loss in a larger majority of very young humans. Until that occurs, as it should and could, the potential value of follow-up services will continue to be grossly restricted.

Audiology, a relatively young professional discipline, has contributed widely and in-depth to better management of hearing impairment. It has done so at levels of research, in standardized testing, in brainstem evoked response audiometry, and in conjunction with early aural rehabilitation.

Audiologic competence plays a leading role in early identification, in follow-up selection and fitting of hearing aids/
auditory trainers, in supervision of auditory functioning
under various environmental conditions, in activating provision of better listening conditions, and in conjunction
with the early learning process inclusive of parent counselling. Superior audiological services, particularly under
conditions of early identification, have identified middle
ear health problems which, when followed by referral to the
otolaryngologist, have resulted, in many instances, in prevention of further hearing loss. In view of the irreplace-
able role of audiology in the betterment of mankind, more
and stronger support must be given to establishing more
centres in the many areas where they are needed. Staffing
must be adequate to meet the demands of new referrals, as
immediately as possible, and to allow follow-up attention
when it is needed. Until audiological services are extended,
in depth and in number, restrictions will continue to be
imposed upon the excellent work which has been done to date,
upon much needed research and application, and upon early
identification and intervention and, thus, of course, upon
human functioning towards the "norm".

    Inventors and technologists have earned recognition
through their development of increasingly effective and
selectively useful hearing aids, auditory trainers, vibratory
systems, "loop" systems, and other amplifying devices, some
with accompanying visual units. Improvements such as sizes
more applicable to use by babies, clarity at more advanced
levels of amplification, sound reception and reproduction
across a broader frequency range at various levels of amplification, and many others, have contributed significantly to
better use of residual hearing, even when it is minute.
Even as the aforegoing, sound-proof audiometric booths and
accompanying equipment and hearing aid test equipment also
represent outstanding progress. It is not unrealistic to
anticipate invention of even more effective systems, perhaps
even more individualized to each hearing impaired person.

    A major gap, which has been allowed to "reign supreme"
through the years and even to this day, is that created
through delays in the proper fitting of the hearing impaired
child with the most appropriate amplifying device. Factors
such as under-staffed and over-scheduled audiologic centres,
distances from required services, and fragmented services,
create great difficulty in appropriate early management.

It is a shame that to procure one small hearing aid unit - a unit which could make the difference between a successful future or an unnecessarily imposed failure - a parent and child may have to travel great distances to various centers. The great distances between repair centres, the frequent lack of appropriate loaner aids during repair periods, the high cost of units for which the expense is not yet covered, or only partially covered by our health care systems, are problems which must be resolved beyond self and with humanity.

Training programs which provide both the infant and the young child guidance towards the "norm", were actually in operation in a few places of the world many years ago, when many of the excellent services of today were not available. Early training programs have increased in number during the last 40 years, more so in the last 25 years. The well-confirmed success stories resulting from some of those programs are reminders of the continuing need for highly qualified personnel to be in direct charge of the learning process.

Some centres provide "clinical" services only, child and parent/guardian exposed to training by teacher/clinician for one or more periods per week. Peer group involvement occurs when the child is ready and can be placed with hearing children in selected nursery schools. There are other centres which provide individualized infant/baby training, and follow-up nursery and kindergarten programs with special services and parent participation continuing throughout. Some peer groups are composed only of hearing impaired children, while in other centres they consist of hearing and hearing impaired children. Integration is becoming more successful, at earlier ages, under conditions in which all the required services are provided and correlated, and the teaching/learning standards of the "norm" are maintained for hearing children (if they are included), as well as for those with hearing losses. Success is measured by the on-going educational and social functioning of those children.

Involved professional personnel in any given early training centre, however "successful" that program may be considered, must always take responsibility on behalf of each child at both individual and "team" levels for action which improves and moves towards prevention and elimination of derogatory factors. Included in that responsibility is:

1) continuing evaluation and monitoring of services in
   operation;

2) recognition and spanning or filling of voids in services
   which restrict a child's functioning;

3) systematic evaluation of each individual child's functioning by observation and written record. This is necessary
   so that the various standardized test findings (audiologic, developmental, psychological, language, speech, etc.),
   can be more realistically interpreted and, as a result,
   information can be more effectively utilized to the
   child's advantage;

4) avoidance of setting restrictive standards for the
   handicap;

5) avoidance of centering "deaf" services so that all children, regardless of their various cultural and family
   backgrounds, and on the basis of audiologic findings only,
   must be trained the same way under one roof.

Earliest identification of hearing loss and the best of
follow-up intervention by professional personnel will be
effective only on the condition that the involvement of
parents/guardians is strongly and healthfully included in
the operations. Counselling (medical, audiologic, genetic,
psychological, family, information-training, etc.), more
often than not must be a continuing service through the
child's early years. It requires close "team" management to
avoid conflicting opinions being put to parents. Good relationships between professionals and parents have resulted,
not only in better parent-child functioning, but additionally
in parents establishing associations with well-defined goals.
Those associations have become a positive force leading
toward better and more needed services for children, more
and better public education, and further, to positive
governmental and administrative support.

Societal changes not restricted to any one part of the
world have resulted in many more mothers working outside
their respective homes. Some do it by choice, but many
more do so through a need for additional family support.
Thus, many more children are being placed in day care and
nursery settings, which vary greatly in "character." It is

indeed an obligation for the future, which should go into action immediately, to initiate coordination between personnel in nursery centres and those providing special services. In addition, there needs to be greater ongoing contact with "working" parents of hearing impaired children and, indeed, with their respective employers. Avoiding that responsibility can, in a short time and far too easily, result in a return to isolated segregation and gross underfunctioning for many hearing impaired young children and, thus, affect them throughout their lifetime.

Progress has been made in the early identification of a hearing loss in children with less severe losses; in identification of those other simultaneously present difficulties not attributable to hearing loss; and in recognizing other related areas. On the basis of information available to date, it has become apparent that more disciplines must become involved and that services within disciplines already in operation for the hearing impaired young population may require extension within one or another area.

Through the years, growth towards earlier and better management of hearing loss has been encouraging. This should be an incentive, both to those presently at work and those in the future, for their effort is not only on behalf of the hearing impaired, but on behalf of mankind at large.

REFERENCES

Abrahamsen, A. Child Language: An Interdisciplinary Guide To Theory and Research (Baltimore: University Park Press), 1977.

Ayres, A. Development Of Sensory Integrative Theory And Practice (Iowa: Kendall/Hunt), 1974.

Bender, R. The Conquest Of Deafness (Cleveland: Case-Western Reserve University Press), 1965.

Cairini, P. "Building A Curriculum For Young Children From An Experiential Base" Young Children, Vol. 32, 1977.

Calvert, D. and Silverman, S.R. Speech And Deafness (Wash-
    ington, D.C.: Alexander Graham Bell Association), 1975.

Cherry, C. On Human Communication (Cambridge, Mass: M.I.T.
    Press), 1968.

Cohen, L. and Solapatek, P. Infant Perception: From Sensa-
    tion To Cognition (New York: Academic Press), 1975.

Crystal, D. "Linguistic Mythology And The First Year Of
    Life" British Journal Of Disorders Of Communication Vol.
    8, 1973.

Curtiss, S., Prutting, C. and Lowell, E.L. "Pragmatic And
    Semantic Development In Young Children With Impaired
    Hearing" Journal Of Speech And Hearing Research Vol. 22,
    1979.

Davis, H. (ed.) "The Young Deaf Child: Identification And
    Management" Acta Otolaryngology 1965.

Davis, H. and Silverman, R.S. Hearing And Deafness, 4th
    edition (New York: Holt, Rinehart and Winston), 1978.

Deutsch, M. "The Role Of Social Class In Language Develop-
    ment And Cognition" American Journal Of Orthopsychiatry
    Vol. 35, 1965.

Eisenberg, R. "The Development Of Hearing In Man: An
    Assessment Of Current Status" ASHA Vol. 12, 1970.

Ewing, E. Hearing Impaired Children Under Five (Washington,
    D.C.: The Volta Bureau), 1971.

Fry, D. Development Of The Phonological System (Cambridge,
    Mass: M.I.T. Press), 1966.

Gerber, S. and Mencher, G. (eds) Early Diagnosis of Hearing
    Loss (New York: Grune & Stratton), 1978.

Gerwin, K. and Glorig, A. (eds.) Detection Of Hearing Loss
    And Ear Disease In Children (Springfield, Ill: C. C.
    Thomas), 1974.

Goldberg, S. "Social Competence In Infancy" (A Model Of Parent-Infant Interaction), Merrill-Palmer Quarterly Vol. 23, 1977.

Goldstein, M. Problems Of The Deaf (St. Louis, Mo: The Laryngoscope Press), 1933.

Greenberg, M. and Marvin, R. "Attachment Patterns In Profoundly Deaf Preschool Children" Merrill-Palmer Quarterly Vol. 25, 1979.

Harris, G. Language For The Preschool Deaf Child (New York: Grune & Stratton), 1971 (3rd ed.).

Harris, G. "Parent Counselling By Educators Of Hearing-Impaired Young Children" Proceedings Of Pacific Northwest Conference, Prince George, B.C., 1975.

Harris, R. "The Speech Pathologist As Counsellor" Australian Journal Of Human Communication Disorders Vol. 5, 1977.

Hubell, R. "On Facilitating Spontaneous Talking In Young Children" Journal of Speech and Hearing Disorders Vol. 42, 1977.

Jarvella, R. and Labinsky, J. "Deaf and Hearing Children's Use Of Language Describing Temporal Order Among Events" Journal Of Speech And Hearing Research Vol. 18, 1975.

Jedrysek, et al. Psychoeducational Evaluation Of The Preschool Child (New York: Grune & Stratton), 1972.

Katz, J. (ed.) Handbook Of Clinical Audiology (Baltimore: Williams and Wilkins), 1972.

Kavanagh, J. and Mattingly, I. (eds.) Language By Eye And Ear: The Relationship Between Speech And Reading (Cambridge, Mass: M.I.T. Press), 1972.

Ling, D. Speech And The Hearing Impaired Child: Theory And Practice (Washington, D.C.: Alexander Graham Bell Association), 1976.

McConnell, F. "The Parent Teaching Home" Peabody Journal Of Education Vol. 5, 1974.

Mencher, G. "Early Detection Of Hearing Loss In Children"
CCCD Newsletter on Communication Vol. 4, 1979.

Mencher, G. "Infant Hearing Screening: The State Of The
Art" Maico Audiological Library Series Vol. 12, 1974.

Magian, V. deC., Anderson, G. and McKenzie, E. "Mobile
Hearing Program In Central Rural Manitoba" Journal of
the Canadian Medical Association Vol. 115, 1976.

Northcott, W. The Hearing Impaired Child In The Regular
Classroom (Washington, D.C.: Alexander Graham Bell
Association), 1973.

Northern, J. and Downs, M. Hearing In Children (Baltimore:
Williams and Wilkins), 1974.

Oyer, H. and Frankman, J. The Aural Rehabilitation Process
(New York: Holt, Rinehart and Winston), 1975.

Phillips, A. and Ling, D. Aural Habilitation Process
(Washington, D.C.: Alexander Graham Bell Association),
1978.

Pollock, D. "Development Of An Auditory Function" O.C.N.A.
Symposium On Congenital Deafness Vol. 4, 1971.

Pollock, D. Educational Audiology For The Limited Hearing
Infant (Springfield, Ill: C.C. Thomas), 1970.

Ruben, R. and Daly, J. "Neomycin Ototoxicity And Nephrotoxi-
city. A Case Report Following Oral Administration"
Laryngoscope Vol. 78, 1968.

Schulte, K. "Mini-Fonator - Development Of Speech For Deaf
And Hard Of Hearing Children" International Journal Of
Rehabilitation Research, Heidelberg, Germany, Vol. 1, 1978.

Streng, A. Syntax, Speech And Hearing (New York: Grune &
Stratton), 1972.

Taylor, I. Neurological Mechanisms Of Hearing And Speech In
Children (Manchester, England: University Press), 1964.

Wedenberg, E. "Hearing Measurement Of Infants" Nord Psychiat
Tidskr Vol. 191, 1961.

Wong, D. and Shah, C. "Identification Of Impaired Hearing In Early Childhood" <u>Journal Of The Canadian Medical Association</u> Vol. 121, 1979.

THE TEAM APPROACH TO CONGENITAL DEAFNESS

Marion P. Downs

University of Colorado, Denver, Colorado

The involvement of many specialists in the diagnosis and management of the hearing impaired child provides an invaluable system to the child and his parents. In our experience, there is no substitute for a team approach to congenital deafness, and we strongly recommend its formation wherever possible.

The congenital deafness team is best centered in a pediatric clinic and basically includes an otologist, a geneticist, an audiologist, a speech pathologist, an educator of the deaf, a developmentalist, and a social worker, as well as a pediatrician. When needed, consultants are obtained from ophthalmology, neurology, cardiology and any other specialities that may be indicated for an individual diagnosis.

The four part program of the congenital deafness clinic of the University of Colorado Health Sciences Center spans the period almost literally from birth to death. This clinic, headed by a pediatrician, Dr. Janet Stewart, is involved in the newborn high risk screening program, so its first contact with a hearing impaired child is shortly after birth. The contact continues, in many cases, to adulthood. The four part program of this clinic includes Diagnosis, Placement Counselling, Monitoring and Advocacy. Although diagnosis is often considered the most important aspect of any program, we have found that all four aspects are equally vital to the child's welfare.

Diagnosis

Diagnosis is a cooperative effort of all the specialists involved, but the pediatrician is the primary manager of the case. The pediatrician cannot only determine the etiology, but also can identify other associated anomalies and can suggest a myriad of laboratory tests that will contribute to the diagnosis. The pediatrician also assesses the overall

development of the child and, in our case, provides genetic
counselling once the etiology is determined. In this, she
is assisted by the otologic expertise of the otolaryngologist
who may request other information, such as polytomography,
CT-scan, or brain stem evoked response audiometry.

The audiologist not only contributes baseline audiometry,
but evaluates the relationship of the child's functioning to
the degree of hearing loss, thus giving information relevant
to the diagnosis. The speech pathologist provides a baseline
speech and language evaluation which will be used to compare
later functioning. During the diagnostic workup, the social
worker becomes involved in helping determine where parents
are in their process of accepting the problem of the deaf
child. Are they in the denial stage, the anger stage, the
mourning stage -- and how can they be helped to an acceptance
of the problem which will allow them to best nurture the
child? It may be necessary at any given point, to bring in
a psychologist for some detailed psychological counselling.

The ophthalmologist is always called in in such cases as
congenital rubella syndrome and any of the associated eye
abnormalities. A renal consultant is obtained in such cases
as hereditary chronic nephritis, Alpert's syndrome, etc.
Cardiologists and neurologists are called in as indicated,
and it is found that in such complex cases as Hunter-Hurler
syndrome, the entire roster of specialists at the hospital
are usually involved.

Placement Counselling

The decision as to the placement of the child in an
educational program must be the parents' prerogative. Unless
the parents have made the decision, there will be second
thoughts and possibly recriminations at a later date. The
parents' decision is based on the following contributions
from the congenital deafness team: (1) information as to the
degree of loss;   (2) the results of the speech and language
evaluations, if relevant;   (3) an introduction to the types
of education available in the community. This would include
visits to each of the facilities that are offering programs
for the deaf and hard of hearing;   (4) encouragement to
choose freely and to feel comfortable with making a change at
a later date if, at any time, it appears that another program
will better benefit the child.

It is essential at this point that advice be given by persons who are not involved in the therapeutic process or the educational system. Here the managing physician – the pediatrician – may be the most effective and objective in guiding the parents.

Monitoring

In the first year or two, the child will be seen at least every six months for the following kinds of evaluations:

1) Medical second looks: Periodic reassessment of the etiology is of the essence in congenital deafness. Even when the etiology has been fairly certainly determined, it is necessary to take another look. Bergstrom has outlined specific reasons for re-evaluation, as follows:

    (1) Repeat audiometry may reveal progression of loss or unsuspected opposite ear involvement;

    (2) Case history review may reveal overlooked historical items such as early history of disease;

    (3) Physical examination may reveal overlooked physical findings or newly developed symptoms, such as thyroid problems, renal problems, night blindness, etc.;

    (4) Repeat family history may show suppressed information. For example, in one case, the father – a physician - was found later to have a hearing loss which he had not reported previously;

    (5) Repeat family history can reveal false-positive items. For example, a parent's report of childhood deafness in the family was found to refer only to episodes of otitis media, rather than familial deafness;

    (6) Red herrings in the physical and historical evaluation may show up with repeated evaluations;

    (7) An incorrect initial diagnosis may be corrected by re-evaluation;

(8)   Mental block phenomenon (Dr. Bergstrom refers here to human failure to think of all the possibilities in a diagnosis);

(9)   Progressive concommitant disease may be identified by follow-up evaluations;

(10) Completion of the workup, including all the laboratory tests that are relevant;

(11) Second thoughts;

(12) New information from a consultant;

(13) New scientific knowledge;

(14) New technology; and,

(15) To determine how the child is doing.

Speech and language evaluations are given to monitor the performance of the child in the particular program in which he has been entered. Again, it is important to have someone who is not involved in the therapeutic process evaluate the ongoing improvement of the child or his lack of improvement. Here the policy of flexibility in placement will be useful. If at any point it is obvious that the child is not making reasonable progress in the system in which he has been placed, consideration can be given to looking at a change of program.

Psycho-social re-evaluation and monitoring is extremely useful to determine whether or not any help should be given the family in psychological or social matters. It may be necessary to solicit public funds to help the family's finances in supporting the child in the particular program in which he is functioning. At any time in the program, public health support for purchase of a hearing aid can be enlisted.

Advocacy

In the team's function as an objective advocate of the child, apart from the methodology or the program the child is in, it may be necessary to arbitrate between the family and the system in the following ways:

(1)   If parents feel that the school system has mis-
      managed the child's placement, it may be necessary
      for the team to represent the family at hearings
      called to evaluate the disagreement. Federal law
      now mandates hearings that the parents can request
      whenever they feel a change is indicated. For
      example, in a public school system where only
      total educational programs were available for hear-
      ing impaired children, the team sent a representa-
      tive to present the case for the child's best
      interests being served by placement in an aural
      program.

(2)   When college age is reached, the team may be called
      upon to support the special interests of the stu-
      dent in obtaining a certain type of education.
      For example, a very bright, hearing impaired stu-
      dent wished to attend an out-of-state college which
      she felt would be more suitable for her particular
      skills and goals. However, the social rehabilita-
      tion service rules stipulated that the stipend was
      only available for in-state colleges. It was
      necessary for doctors, audiologists, and speech
      pathologists to present the case of students being
      supported for the out-of-state college placement.
      The case was eventually decided in the student's
      favor.

(3)   The interpretation of new advances, new technol-
      ogies or new surgeries can better be done by an
      objective team in which the parent has confidence.
      For example, our team has saved many a large
      expenditure for such useless treatment as acupunc-
      ture during its heyday; it has prevented expendi-
      tures for unnecessary hearing aids that will be
      urged by unethical salespersons. Further, in this
      day of micro-surgery of the ear and electrical
      implants, the team must again act as advocate for
      the child's best interests in helping to determine
      whether the innovations in surgery and implants
      may be applicable to the individual child.

It is evident that the work of a congenital deafness
team may be never-ending. It will continue until the client
is fully achieving and completely comfortable in the environment that has been chosen.

THE HEARING IMPAIRED INFANT: "PRIMARY CARE"*

D. Robert Shea
Glenrose Hospital, Edmonton, Alberta

"Deafness never killed anyone -- but who can count the lives it has wasted?" (Jaffee, M.D.)

The primary care physician, whether family physician or pediatrician, comes in contact with a hearing impaired infant or child in various ways. The infant may be referred or returned to him from an intensive care nursery (ICN) setting for continuing care with the presence of hearing impairment already established by specific audiology screening and confirmatory auditory brainstem response (ABR) or, hearing impairment may become apparent in an infant or child already under care. In either situation there are factors with which the physician should be familiar to facilitate appropriate medical management of that infant or child. As stated in the foreword to the text Childhood Deafness, Causation, Assessment and Management (Bess, 1976), "The management and care of deaf children is a combined operation calling for the whole hearted cooperation of many disciplines -- one that does not delegate to any discipline the automatic right to leadership" (Sir Terrance Cawthorne, 1966). This is certainly true and the primary physician with a hearing impaired child in his practice needs to have a close working relationship with the child's otologist and good communication with the assessment and rehabilitative facilities serving that child. In large urban centers the family will often contact members of the team working with the child when confronted with a problem pertaining to the ears or, at times, concerning behaviour problems. Often members of the team are in a position to meet these needs. In smaller centers and rural communities the first person approached when a problem arises is usually the physician. For that physician, the following factors and information are felt to apply in the primary medical management of hearing impaired children.

---

* Dr. Shea has directed this paper specifically to Primary Care Physicians.

Known Hearing Impairment

In this situation the nature of the hearing loss has
probably been defined or is under continuing otological
and audiological review. If hearing loss has been defined
as bilateral and moderate to severe, or severe to profound,
the child will likely have been fitted with hearing aids or
is in the process of being appropriately aided. If the
hearing loss is unilateral and normal hearing is present on
the other side, it is unlikely an aid would be utilized.
Even in cases of severe to profound bilateral hearing loss,
there is always the possibility of residual hearing being
available with appropriate amplification and auditory training. It is, therefore, important that any residual hearing
be prevented or minimized. It must be remembered that the
child with sensory-neural hearing loss is not immune from
middle ear disorders that also affect children with normal
hearing. Five studies involving severe to profound hearing
impaired children agreed that around 20% have a superimposed
conductive hearing loss that requires detection and treatment
to facilitate better function and benefit from amplification.
(Brooks, 1979).

Conductive hearing loss occurs with middle ear disease
arising through infection of the middle ear or through anatomic dysfunction as with eustachian tube obstruction. The
young infant cannot say, "Doc, it's my ears!" It helps to
be suspicious. Earlier pediatric clinicians used to teach
that there are three things that will cause a baby to waken
at night, screaming. These are earache, colic, or a fissure-
in-ano. Tugging at an ear while crying or rolling the head
from side to side and fussing may be an indicator of earache.
We tend to get very casual and sometimes careless in our
acceptance of colic as a cause of discomfort. Levin (1975)
describes how, "many doctors and mothers, when presented with
a baby, healthy or ill, contented or crying, tend to interpret situations in terms of the infant's abdomen, and noise
from either end is believed to indicate something wrong
within the gut, rather than within the brain or ear." He
found, of 66 infants less than 12 weeks of age presenting
with unusual or excessive crying, 9 had otitis. Three had
other conditions that might have contributed to their distress, but 6 were otherwise normal. All 66 mothers had
suspected a stomach disorder; none had suspected the middle
ear (Brooks, 1979).

The medical management of otitis media is based upon the infecting organism. Howie (1977) in a cohort from his own practice followed from birth, found that 63% had otitis media within the first 2½ years of life and those whose initial infection was from Streptococcus pneumoniae were two and one half times more likely to go on to have six episodes within those first 2 years. S. pneumoniae ranks as the major pathogen with the second most common organism isolated from middle ear disease Hemophilus influenzae. Some immune factors are of note. Specific antibody to the respective bacterium isolated from the middle ear fluid existed in both the acute serum and middle ear fluid in 50% of patients. In 10% of the patients under one year of age, there was an increase in specific antibody in convalescent serum 2 weeks later. This 10% increased to around 50% between ages 1 and 3 years. Most patients "outgrow" the otitis media stage of life by age 6 to 10 years, which is perhaps a reflection of the maturing immune system. Some (Lim, 1977) feel the early use of antibiotics reduces the ability to generate specific antibody, but I doubt many of us would withhold antibiotic treatment in the face of obvious infection. While vaccines against both S. pneumoniae and H. influenzae have been developed, they are not yet in common use. Optimal antibiotic therapy of acute otitis media currently consists of combinations of the sulfonamides and Penicillin V or Erythromycin for a period of 10 to 14 days. Ampicillin utilized earlier in otitis media in infancy because of its coverage of both of the above infecting agents, now finds less usage because of increasing incidence of H. influenzae resistance to Ampicillin. If middle ear fluid persists beyond 4 to 6 weeks, myringotomy with aspiration and culture should be undertaken together with insertion of ventilation tubes. The same should also be done for those experiencing their third bout of otitis media within a 12 month period. If mastoiditis or labyrinthitis is associated with the otitis media, the child should be hospitalized, myringotomy performed, and I.V. antibiotics instituted (Ruben, 1977).

The management of serous otitis is variable. The use of nasal decongestants for 5 days is usually not successful as most are due to anatomic or functional disturbance at the eustachian tube. Most physicians will use oral decongestants but if the fluid persists beyond 3 weeks, or if its appearance is repeated and recurrent, then consideration should be undertaken regarding the placing of ventilation tubes. Otological opinions vary on the value of adenoidectomy or adenoid-tonsillectomy.

Other childhood illnesses thought to be benign, but
which are of concern both to normal children and to those
who are hearing impaired, must include measles (Rubeola),
mumps and meningitis. Measles, in addition to its association
with otitis media, can cause a labyrinthitis. Mumps damages
hearing in up to 5% of cases and is considered to be the
leading cause of acquired unilateral, sensory-neural hearing
loss in children. This deafness may be profound and permanent, but some show less severe loss and partial recovery in
50% to 90% of cases (Wong and Shah, 1979). In an individual
with congenital unilateral hearing loss, the added insult of
unilateral deafness in the hitherto normal ear would be hard
to defend morally, if not legally, with the current availability of mumps vaccine. On the same grounds, with the
increasing availability of vaccines against S. pneumoniae
and H. influenzae -- organisms also involved in meningitis
in infants and children, there is a need to consider vaccina-
tion of hearing impaired children less than 2 years of age to
try to avoid further insult to already impaired hearing. The
incidence of hearing loss with meningitis is reported to be
6% with the highest incidence in the first year with the
majority occurring between age 3 months and 3 years (Keane
et al, 1979). Male to female ratio was 1.4 to 1 and involved
agents were H. influenzae, S. pneumoniae and N. meningitis,
in that order. The mechanism of the hearing loss with meningitis is believed to involve the arachnoid in the region of
the internal auditory canal producing a neuritis or peri-
neuritis of the VIII nerve. Small vessel thrombophlebitis
and increased intracranial pressure may interfere with cerebral circulation, leading to cortical anoxia and necrosis
which may damage central auditory pathways resulting in
auditory processing problems. These are complications beyond
those associated with the more common mechanism of hearing
involvement by spread of infection or bacterial toxin directly
through the internal auditory canal or cochlear aqueduct
(Lindsay, 1973; Igarishi and Schuknecht, 1962). Serous or
purulent labyrinthitis may ensue, causing partial or complete
destruction of the VIIIth nerve elements.

From the above discussion pertaining to the risk of
hearing loss as sequellae from measles, mumps and meningitis,
auditory evaluation should be undertaken early in the
recovery period, particularly with meningitis.

No Hearing Impairment Evident

To what should the primary physician be alert in the
care of infants and children in the absence of known hearing
loss? Many are aware, but all need to be reminded, about the
incidence of hearing loss in specific populations. Approximately 10% of all pregnancies are "high risk" and statistically, 3% of the babies in that at-risk group will have
significant hearing loss. One out of 50 ICN graduates will
be deaf (Galambos and Galambos, 1979). In most ICN settings
there are now routine screening procedures utilizing such
methods as the Crib-o-gram (Simmons, 1979), or similar
systems, or else there is follow-up by behavioural audiometry
or ABR studies. Many of us are concerned about the other 90%-
those who are born outside that 10%' "high risk" designation.
Though they may appear to be normal, one in every 1000 will
be deaf. Congenital deafness in the absence of other prenatal or perinatal causes, excepting family history of early
severe deafness of unknown cause, accounts for 20% to 50% of
the cases of profound deafness in children. Hereditary
nerve deafness is usually bilateral; if unilateral, it is
inherited as an autosomal dominant trait that is not always
penetrant (Wong and Shah, 1979).

Fifty per cent of asphyxia in newborns occurs in "low
risk" pregnancy and thus, is not anticipated as it would be
in the "high risk" group. Neonatal sepsis with gram negative
organisms, either of itself or when treated with ototoxic
drugs where renal function is impaired, it must be remembered,
is also potentially causative of deafness.

At this date, the list of potentially ototoxic drugs
would include:

Antibiotics	Diuretics
Streptomycin	Furosemide
Kanamycin	Ethacrynic Acid
Gentamycin	
Tobramycin	
Amikacin	
Neomycin	

For protocols regarding identification and diagnosis of
children in whom there is suspicion of congenital or acquired
hearing loss, the reader is referred to the front of this
book where the "Recommendations of the Saskatoon Conference
on the Early Diagnosis of Hearing Loss" and the

"Recommendations of the Nova Scotia Conference on the Early
Identification of Hearing Loss" are listed.

Rehabilitation

     Part of early management is rehabilitation. The primary
physician must know what is available in his own area regarding the assessment of a child found to be hearing impaired.
In most provinces there are centralized facilities embodying
Otologists, Pediatricians, Audiologists, Speech Pathologists
and often Psychologists, Social Workers and Educators of the
Hearing Impaired who, as an interdisciplinary team, assess
the child and in the light of their findings, recommend a
rehabilitative program. This program requires close monitoring regarding progress. Not many physicians are in a position
to advise on educational methods indicated for a specific
child. This is often difficult for experienced assessment
teams. A physician does no harm in suggesting to parents
that they find out as much information as possible about the
available and alternative programs provided in the area.
Auditory-oral programs depend on the use of residual hearing
with the assistance of amplification, plus training to learn
to listen, to hear and to speak by means of the auditory
channel. Here the emphasis is on listening, rather than
looking. Total communication programs utilize auditory
training along with the amplification, together with speech
reading and manual communication expressed through signs and
finger spelling. Total communication utilizes the simultaneous use of manual and spoken words to stimulate speech.
Once the decision is made, the parents, though committed to
that program, should try not to close the door on other
alternatives. With further development and maturation there
may be a need for a change to a different setting. Parents
should be flexible enough to accept the evidence for the
need for change in the interests of the child.

     A physician may find that on-going medical exams of
hearing impaired infants and children can be facilitated by
first taking the time to demonstrate examination procedures
on a toy animal with obvious anatomic parts. The few seconds
taken to look and let the child look into the ears, nose and
mouth of a plastic bunny, lamb or deer, plus showing how to
listen with a stethescope and how to palpate the abdomen pays
off in decreased physical and behavioural resistance to the
examination. Handing the child the toy to hold, which
occupies the hands, also helps the physician obtain better

clinical information.

The following summary of information for parents made
available by the Canadian Hearing Society may be useful in
contacts with parents who confront the physician with their
day to day problems and concerns. A list of information
sources for parents is also appended.

"All children, deaf or hearing, go through similar
stages. Deaf children tend to demonstrate more frustration
because of the lack of communication.   All children need
love. The deaf child cannot hear affection in a voice, but
he can see it in your face and in your actions. Extra cuddling and warmth needs to be demonstrated. Some resist cuddling but an approving pat on the head or a brief caress will
often suffice. Routines are helpful so that such a child can
learn to anticipate by repetition from day to day. Consistent and loving "limits" are also required which are really
lessons in living rather than punishment. Snap-shots are
useful in explaining where he is going or what he is going
to be doing, and in the absence of snap-shots, drawing little
stick figures will often convey what is intended. Positive
reinforcement on completion of the desired activity promotes
better compliance with subsequent similar activities. All
children have fears and deaf children are no exception.
Being deaf in a dark room is not pleasant -- a night light
helps. Demonstrating that when you have to leave you will
return can be done by starting off with a ten or fifteen
minute absence and then extending it to hours, having reassured him that you will, in fact, return. The expression
of his emotions should be encouraged: happy, sad, angry,
scared, so that these can be conveyed meaningfully to you for
your appropriate response. Deaf children need to play with
other children who serve as models for the deaf child's
behaviour and sandbox activities in your own or neighbor's
yard should be encouraged. Dads are essential components in
all of the above, as well as in spelling mother off and
relieving her of her constant role of mother, teacher and
playmate."

Advocacy

Someone must act as an advocate for the hearing impaired
child. Too often parents are inadequately informed as to the
needs for their child and how these needs may best be met.

There is a specific need for physicians to advocate surveillance in delivery rooms and nurseries for babies who are at
risk for hearing loss. Provincial and State Departments of
Health need to be encouraged to establish programs for early
identification of hearing loss in infancy. Such programs
should be incorporated into existing health care systems and
the selected identification system should be applied universally to the whole infant population. A revised "Physician's
Notification of Birth" form should be adopted incorporating
high risk factors and a single provincial or state agency
should be identified as being responsible for maintenance of
this data.

There is a need for advocacy regarding the teaching of
early identification, diagnosis and management of hearing
impaired children into the curriculum of the Schools of
Medicine and Nursing. Colleges of Education should be
encouraged to include in the curriculum information on the
implications of hearing loss and the management of the hearing impaired child in the classroom. Such information should
be provided by trained educators who, themselves, are working
with hearing impaired children in the regular classroom. A
spectrum of generally accepted rehabilitative teaching programs in educational systems should be available to meet the
specific needs of each individual child.

Rubella immunity should be mandatory as a condition for
employment in public institutions dealing extensively with
children, such as in Children's Hospitals and Schools. Close
liaison should be advocated among physicians, audiologists,
speech pathologists, educators and parent groups to provide
accurate information and continuing support for families of
hearing impaired children. The above resolutions were
adopted by the Canadian Advisory Coalition on Childhood
Hearing Impairment (CACCHI), a coalition representing Canadian
otologists, pediatricians, family physicians, audiologists,
speech pathologists and educators of the hearing impaired.

Empathy

In all handicapping conditions in infancy and childhood
there is a need for empathy on the part of the attending
physician. Many handicapping conditions are outwardly and
physically obvious. Though often associated with recognizable abnormalities, deafness does occur alone and is outwardly unrecognizable. Unlike meningomyelocoele, cerebral
palsy, mental retardation and epilepsy, it is a low profile

disorder. There isn't much status in being deaf. The hearing impaired miss a lot of the nuances within their own family, let alone in the classroom, on the playing field, or elsewhere in the community. Is it any wonder there are behaviour problems that have their origins in frustration at not understanding or being understood? -- at being chastised for not doing the assignment because the teacher mumbled or didn't think to write the assignment on the blackboard? No, deafness never killed anyone. But rather than contributing to the waste occurring in the lives of the hearing impaired, we can, as primary physicians, enhance those lives by better awareness of their needs and our individual preparation or preparedness to meet and serve those medical needs as well as advocating those measures and facilities so necessary for the management of the hearing impaired.

Sources of Information for Parents

The Canadian Hearing Society
60 Bedford Road
Toronto, Ontario, M5R 2K2

The Alexander Graham Bell
  Association for the Deaf
1537 Thirty-fifth Street N.W.
Washington, D.C., 20007, U.S.A.

The John Tracy Clinic
806 West Adams Boulevard
Los Angeles, California
90007, U.S.A.

International Association
  for Parents of the Deaf
814 Thayer Avenue
Silver Spring, Maryland
20910, U.S.A.

REFERENCES

Brooks, D.N. "Design factors in the identification and assessment of hearing loss" Annals of Otology, Rhinology, and Laryngology, Suppl 60 Vol 88, 1979.

Downs, M.P. and Hemenway, W.G. "Report on hearing screening of 17,000 neonates" International Audiology 8:72 - 76, 1969.

Downs, M.P. and Silver, H.K. "The A B C D's to H.E.A.R." Clinical Pediatries 11:643 - 566, 1972.

Galambos, C. and Galambos, R. "Brainstem Evoked Response
    Audiometry in Newborn Hearing Screening" Archives of
    Otolaryngology 105:86 - 90, 1979.

Gerber, S.E. and Mencher, G.T. (eds.) Early Diagnosis of
    Hearing Loss (New York: Grune & Stratton), 1978.

Howie, V.M. "Acute and recurrent otitis media" in Jaffe, B.F.
    (ed.) Hearing Loss in Children (Baltimore: University
    Park Press), 1977.

Igarishi, M. and Schuchnect, H.F. "Pneumonoccocci otitis
    media, meningitis and labyrinthitis, A human temporal
    bone report" Archives of Otolaryngology 76:126 - 130,
    1962.

Jaffe, B.F. (ed.) Hearing Loss in Children (Baltimore:
    University Park Press), 1977.

Keane, W.M., Potsic, W.P., Rowe, L.D. and Konkle, D.F.
    "Meningitis and Hearing Loss in Children" Archives of
    Otolaryngology, Vol 105:39 - 44, 1979.

Levin, S. "Infants with earache" South African Medical
    Journal 49:1530 - 1532, 1975.

Lindsay, J.R. "Profound childhood deafness: Inner ear
    pathology" Annals of Otology, Rhinology and Laryngology
    82:88 - 102, 1973.

Lim, D.J. "Infectious and Inflammatory Auditory Disorders"
    in Bess, F.H. (ed.) Childhood Deafness: Causation,
    Assessment and Management (New York: Grune & Stratton),
    1977.

Ruben, R.J. "The ear" in Rudolph, Barnett, Einhorn (eds.)
    Pediatrics (New York: Appleton, Century, Crofts), 1977.

Simmons, F.B., McFarland, W.H. and Jones, F.R. "An automated
    hearing screening technique for newborns" Acta Otolaryn-
    gologica 87:1 - 8, 1979.

Wong, D. and Shah, C.P. "Identification of impaired hearing
    in early childhood" Canadian Medical Association Journal
    121:529 - 542, 1979.

EARLY DETECTION AND TREATMENT OF DEAF CHILDREN: A EUROPEAN CONCEPT

Ole Bentzen
Janne Hartvig Jensen
The State Hearing Institute, Denmark

The Joint Expert Committee on the Physically Handicapped Child of the World Health Organization indicated (1958): Primary prevention relates to measures which prevent the initial occurrence of the handicap. Secondary prevention relates to early detection, early diagnosis and early aid, continuous treatment and rehabilitation, so that the extent of the impact of the disability will be mitigated as much as possible. For historical reasons, secondary prevention is dealt with first.

Early Detection

Modern rehabilitation of children with handicaps has shown that 30% have more than one defect, and that each is the nucleus for that chain reaction where handicap number 1 compounds the effect of handicap number 2, and so on. Taking an undiagnosed and, therefore, untreated deaf child as an example, the chain reaction could be:

1) bilateral severe hearing defect results in a lack of language development and the child becomes deaf-mute;

2) not being able to follow the ordinary school system, the child has to join the school for the deaf as a boarder and must leave parents and siblings;

3) the child becomes a pupil at the deaf school, together with other pupils with the same hearing and language handicap, and has to communicate through sign language, thus becoming a signing-deaf;

4) the child leaves the school as an adult without the ability to communicate with oral language, joins the club for the deaf, may be in sheltered workshops for the deaf, and becomes a member of the deaf minority in his homeland;

5) the deaf youngster may choose his partner among the deaf,
    being parents with a risk of about 10% deafness in their
    offspring.

        The figures in brackets not only list the problems, but
indicate the possible compounding handicaps forming the chain
reaction developing from undetected deafness in the newborn
or very young baby. In order to stop or minimize the elements
of this negative chain reaction, early detection, diagnosis
and treatment of the deaf, and of any other child with a
defect, including some sort of "at risk children" programme
is essential.

        Should the risk and high-risk register only cover the
deaf? The answer is simple: Never! This statement is based
on the experiences by Downs (1971), Egan (1977) and Rosen and
Austin (1979) who concluded that neonatal testing techniques
in their then present form could not be considered to validly
identify infants with hearing loss. The method might
actually become counter-productive by promoting false complacency in key personnel. The fact that children with a
handicap, quite apart from the nature of the defect, have
more in common than in difference, also supports the concept
of the risk registration.

Risk Children

        The first risk children programme was introduced in our
country in 1965, in the County of Ringkøbing (see later) with
about 4000 births per year. The registration used a reference form with the headlines:

Name: Mother and Father:
                                    Names:
                                    Occupations:
Birth position:

Sex, weight, length, screened at once or later:

Twin: Was the child helped to breath:

Icterus: none-slight-severe   Complications: which

1. Conditions during and after the birth;

2. Hereditary elements in the family;

3. Influences in intrauterine period;

4. Malformation of the child;

5. The child's diseases;

6. A child who did not develop normally;

7. Conditions in adolescence.

    The registration of these children to a central board of
doctors, health nurses and social personnel should be made
immediately after defects and/or diseases are suspected. In
most cases, it was done by the midwife or the doctors at the
hospital. The small staff of health nurses was reserved for
the visits to the homes and the guidance of parents of children at risk. This contact by the health nurse was established
after her contact with the family doctor. Experience has
demonstrated that 63% of the mothers with diseases during
pregnancy, who gave birth to children with handicaps, were
registered by the Mother Welfare prior to the births. The
mothers belonged to homes with chronic diseases in the family
or were known as socially insufficient parents; 54 of 202
homes (27%) were strained by insufficient economic and/or
housing problems. Forty per cent of all cases of asphyxia
occurred in children from such homes (Nørrelund, 1971). As
regards lack of antenatal examinations, 46% of these mothers
belonged to this milieu. The health nurses indicated that
64% of the families fully accepted the visits of the nurses.
Among the families less positive or finding the service need-
less, were 43% of all complications at birth, 44% of all
cardiac abnormalities and 56% of all rachitic children. These
facts stress the importance of the establishment of Risk-
children Registration as the basis on which the health nurse
service can operate in the search for such children. The
frequency of risk children is about 10%.

    In spite of the fact that such a program of registration
and health visiting never fulfills the optimal requirements,
its value has been demonstrated. The demand for closer co-
operation between the health visitor and the general

practitioner has provided an additional benefit to the early
detection of defects in children. The doctors gained an
increasing understanding of the value of health visitors and
their capacity to provide assistance to the general
practitioner.

High-Risk Children

     In 1979, another programme for the registration of
children with defects and/or social handicaps was established
in a town with 63,000 inhabitants. The birth rate is 950
babies a year. This programme only covers children up to the
age of 7 years; children with chronic diseases, defects and
handicaps; or children growing up in an insufficient social
environment. Only the severe cases are reported to the Board
of Pediatricians, health nurses and social administrators.
For the year 1979, high-risk children were registered as
follows: 19 cases suspected of retarded development and
speech retardation, 15 cases with social problems, 4 cases
with problems of the parents, and 9 cases of defects and
chronic diseases. The main purpose of this registration, in
close contact with the pediatric department of the hospital,
is to streamline the collaboration between any type of expert
and any sort of requirements needed for the sake of the child
and its family.

The BOEL Test

     The BOEL screening test devised for the early discovery
of communication disorders in infants (Stensland-Junker, 1976;
Barr et al. 1978), has been used in the County of Århus,
(pop. 560,000), during the past 3 years. Children aged 7 - 10
months have been tested by their regular health visitors,
and the children who failed the primary screening were
referred for further evaluation at the State Hearing Centre
Århus. Out of a total of 12,000 infants tested by 120 health
visitors during the period of March 1, 1977 - March 31, 1980,
167 children (1.4%) did not respond properly to the sound
signals.

     In the following, we are only looking at the results
concerning the detection of hearing defects (Table I).

TABLE I: DISTRIBUTION OF HEARING LOSS IN 202 CHILDREN
DERIVED FROM A POPULATION OF 12,000 CHILDREN

	No.	Per Cent
Children Examined	12,000	100%
Hearing Loss Suspected	167	1.4%
Hearing Loss Confirmed:		
Middle Ear	27	
Sensory-neural	2	
Hearing loss not suspected with BOEL test	2	
Total number of sensory-neural cases	4	0.033

In conclusion, we must say that the BOEL test has not
provided us with a new and simple hearing test. It never
claimed to be one, but as the sound makers play an important
role, many parents may be given a false security if the child
passes the test. The intensity of the bells is too high to
reveal even moderate hearing losses, and lack of interest in
the sound may be a sign of understimulation or of chronic
middle ear problem. The BOEL test, however, has given us a
very close contact with the health visitors. The test has
made them more aware of probable hearing losses, and the
importance of finding them as early as possible. Many
children have been referred before the BOEL test age because
the health visitor found the child at risk at an early age.

Risk Parents

It should be noted that, in general, virtually no
disease or acquired defect is entirely of exogenous origin;
genetic factors always play some role. Rubella embryopathy,
being by far the most important prenatally acquired cause of
profound childhood deafness, was studied in relation to
juvenile diabetes by Forrest et al. (1969), and Johnson and
Tudor (1970). They postulated that the association of
rubella embryopathy with juvenile diabetes was more frequent
when there was a genetic predisposition to diabetes. Andersen et al. (1970), found a genetic predisposition to noxious
effects on hearing of the fetal viral infection. In relatives of children with deafness due to rubella, they found,

by refined testing involving the use of Bekesy audiometry and measurement of the stapedius reflex, subclinical abnormalities in the parents.

Both the mother and the father play a role in the production of a defective child. The chromosomal studies of fathers of mongolic children have shown that it is their genetic responsibility alone in some cases. The well-known fact that diabetic mothers give birth to over-weight babies with an increased incidence of congenital malformations (Pedersen et al. 1964), is now supplemented by the knowledge that even in couples in whom only the father has diabetes, their children can be over-weight at birth by 10% of the normal birth weight.

Otosclerosis

As a consequence of our examination of about 500 patients with otosclerosis, skin biopsies in these individuals demonstrated abnormalities indicating that this disease could be part of a generalized connective-tissue insufficiency (Bentzen 1961; 1967). The same abnormalities are found in individuals with osteogenesis imperfecta (Stadil, 1961). Analysis of the birth weight of neonates born to otosclerotic mothers with no diabetes in the family seems to indicate that these females may also be risk mothers. In our studies, 675 children of otosclerotic mothers had birth weights compared with a normal population of babies (Table II).

TABLE II: DISTRIBUTION OF BIRTH WEIGHT IN NEONATES OF OTO-
           SCLEROTIC MOTHERS, COMPARED WITH STATISTICS OF THE
           NEWBORN, 1964, ÅRHUS, DENMARK

Birth Weight	Normal Population	Mothers with Otosclerosis
More than 4,500 grams	2.2%	9.7%
Under 2,600 grams	6.4%	8.4%
Number of children	1,369	675

Cornea-positive Mothers With X-ray
Positive Cochlear Otosclerosis

In a series of patients with pure bilateral sensory-
neural hearing loss examined by x-ray and semi-axial tomo-
graphy, (Sindrason et al. 1980), pregnancy and birth have
been studied in 10 mothers. They were primarily not selected
for this purpose. The values from corneometry in 7 women
were between 0.595 mm and 0.560 mm and in 3 between 0.555 and
0.540 mm. The x-ray examination demonstrated different
degrees of sclerotic processes at the oval window and/or
cochlea for both ears in 8 women; in a single ear only in 2
women.

They had a total of 32 pregnancies resulting in 29
births (Table III).

TABLE III: PREGNANCIES AND BIRTHS IN A SERIES OF 10 WOMEN,
            ALL CORNEA-POSITIVE WITH X-RAY-POSITIVE COCHLEAR
            OTOSCLEROSIS INDICATING INSUFFICIENCY OF THE
            ORGAN OF CONNECTIVE TISSUE

Pregnancies

32 cases   Abortion: 1   Extra-uterine: 2 (same mother)

Births

29 cases	Under 2600 g	2600-4500 g	Over 4500 g	Girls	Boys
Single-28:	1	26	1	17	11
Multiple-1:	1	1		1	1

Postpartum Complications

Severe haemorrhages: 4 cases (same mother)

Children with a defect: 3

Rubella embryopathy: 1 girl

Unilateral deafness: 1 boy (twin)

Micrognathia, etc.:   1 girl (twin)

The two pregnancies with extra-uterine localization
occurred in the same mother. Giving birth to 3 normal children resulted in her sterilization.

In one mother, all 4 births were complicated with severe
postpartum haemorrhages. After the first birth, her doctor
advised against being pregnant again. Later, a diagnosis of
pernicious anaemia was made (HCA 19.413). The pregnancies
by 2 women in whom examination with both x-ray of the pars
petrose and corneometry supported the suspicion of the
existence of an insufficient connective-tissue organ are
supplemented by Table IV. The table illustrates what
happened to the offspring of 5 mothers with otosclerosis and
2 mothers with normal hearing, all cornea-positive. Shown
are birth weight, complications at birth, hearing ability and
the results of corneometry. The influence of the cornea-
positive father on the offspring indicated by birth weight,
defects, hearing ability and results of corneometry is shown
in Table V. In the 12 couples of parents (Tables IV and V)
5 had a child with juvenile otosclerosis and 2 couples had
more than 1 child with sensory-neural hearing defect. The
case described below in Table IV as HCA 63.107 is shown in
the corneogram seen as Figure 1.

Twenty-five Years of Experience
in the Treatment of Deaf Children

The first school in Denmark for the instruction of deaf
children was started in 1806. It was Peter Castberg, a
general practitioner, who inspired by his travels abroad,
founded the school. He was particularly interested in the
French method, the sign-language method, which he had studied
in Paris. Sign language was, in his opinion, the "mother
tongue of the deaf."

In 1945, the speech method was introduced into this
country by A. Dahlerup, a clergyman who had studied abroad,
notably Germany, among other places. He repudiated the sign
method and believed that "sound language" could also, for
the deaf, be "a conversation with oneself," for which reason
the language should be learned directly and the translation
process avoided. In 1950, Dahlerup started a private school
where the pupils were instructed according to the speech
method.

TABLE IV: FIVE CORNEA-POSITIVE MOTHERS WITH OTOSCLEROSIS AND TWO CORNEA-POSITIVE MOTHERS WITH NORMAL HEARING. THEIR CHILDREN INDICATED BY BIRTH WEIGHT, COMPLICATIONS AT BIRTH, HEARING ABILITY AND RESULTS OF CORNEOMETRY

Diagnosis	Mother Cornea	Father Cornea	Children Cornea	Birth Weight	Diagnosis
Coch. otosclerosis bilat. 66.153	0.580			B 3.0	dyspepsia, sevr. died
				F 3.5	" " "
				M 3.5	" mod. living
Otosclerosis bilat. 62.279	0.550	0.520	0.565	F 3.2	hi. freq. loss bilat.
			0.605	M 4.0	" " " " "
			0.550	F 3.2	" " " " "
			0.580	F 2.3	" " " " "
			0.550	F 3.0	" " " " "
			0.560	F 4.2	normal
Otosclerosis bilat. 1463	0.545			F 3.6	par. placenta acreta
				F 3.7	total placenta acreta
Otosclerosis bilat. op. 30.888	0.545	0.550	0.540	F 4.0	otosclerosis
			0.535	F 4.0	normal
Otosclerosis bilat. 64.991	0.545	0.570	0.570	F 3.3	normal
			0.540	B 3.5	"
			0.560	B 4.0	"
			0.565	B 3.5	"
Normal hear. neuritis optic 63.107	0.605	0.550	0.580	B 5.0	Normal
			0.545	G 3.5	skin biops. abn.
			0.600	G 4.7	
			0.565	G 4.8	
normal hear.	0.545	0.510			abortion
					abortion
					abortion
					abortion
				M 1.4	asphyxia with hear. loss

TABLE V: FIVE CORNEA-POSITIVE FATHERS. THE OFFSPRING, INDICATED BY BIRTH WEIGHT, DEFECTS, HEARING ABILITY AND RESULTS OF CORNEOMETRY, FROM FIVE CORNEA-POSITIVE FATHERS.

Number	Father Cornea	Mother Cornea	Children Cornea		Diagnosis
Neuromusc. disease perc. deafn. right ear 58.754	0.620	0.550	0.595	F 3.7	normal
			0.595	M 4.3	hi. freq. loss bilat.
			0.595	M 3.0	hi. freq. loss bilat.
					neuromuscl. disease
normal 50.666	0.580	0.530	0.560	G 3.5	otosclerosis bilat.
			?	F 3.5	ano-vaginal fistula
			?	M 3.5	
Perc. hear. loss bilat. 50.449	0.590	otoscl.	0.565	M 2.4	cochl. otoscler. bilat.
			?	M 2.4	art. hyperten.
			?	F 2.7	
otoscler. bilat. 50.232	0.565	0.565	0.540	F 3.2	otoscler. bilat.
			0.540	F 3.4	cholesteatoma
perc. hear. loss bilat. 50.465	0.555	0.520	0.575	M 3.5	otosclerosis

FIGURE 1:   RESULTS OF CORNEOMETRY PLOTTED IN A CORNEOGRAM
             FOR A BLIND MOTHER AND HER 4 HEALTHY CHILDREN
             (CASE HCA 63.107)

A 48 year old woman with acute bilateral optic neuritis
causing blindness appeared to be cornea-positive;
corneometry: 0.605 mm. Light-microscopic examination of the
skin showed atrophy of the epidermis and degeneration in the
collagen and elastic fibres.   All four children were examined
for birth weight and results of corneometry.   Examination of
the skin in all four children showed mild degenerative abnormalities in the collagen.   All were healthy, and all had
normal hearing, as did the mother.   Their father had normal
hearing, and corneometry was within normal limits.

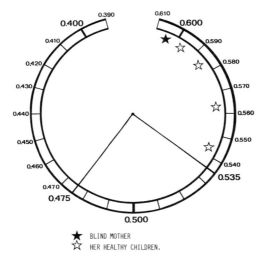

The occurrence of otosclerosis as a manifestation of
insufficiency of the connective tissue organ, and the demonstrated abnormal incidence of birth weight in children borne
by mothers with otosclerosis, seems to indicate that they
can be risk mothers.   This hypothesis is further supported
by the findings of abnormal pregnancies and births, and
children born with congenital defects in cornea-positive
and x-ray-positive otosclerotic mothers.

The objective method for the diagnosis of connective-
tissue insufficiency by corneometry seems to be helpful in
the screening of risk parents, mothers as well as fathers.

The first classes for hard-of-hearing children were
started in Copenhagen in 1916. In 1954, the first centre
for special educational treatment under the administration
of the primary school was opened in Århus. The school system
for deaf and hard-of-hearing children in Denmark (population
of 5 mill) today includes 3 day- and boarding-schools for the
deaf, one boarding school for further education and 12 centres
for special education situated in the ordinary primary school.
The "Folkeskoleloven (Primary Education Act) of June 7, 1958"
and subsequently issued government circulars of 1961 and 1965
require the local authorities to provide special schooling
for those pupils, quite apart from the nature of their
handicap, who are unable to follow the ordinary curriculum.

Hard-of-Hearing and Deaf
Children in a County of Denmark

To illustrate the educational task that hearing-defective
children present, conditions in one county of this country
have been chosen for examination. In the county of Ringkøbing
(population approximately 250,000), the primary school's
centre in Herning is responsible for hard-of-hearing and deaf
children. That county does not have a specific school for
the deaf. One of the authors (OB) has been the otological
and audiological officer to the area, paying regular visits
to the primary centre in Herning, since its establishment in
1961. A summary of the results of our work indicates the
following. In 1974, within a population of 250,368, 4,056
children were born. The hearing status of hard-of-hearing
and deaf children in the county born between 1959 - 1969
shows 120 children with a hearing loss equal to, or greater
than 40 dB. Among them, 40 children have a monaural hearing
loss with normal hearing in the other ear. They all attend
the normal school. There were 80 children with a binaural
hearing loss equal to, or greater than 40 dB in the better
ear. Of these, 45 are pupils in the ordinary school, 31
attend the centre for special education in the ordinary
school, and 4 stay at the boarding school for the deaf in
another county. The distribution of the degree of their
hearing losses appears in Table VI, where the hearing loss
in dB is measured as Threshold Carhart (TC). That is, the
average of the thresholds at 500, 1000 and 2000 Hz in the
better ear is used for comparison of the degree of the hearing defect.

TABLE VI: HEARING STATUS OF SCHOOL CHILDREN WITH BINAURAL
            HEARING DISORDERS LIVING IN THE COUNTY OF RINGKØ-
            BING AND BORN BETWEEN 1959 – 1969. DISTRIBUTED
            ACCORDING TO SCHOOL PLACEMENT IN NORMAL PRIMARY
            SCHOOL OR SPECIAL CENTRE CLASSES.

Hearing loss is reported in decibles measured as Threshold
Carhart (TC). There are 45 pubils in a normal school and 31
in a special education centre.

School Placing	Primary		School		
dB Level:	40–70 dB	80–110 dB	40–70 dB	80–110 dB	Total
Type of Loss:					
Conductive hearing loss	8			1	9
Sensory-neural hearing loss	28	9	9	21	67
TOTAL	36	9	9	22	76

        We have chosen a hearing loss equal to or greater than
40 dB in the better ear to indicate the children in question.
A hearing loss of this dimension is so obvious a handicap
that parents will consult a doctor and/or the school teacher
will refer the child to the school medical officer for examination. Despite hearing aid treatment, a hearing defect of
this dimension often calls for supportive measures from the
educational authorities.

        Since 1950, all hard-of-hearing and deaf individuals in
Denmark, children as well as adults, get free aids. All 80
children have been treated with binaural hearing aids from
their first years of life, and most of them have attended

normal kindergarten. As appears from Table VI, a little over
half of the children, 45 pupils, are attending classes in
the normal school, 9 of these have hearing defects greater
than 80 dB. The rest, 31 pupils, are in a special school,
22 of whom have hearing defects greater than 80 dB.

The survey shows that the speech of one-third of the
hard-of-hearing and deaf children can only be understood by
their families. The rest understand and are understood by
strangers. Only 5 of the pupils support their speech by
using sign language. Only 4 children of a total of 80 children were transferred to the school for the deaf, where they
are residential pupils.

The very high frequency of the hard-of-hearing and deaf
children being able to talk is a consequence of their early
start at using aids; their attendance at normal kindergarten;
and their schooling either in normal classes in ordinary
schools or centre classes where their teachers may conduct
20 - 30% of the weekly lessons in ordinary classrooms.

Since 1928, a number of severely hard-of-hearing and
deaf children have been taught by the speech method at a
special private school in Vejle, Denmark. The children who
remained in their homes attended the school daily, where
training was based on education in the understanding of
speech, articulation, lip-reading and training of hearing
itself. In 1954, the systematic use of hearing aids for
all pupils was introduced. A comparison between the hearing
loss of 59 pupils in that group and 43 members of the sign
language deaf society in Denmark shows a similar distribution
of hearing loss in the two groups. While the 43 sign-deaf
all use manual communication and, thus, cannot make themselves understood to strangers, an examination of the 59
former pupils of the school in Vejle shows that 48 of them,
or 80%, speak so well as to be understood by strangers. A
survey of the pupils' later theoretical education shows that
12 men and 2 women from the Vejle program have completed
secondary school without any form of special aid or the use
of an interpreter. The oral training has, thus, enabled
them to communicate with normal-hearing people.

Treatment with hearing aids has, in this study, only
played a secondary role. There are only 5 of the 59 who
used hearing aids before they entered school at the age of
7 years. This fact clearly demonstrates the effectiveness

of the speech method, as the utilization of this teaching,
together with the child's staying in its own home, has
primarily enabled these children to learn to speak.

In experiences both from a Danish special school started
1928 with education of the deaf based on the speech method,
and the results from a Danish county where nearly all hard-
of-hearing and deaf children are kept at home attending
either the ordinary school in normal classes or the centre
classes, the fundamental importance of the language milieu
is demonstrated. In both examples, a high frequency of
hearing-defective children achieve the ability to communicate
with strangers by intelligible speech.

This standard for the rehabilitation of the deaf has
been used in a survey of a large number of hard-of-hearing
and deaf children in Europe in which 3,462 children with
hearing loss of 50 dB or worse in the better ear have been
studied in their eighth year of life.

Childhood Deafness in the
European Community

In 1972 - 1973, the Commission's Medical Research
Committee (CRM) of the European Community set up an ad-hoc
Working Group on Deafness. It was decided to study the
incidence of deaf children, the etiology of hearing defects,
hearing aid usage and the results of different teaching
methods in the nine countries in the European Community
(total population approximately 250 mill). The research
started in 1974 with the objective: "To determine the prevalence of hearing loss of 50 dB or worse in all children
born in 1969 in the nine countries of the Community and to
obtain information on the cause of deafness, the type of
education and the communication ability of each child."
Using questionnaires, information about 3,462 children has
been obtained from the total of 4,126,466 live births in
1969.   The children having a hearing loss of 50 dB or worse
in the better ear were born in 1969 in Belgium, Denmark, Eire,
France, Italy, Luxenburg, the Netherlands, United Kingdom
and Western Germany. The data were collected in 1977 and
focus on the situation of eight year old children in the
study area.

The study of etiology shows that at least two-thirds of
the children are congenitally deaf. For all member countries,
the hearing defects for half the children are confirmed by
their third birthday. By six years of age, 90% have been
diagnosed as deaf. These results stress the importance of
early diagnosis through the establishment of programmes for
high-risk children.

The distribution of hearing loss for all children shows
that 40 - 50% have a hearing loss of 90 dB or more in the
better ear, a fact which indicates the possibility of finding
children early in their lifetime. Treatment with hearing
aids has been prescribed for half the children by the time
they reach their fourth birthday, and in 90% before they are
six years old. The type of hearing aid chosen (ear level or
body aids) is about 50-50. Binaural aids are used with about
three-quarters of the children in four countries, and with
about two-thirds in four other countries. In one country,
only one-third of the children use binaural aids. Binaural
aids or body aids with Y-cord are used in 69% of all children.

In the European Community, approximately two-thirds of
the children attend special schools for the deaf, the
remainder attend ordinary school. Manual communication is
used by 35% of all children.

Twenty-nine per cent of all children are reported to
have associated handicaps, with 9% of the children in the
study reported as below normal intelligence. It would
appear from the results that, making due allowance for
hearing loss, the reading capacity of pupils in special
schools for the deaf is of a lower standard than those in
the ordinary schools.

Less than half of the children (47%) have the ability
to communicate with speech which is intelligible to strangers.
A quarter of the children were able, at best, to speak in
single word utterances. This places them as developmentally
equivalent to a child of less than 2 years old. The ability
to speak intelligibly to strangers ranges from two-thirds
in some countries to one-third in other countries, notably
where only about 40% of the children always use hearing aids
out of school.

Conclusion

Early detection of deaf children, as well as other
children with congenital or early acquired defects, is of
paramount importance for the rehabilitative programming of
the child. Experience from different studies concerning
the screening of neonates for hearing defects indicates that
earlier methods cannot be considered valid to identify
infants with hearing loss. Programmes for risk children
and high-risk children covering all sorts of defects and
handicaps have to be established for the safety of early
detection. The BOEL test, performed by the health nurse
with suspected children examined by a trained medical doctor
and a speech and hearing therapist, appears to be able to
find the unstimulated child in the first year of life.

Methods should be evaluated for the screening of risk
mothers and fathers. For example, screening for insufficient
connective tissue in the parents seems, to some extent, to
be possible by corneometry, an optical, harmless examination
of the cornea.

The situation of the deaf child in Denmark, detected
early and treated early with binaural aids, is shown in a
country where nearly all of the deaf and hard-of-hearing
children attend the ordinary school.

The aim in all rehabilitation of deaf children is the
development of the ability to speak to strangers intelligibly,
or at least to parents and other members of the family.
Premise number 1 is there should be early detection of these
children; premise number 2 is that early and continuous
treatment by binaural hearing aids and the ability to grow
up in milieu of speech should continue during schooling.

The situation for hearing impaired children born in
1969 in 9 European countries was analyzed at their eighth
year of life in a study done by an ad-hoc Working Group on
Deafness in the European Community. The European report on
3,462 children, of whom about half have a hearing loss greater
than 90 dB in the better ear, shows the degree to which the
deaf children have been rehabilitated. These children's
ability to speak intelligibly to strangers differs from two-
thirds in some countries to one-third in other countries.
The European report came to the conclusion that the earliest
possible provision of hearing aids is important; that further

work has to be carried out on the type of school placement;
that the degree of integration with normally hearing and
speaking children is critical; and that the efficiency of
specialized teaching techniques have to be studied in the
future. These points are valid for any deaf child in the
world and, therefore, guidelines for the future management
of the deaf child from a global point of view.

REFERENCES

Andersen, H., Barr, B. and Wedenberg, E. "Genetic disposition of prerequisite for maternal rubella deafness"
Archives of Otolaryngology 91:141, 1970.

Barr, B., Stensland-Junker, K. and Ovard, M. "Early Discovery of hearing impairment: A critical evaluation of
the BOEL test" Audiology 17:62 - 67, 1978.

Bentzen, O. "Les anomalies de la peau chez les otospongieux"
Excerpta Int. Congr. Serv. 35:40 - 41, 1961.

Bentzen, O. "The otosclerotic syndrome" Acta Otolaryngologica
suppl. 224:124 - 132, 1967.

Bentzen, O. and Knudsen, V. "Taleoplaering af døve og svaert
tunghøre børn" Ugeskr. Laeg. 130:1990 - 1994 (with English
resume), 1968.

Downs, M.P. "A current overview of newborn hearing screening"
in Cunningham, C.C. (ed.) Conference On Newborn Hearing
Screening (Washington, D.C.: Alexander Graham Bell
Association for the Deaf), 1971.

Egan, J.J. "A survey of the use of high-risk registers in
the United States" ASHA 19:320 - 322, 1977.

Forrest, J.M., Menser, M.A. and Harley, J.D. "Diabetes
mellitus and congenital rubella" Pediatrics 44:445, 1969.

Johnson, G.M. and Tudor, R.B. "Diabetes mellitus and congenital rubella infection" American Journal of the
Disabled Child 120:453, 1979.

Joint Expert Committee on the Physical Handicapped Child. WHO techn. Rep. Ser. 1958, 58, 8.

Martin, J.A.M., Hennebert, D., Bentzen, O., Morgon, A., Holm, C., McCullen, I.S., Meyer, M.L. and deJonge, G.A. Childhood Deafness in the European Community, Contract N. 359-77-9 EC.I.U.K., in press.

Mencher, G.T. "A program for neonatal screening" Audiology 13:495 - 500, 1974.

Nørrelund, N. "Mødrehjaelpen og sundhedsplejerske" Ugeskr. Laeg. 133/18:900 - 904, 1971 (English resume).

Pedersen, L.M., Tygstrup, I. and Pedersen, J. "Congenital malformations in newborn infants of diabetic women" Lancet 1:1124, 1964.

Rosen, K. and Austin, A.M. "The high-risk register for neonates at risk of deafness: Limitations of presently recommended procedures" Australian Journal of Audiology 1:67 - 71, 1979.

Stadil, P. "Histopathology of the Corium in Osteogenesis Imperfecta" Danish Medical Bulletin 8:131 - 134, 1961.

Stensland-Junker, K. "BOEL - a child welfare program for early screening of communication abilities" in Mencher, G.T. (ed.) Early Identification of Hearing Loss (Basel: Karger), 1976.

OTOLOGICAL CARE OF THE HEARING IMPAIRED CHILD

Robert J. Ruben
Gary Fishman
Albert Einstein College of Medicine, Yeshiva University, New York

Introduction

Continuous otological care of the hearing impaired child has been traditionally practiced for almost two centuries. One of the earliest examples of continuing otological care is to be found in the appointment in 1800 by Abbee Sicard of Dr. Jean-Marc-Gespard Itard as resident physician to the institute of the deaf mutes (Lane, 1976). Since then, throughout the world there have been many otologists who have participated in the continued otological care of the hearing impaired child. This has occurred either within an institution or in an ambulatory center within clinics or private offices. Continued otological care would appear to be appropriate in that the disease processes which cause hearing impairment are not static; new disease processes may, and do occur; and the child is a developing organism in which processes will have different effects at different times of the child's life.

This report will examine the findings of continuing care examinations of a population of hearing impaired children. The findings of other studies of acquired otological diseases affecting the child will be analyzed. This data will then be discussed in terms of the type of program which is needed to promote optimal otological care for the hearing impaired child.

The Population

The City of New York has an established program for the diagnosis and care of hearing impaired children. This program in part consists of several hospital based diagnostic and follow-up centers for the hearing impaired children. The program mandates that each child who has been diagnosed as having significant hearing impairment, usually a severe to profound hearing loss, must have an annual examination performed by a board certified otolaryngologist. Entrance into this follow-up program is essentially restricted to families with limited economic resources. The follow-up population includes child-ren with severe to profound hearing loss who are from econom-ically deprived or depressed families, or those who are in foster homes. Children remain in the program until 21 years of age.

The follow-up examinations of 212 different children in the program at the Bronx Municipal Hospital Center from 1976 to 1979, with an age range from 2 to 20 years, with an aver-age age of 9 years 4 months, were analyzed to determine the incidence of significant findings at the time of the examina-tion (Tables I and II). The index visit was the last recorded follow-up for each child. Data was taken from the notes recorded by the attending otologist. There was no uniform assessment of the various conditions which occurred and various otologists would seek different types of informa-tion. This study is retrospective and will only give an approximation of conditions which can be assessed.

TABLE I

INCIDENCE OF SIGNIFICANT FINDINGS IN THE ANNUAL OTOLOGICAL
EXAMINATIONS OF 212 HEARING IMPAIRED CHILDREN

Findings	% of Total Population*	% of Significant Findings **
Hearing Aid	29.0	57.0
External Auditory Canal	6.0	11.0
Middle Ear	6.0	11.0
Inner Ear	3.0	7.0
Otorhinolaryngological Disorder other than ear	3.5	8.0
Other	2.5	6.0
Total Incidence	50.0%	

*   Denominator = 212 examinations
** Denominator = 107 significant findings.

TABLE II

INCIDENCE OF SIGNIFICANT FINDINGS IN THE ANNUAL OTOLOGICAL
EXAMINATION OF 212 HEARING IMPAIRED CHILDREN

Finding		N	% *
Hearing Aid:			
Malfunction		36	17.0
Misfit of mold		14	7.0
Poor acceptance		11	5.0
	Total	61	29.0
External Auditory Canal:			
Impacted cerumen		6	3.0
External otitis		6	3.0
	Total	12	6.0
Middle Ear:			
Middle ear effusion		11	5.0
Tympanic membrane perforation		1	0.5
	Total	12	5.5
Inner Ear:			
Increased threshold		7	3.0
	Total	7	3.0
Otological Disorders Other Than Ear:			
Upper respiratory infection		3	1.0
Tonsillar hypertrophy		3	1.0
Velopharyngeal insufficiency		1	0.5
Pharyngeal papillomata		1	0.5
Bronchial cleft fistula		1	0.5
	Total	9	3.5
Other:			
Neurological disease		5	2.0
Spontaneous nystagmus		1	0.5
	Total	6	2.5

* Denominator = 212 Examinations

The population has several biases and does not represent
a total universe of hearing impaired children. The first is
in the economic selection of those children which are included.
The children were, for the most part, medically indigent. In
addition, the social problems of this group were significant
in that many of the appointments were not kept because of lack
of funds for transportation, overriding family problems, lack
of understanding the reasons for follow-up (many are Spanish
speaking), and the moving of a family from one part of the
city to another or from one region to another (e.g., Puerto
Rico). It is also felt that many of the visits were
initiated because of the crises which had occurred. This
population does not reflect what the true incidence and prevalence would be if all children could have been examined
each year. There are factors in selection which could cause
either an increase or decrease of incidence.

Data

The incidence of the types of significant findings are
to be found in Tables I and II. It is noted that 29% of the
total population of 212 children have difficulty with the
hearing aid. These were either hearing aid malfunction or
loss, molds that did not fit, or there was poor acceptance of
the hearing aid. Diseases of the external auditory canal
accounted for 6% of the significant findings in the total
population, and included impacted cerumen and external otitis.
Diseases of the middle ear, including middle ear effusion and
a perforation of the tympanic membrane, accounted for 6% of
the significant findings. Otorhinolaryngological disorders
other than the ear accounted for another 3.5% of the problems,
and other disorders were noted in 2.5% of the population. The
overall incidence of significant findings for the entire population was 50%.

The twenty-one children, for which the yearly visits
were analyzed, were followed for 1 to 12 years with an average of 6 years' follow-up. The actual number of examinations
was 83, or approximately 4 per child. This averaged about
1.5 years between examinations for each child. This group
missed 58 of a theoretical total number of 141 examinations.
In other words, only 59% of the examinations were actually
made.

TABLE III

PREVALENCE OF A SIGNIFICANT FINDING IN THE ANNUAL OTOLOGICAL
EXAMINATIONS OF 21 HEARING IMPAIRED CHILDREN

# of Findings	# of Children	%
0	6	29.0
1	2	10.0
2	4	19.0
3	4	19.0
4	5	24.0

Prevalence of 1 or more significant findings = 71%

A total of 21 children or every 10th child, was selected
for our study of the prevalence of the significant findings
which had occurred at the annual examinations, each of which
those children had attended (Tables III and IV).

TABLE IV

PREVALENCE OF SIGNIFICANT FINDINGS IN THE ANNUAL OTOLOGICAL
EXAMINATIONS OF 18 HEARING IMPAIRED CHILDREN WITH TWO OR MORE
EXAMINATIONS

# of Findings	# of Children	%
0	3	17.0
1	2	11.0
2	4	22.0
3	4	22.0
4	5	28.0

Prevalence of 1 or more significant findings in children with
two or more examinations = 83%

The number of significant findings per child is noted in Table III. Six children (29%) did not have a significant finding. The remaining 71% had a specific finding at least once. The frequency of specific findings were 2 children with one finding; 4 children with two findings; 4 children with three findings; 5 children with four findings. Again, the total prevalence of one or more significant findings in this population was 71%.

Table IV shows that the prevalence of significant findings was greater when the three children who were not followed up for more than one year were omitted. This increases the prevalence of one or more significant findings to 83%.

The types of findings in this group of 21 children are tabulated in Tables V and VI. No significant findings were found in 41 of the 83 examinations. Significant findings were observed 45 times (3 of the children were noted to have 2 significant findings at one visit). The incidence of significant findings of this group was 58%. This is similar to the incidence of 50% which is found in the overall population of 212 children.

TABLE V

INCIDENCE OF SIGNIFICANT FINDINGS IN THE ANNUAL OTOLOGICAL EXAMINATIONS OF 21 HEARING IMPAIRED CHILDREN

Findings	% of Total Findings *	% of Significant Findings **
Hearing Aid	19.0	35.0
External Auditory Canal	8.0	16.0
Middle Ear	13.0	24.0
Inner Ear	1.0	2.0
Otological Disorders other than ear	7.0	13.0
Other	5.0	9.0

Incidence of Significant Findings = 58%

* Denominator = 86 Examinations of which 41 were normal.
** Denominator = 45 Significant findings.

TABLE VI

INCIDENCE OF SIGNIFICANT FINDINGS IN THE ANNUAL OTOLOGICAL
EXAMINATIONS OF 21 HEARING IMPAIRED INFANTS

Findings		N	% *
Normal Examination		41	48.0
Hearing Aid			
Malfunction or lost		11	13.0
Misfit mold		2	2.0
Poor acceptance		3	3.0
	Total	16	19.0
External Auditory Canal			
Cerumen		6	7.0
Otitis external		1	1.0
	Total	7	8.0
Middle Ear			
Middle ear effusions		9	10.0
Tympanosclerosis		1	1.0
Middle ear malformation		1	1.0
	Total	11	13.0
Inner Ear			
Improvement of discrimination		1	1.0
	Total	1	1.0
Otorhinolaryngological Disorders Other Than Ear			
Upper respiratory infection		2	2.0
Tonsillitis		2	2.0
Pharyngeal papillomata		1	1.0
High arch palate (?submucosal cleft)		1	1.0
	Total	6	7.0
Other			
Visual perceptual abnormality		1	1.0
Failure of expected language development		2	2.0
Significant linguistic improvement		1	1.0
		4,	5.0

* Denominator = 86 Examinations

The incidence of significant findings in the group of 21 children included:

1) hearing aid problem - 19%;
2) external auditory canal disease - 8%;
3) middle ear disease - 13%;
4) inner ear disease - 1%;
5) otorhinolaryngological disorders other than ear - 7%; and,
6) other - 5%.

A comparison of the incidence of significant findings for the long term group of 21 children and the entire subject group of 212 children shows two interesting differences (Table VII). The first of these is that difficulty with hearing aids was reduced by 22% for the 21 children for which all visits were tabulated. The incidence of middle ear effusion was increased by 13%, which was more than double that reported when only one visit per child was assessed.

TABLE VII

COMPARISON OF THE INCIDENCE OF SIGNIFICANT FINDINGS IN AN
ANNUAL OTOLOGICAL EXAMINATION OF 212 HEARING IMPAIRED CHILDREN
WITH THE INCIDENCE OF SIGNIFICANT FINDINGS IN ALL THE
EXAMINATIONS OF 21 HEARING IMPAIRED CHILDREN

Incidence at Annual Examination*			Incidence at all Examinations**	
Findings	N	%	N	%
Hearing Aid	61	57.0	16	35.0
External Auditory Canal	12	11.0	7	16.0
Middle Ear	12	11.0	11	24.0
Inner Ear	7	7.0	1	2.0
Otorhinolaryngological Disorders other than ear	9	8.0	6	13.0
Other	6	6.0	4	9.0

*   Denominator = 107 Significant Findings
** Denominator = 45 Significant Findings

Discussion

The data presented in Tables II and IV show the types of significant problems which were recorded. The most frequent occurrences were problems with the hearing aid, previously either not worn or lost. A number of patients had hearing aid molds which did not fit. The detection of these conditions is important in that they prevent the child from receiving optimal habilitation. Children in schools for the deaf will usually, but not invariably, have this problem attended to at the school. However, there is an increase in the number of children who have been mainstreamed into regular schools. Opportunities are quite limited for those children in general educational settings to have their hearing aid problems identified and corrected. There is an apparent need for periodic assessment of the conditions of the hearing aid and the mold by a person outside the educational setting, preferably one who can institute remediation for this type of a problem.

Lack of acceptance of a hearing aid is a problem which is most often encountered in the adolescent. This is a difficult problem, but it can be recognized and treated. The otological setting is one area in which, with understanding, a great deal of acceptance can be achieved.

The problem of external auditory canal disease, either impacted cerumen or external otitis, was relatively common in our study group. Both of these conditions prevent the effective use of a hearing aid and must be treated medically. Impacted cerumen was usually an incidental finding. Otitis externa many times was found to have persisted for a number of months before the child came in for the annual visit. The otologist can both cure the external otitis and initiate proper ear care so as to minimize the re-occurrence of that disease.

Diseases of the middle ear, primarily middle ear effusion, were found to have an incidence of 6% in the total population and found in 10% of the examinations in which all the follow-up data was analyzed. Seven of the 21 children (33%) had at least one documented episode of middle ear effusion during the long term follow-up. This is similar to that found in studies of three different schools for the deaf (Craig, Stool and Laird, 1979; Mehta and Erlich, 1978; and Rubin, 1978). The effect of middle ear effusion in children

with severe to profound hearing loss is to further increase
the threshold of hearing and to decrease speech discrimination (Ruben and Math, 1978).

Craig, Stool and Laird (1979) have reported a one year
prospective study of otological disorders in 446 students
enrolled in a school for the deaf. The findings show that
during the year, 40% of the children had some form of otological disorder, mainly middle ear effusions. The authors
reported data by age, group and season. The incidence of
ear disorders varied by age. Abnormalities were found in
72% of the children aged 2 - 5; 40% of the children aged 6 -
8; 43% of the children aged 9 - 13; and 29% of the children
aged 14 - 21. Seasonal variation between fall, winter and
spring was approximately the same, except for the children
aged 2 - 5 who had almost a three fold increase in ear/
otological pathology in the winter and spring, compared to
that which was found in the fall. Craig and his co-workers
found that 26% of the children aged 2 - 5 had ear disease at
least once during the year, while only 2% of the children
aged 14 - 21 had one episode of ear disease during the year.

The middle ear effusions in 32 - 33% of the children in
the Craig, Stool and Laird and the Mehta and Erlich studies
did not resolve spontaneously and/or were refractory to
medical therapy. These children required myringotomies and
insertion of ventilating tubes. Otological surveillance was
able, in both the studies, to detect otological disease and,
with either medical or surgical intervention, to result in
an attenuation of conditions so that optimal use of hearing
could be obtained.

The threshold of hearing increased in 3% of our population. The causes of these changes in threshold are not known,
but the changes initiated an investigation to attempt to
determine the underlying cause. The change in threshold
resulted in change of amplification and/or the habilitative
program for the child.

Other otolaryngological conditions occurred in 3.5% of
the population, or 8% of the total positive findings. Those
conditions were treated, so as to insure an optimal health
status for each child.

There were a number of other specific findings recorded at the annual examination. The development of, or detection of, neurological diseases was not unexpected in this multi-handicapped population. Additionally, in the total assessment of all follow-up, two other significant observations were made. One child was found to have visual perceptual problems and two children were noted not to achieve their expected language development. This latter finding is import-ant for it illustrated the advantage of having another pro-fessional independently assess the progress which the child is making. In our experience, this has, on many occasions, been important in causing a change in the habilitative pro-gram of the child, or occasionally, a change in the expecta-tions for the child.

Conclusions

The efficacy of routine otological care has been demon-strated from these data. The information reported shows that there is an incidence of 50% and a prevalence of 71% for significant findings to be noted in a scheduled annual otological examination which occurred at approximately 1.5 years. This information was obtained from an economically deprived group of children with many social problems. Whether the incidence would be significantly higher or lower for the total population, with all socio-economic groups who had regular follow-up, is not known. Table VIII offers, on the basis of this study, a minimal list of the problems which should be assessed at each otological examination.

The frequency of each follow-up visit must vary accord-ing to the age and other characteristics of the child. The data from Craig and his co-workers was based on three examinations per year. This frequency resulted in the detection of abnormalities of the ear in 72% of the children aged 2 – 5 and 40% of the children aged 6 – 8.

The frequency of examination every four months appears to detect most of the children with middle ear effusions and diseases of the external auditory canal and middle ear. If the diagnosis is not made at the examination, it is possible for a child to have an ear condition for four months before the next examination. Information which is known concerning middle ear effusion would indicate that for children less than 5 years of age, there should be otological signs and

TABLE VIII

SUGGESTED MINIMAL INFORMATION TO BE ASCERTAINED AT EACH
OTOLOGICAL EXAMINATION

Hearing Aid
    Presence
    Function
    Fit of Mold
    Acceptance of Aid

External Auditory Canal
    Cerumen
    External Otitis

Middle Ear
    Middle Ear Effusion
    Tympanosclerosis
    Tympanomastoiditis

Inner Ear
    Change in Threshold
    Vestibular Function

Otorhinolaryngological Examination Other Than Ear
    Mouth   Pharynx
    Nose   Salivary Orifices
    Palate   Larynx
    Teeth   Neck
    Tongue   Paranasal Sinuses
    Tonsils

Other
    Language Development
    Speech Development
    Voice
    Visual Acuity
    Social Development
    Neurological Development

information derived from electroacoustic impedance bridge
studies which indicate an abnormality in the middle ear
suggestive of the possibility of the development or the resolution of a middle ear effusion. A number of children would
have these types of abnormalities observed and then would
have a more frequent schedule for examinations so as to determine whether or not middle ear effusion was present and what
treatment was required. It would appear that a frequency of
every four months would identify almost all of the children
who have middle ear effusions or would have a propensity for
acquiring a middle ear effusion. If the time period was
extended to 6 months for this age group, then there would be
an increase in the number of children who would not be identified as having middle ear effusions. It would then be possible with a frequency examination every 6 months, for a child
to develop middle ear effusion for several months and have a
resulting increase in the threshold of hearing. Further, if
the disease was not detected and treated within a six month
period, there will be some children who will acquire more
serious middle ear diseases. It is on the basis of the data
from this study and the others reported that we recommend
that the frequency of otological examination for children
less than 5 years of age should be at a minimum of every 4
months. This periodic schedule should be increased in frequency if there is middle ear effusion, or if the signs of
possible development of middle ear effusion are found.

Children older than 5 years of age are less prone to
middle ear effusions and may not need as frequent examinations. The reports of prevalence and incidence for the
entire population are based on approximately one examination
every 1.5 years. This reveals an incidence of a significant
finding in 50% and a prevalence of 73%. If the frequency of
visits was increased by a factor of three, that is, one visit
every 6 months, one might expect a reduction of the incidence
to approximately 18%. Thus, almost one out of every 5 children at each visit would, on the basis of the data, have a
significant positive finding. It is felt that such an incidence of significant findings might even be greater if there
was a 6 month frequency of examinations united by the assessment inventory as suggested in Table VIII. It is also
important to be able to individualize the frequency of the
otological examination for each child. A 6 year old child
with a history of middle ear effusion will need to be evaluated, more than one without such a history. A 10 year old

with an increased hearing threshold will need more frequent
examinations than one without changes in hearing level. A
teenager who has rejected a hearing aid will require more
counselling and, consequently, a greater number of otological
visits than one who is well fit and is integrated in the
public school.

The major effectiveness of such otological care is
dependent upon the cost and the benefits. The costs are
easy to calculate, but the value of the benefits is extremely
difficult to determine. Even though there is a lack of
information in the area of effectiveness, it is perceived
from these observations that the benefits derived from the
otological examination far outweigh its costs.

The information which has been reported and reviewed in
this communication shows the efficacy of ongoing otological
care for the hearing impaired child. The frequency of such
evaluations will be determined to a great extent by the types
of conditions which the child manifests. As a minimum
requirement, each child less than 5 years of age should be
examined every four months, and those over 5 years of age
every six months.

* Acknowledgment of the long-term support of the Manheimer
   Foundation and C.H.E.A.R., Inc., is gratefully acknowledged.

REFERENCES

Craig, H.B., Stool, S.R. and Laird, M.A. "Project Ears:
    Otologic maintenance in a school for the deaf," American
    Annals of the Deaf, 124:458 - 467, 1979.

Lane, H. The Wild Boy of Aveyron (Cambridge, Massachusetts:
    Harvard University Press), 1976.

Mehta, D. and Erlich, M. "Serous otitis media in the school
    for the deaf," Volta Review, 80:75 - 80, 1978.

Ruben, R.J. and Math, R. Serous otitis media associated with
    sensory neural hearing loss in children," Laryngoscope,
    88:1139 - 1154, 1978.

Rubin, M. "Serous otitis in severely to profoundly hearing
    impaired children, Ages 0 - 6," <u>Volta Review</u>, 80:81 - 85,
    1978.

OTITIS MEDIA IN INFANCY

Denzil N. Brooks
Withington Hospital, Manchester, England

The importance of early identification, diagnosis and management of severe hearing loss in infants has been amply demonstrated, not least by the three conferences held here in Canada on these specific subjects. Considerable efforts are now made in the better endowed societies to mitigate the adverse effects that inevitably occur if early and sustained assistance is not provided to the child with this degree of hearing impairment.

There has been very much less recognition of the potentially harmful effects of mild hearing loss arising principally from dysfunction of the middle ear system. One reason for this may be the contrast between the two types of hearing loss. Compared with severe or profound deafness, mild conductive hearing loss seems, superficially at least, to be of much less consequence. It appears to be so much less of a handicap that it can easily be under-estimated or even overlooked. Another reason may be that the majority of children with mild conductive hearing loss (usually otitis media with effusion - OME) appear to recover normal function and normal audition after a period of time. However, there is growing recognition that not all children recover fully from infantile and childhood middle ear dysfunction, and that in some of those who do appear to recover in the short term, there may be sequelae that diminish the quality of life or that persist into and possibly throughout their adult life.

Though in terms of severity of hearing loss, middle ear disorders may be relatively small, in numerical terms they greatly outweigh sensory-neural losses, which occur at the rate of not more than 1 per 1000 live births. Howie and his colleagues (1975) analyzed the records of 488 children in Huntsville, Alabama, who had been followed from birth through age 6 years. Forty-nine per cent of these children had an attack of OME before their first birthday, and over 60% before their second birthday. Kaplan and colleagues (1973) studied a cohort of 489 Eskimo children through the first 10 years of life. Seventy-eight per cent had their first attack of OME before their second birthday. Brownlee et al (1969) found

in a study of 651 children in South Carolina that 84% had
had at least one attack of OME by the age of 5 years. Klein
(1979), in an epidemiological study of more than 2500 children, reported that around 75% had OME in the first 2 years
of life. There is general agreement among these four studies
that from 60 to 80% of all children have at least one episode
of OME before the age of 2 years. Indeed, OME is second only
to the common cold as the most prevalent disease in childhood.
It is almost the exception not to have had at least one
episode of OME by the age of 5 years. This being so, should
we be concerned over the high incidence of OME? Is it not
part of the natural process by which our immunological
defences are developed?

     There are two reasons why we cannot dismiss this condi-
tion so readily. Firstly, though a majority of normal children have OME and progress into adult life with normal middle
ear function, a small but significant percentage fail to
recover and enter adult life with recurrent or persistent
disease. Secondly, the sequelae to persistent OME may be
more profound than has generally been realized heretofore.
Otitis media, treated or untreated, may lead on to atelectasis,
attic perforation with cholesteatoma, tympanosclerosis, and
a number of other complications. These are reviewed by
Glasscock (1972) and present a frightening, though fortunately rare, picture. Brooks (1974) examined the middle ear
function of 1053 school children aged between 4 and 11 years.
Although the percentage of middle ear dysfunction decreased
with age from levels of 40% at age 4 to 20% at age 5, 12% at
age 6 and 8% at age 7, it did not disappear completely. It
appeared to level out by the age of 10 or 11 years to a
constant value of around 2 or 3%. The same author (Brooks,
1976) studied a group of 80 children over a 10 year period
from entry into primary school at an age of around 5 years.
The majority (67 = 84%) had not more than 2 episodes of OME
over the whole period of observation. Thirteen children had
more persistent or repeated bouts of OME, but 9 of these
reverted to normal middle ear function after a period of 1 to
2 years. There were 4 children who, at the age of 15 years,
had tympanograms that still indicated very poor middle ear
function. Perusal of the records of these children indicated
that in each case, there had been multiple episodes of OME
over the period of observation, and a high probability that
the problem had been present before the children entered full-
time education. In a further study (Brooks, 1980), it was
observed that 1 in 6 adult subjects applying for a hearing

aid had evidence of middle ear disorders that could be
traced back to early childhood. A few had obvious conditions such as perforations, discharge or gross tympanic
retraction, but the majority had a mild conductive impairment of the order of 15 dB. However, this was such that
when added to a presbyacusic hearing loss, the need for a
hearing aid was felt some 12 years sooner than was the case
for subjects with no conductive hearing loss or history of
middle ear disease.

     A number of studies suggest shorter term effects attribu-
table to OME or the hearing loss associated with it. One of
the earliest reports was by Bond (1935) who studied a sample
of 128 New York school children. The prevalence of hearing
loss among those with poor reading skills was 15 times
greater than in those with normal reading ability. The
studies of Ling (1959) suggested that losses as small as 15
to 25 dB (such as arise from OME) could lead to educational
retardation in specific areas and that this was unlikely to
be ameliorated without special remedial teaching. Holm and
Kunze (1969) carried out a carefully controlled study in
which children with mild and fluctuating hearing loss commencing before the age of 2 years were matched for age, sex and
socio-economic background with a group having no evidence of
middle ear dysfunction or hearing loss. The language performance of the two groups was compared by means of a large
number of linguistic and vocabulary tests. The group with a
history of OME showed statistically significant delays in all
language skills requiring the receiving or processing of
auditory stimuli or the production of verbal responses.
Hamilton and Owrid (1974) compared the linguistic skills of
a group of 30 children with a history of middle ear dysfunction with a matched group of children having no history of
middle ear disorders. The group with hearing loss showed
appreciable retardation compared both with the norms for the
test used and with the control group. Dalzell and Owrid
(1975) reviewed 24 of the original group of 30 children from
the Hamilton and Owrid study, 5 years after the original
investigation. Their finding was that though the hearing
losses had, in general, improved consistently, for some of
the children there remained a considerable retardation in
linguistic performance.

     Lewis (1976) after studying a group of 14 aboriginal
children with histories of chronic middle ear disease, concluded that "chronic middle ear impairment not only restricts

the development of some auditory processing skills, but dis-
torts the integrational pattern". Zinkus, Gottlieb and
Schapiro (1978) compared 2 groups of children aged approximately 8 years. One group had a history of persistent OME
during the first 3 years of life; the second group had histories of relatively mild OME amounting to not more than one
brief episode a year during the first 3 years of life. The
children in the first group manifested substantial retardation in a number of aspects of communication vital to
learning.

Katz (1978) cites a number of studies to support the
hypothesis that some degree of brain dysfunction may result
from the auditory deprivation arising from early and persistent middle ear disorders. Physiological support for this
hypothesis comes from the work of Webster and Webster (1977)
who demonstrated that mice reared under conditions of auditory deprivation showed central morphological deficits (in
the ventral cochlear nucleus and medial nucleus of the trapezoid body) compared with normal control animals. A similar
picture was observed in the brain of a girl, aged 9 years,
who had suffered from profound sensory-neural hearing loss
from birth. Downs (1977) cites a number of studies which,
taken together, lead to the conclusion that persistent or
episodic OME in the first 2 years of life may give rise to
irremediable condition defined by Downs as an irreversbile
auditory learning disaster (IALD).

Additional to, or possibly arising from, the educational
consequences of persistent OME, there may be psychological
problems. Fisher (1965) observed that children with mildly
impaired hearing showed considerably more maladjusted behaviour than normal children. In boys this manifested principally in demonstrative patterns of behaviour. Struggles
(1975) in his work as an Educational Psychologist, also
found that a history of OME was a common finding in children
referred to him for guidance. Hersher (1978) closely examined
22 hyper-active children referred to him for behavioural
problems. He found a significantly higher proportion had
had more than 6 episodes of OME, compared with a matched
group of normal children. These children had been diagnosed
as having minimal brain dysfunction.

The evidence then is such that there are no grounds for
complacency about the potentially harmful effects of persistent OME. Particularly is this so regarding OME that arises

in infancy. In the studies of Holm and Kunze (1969) and
Zinkus et al (1978), the onset of the disorder was in the
first years of life and persisted through the years when
rapid language development takes place. Downs (1977) additionally points out that although the information content of
speech is largely carried by the consonants, these have a
very small proportion of the acoustic energy. Normal hearing
individuals, therefore, use contextual strategies and a
wealth of experience to build up a complete auditory picture.
The infant or child with mild hearing loss neither hears the
soft components of the consonants, nor has the background and
experience to accurately infer them. In consequence, the
reception of auditory information is, and continues to
develop, in an incomplete form.

Thus, although we are concerned about all children who
have OME, we need to be especially concerned about those in
whom the condition starts at an early age and persists,
possibly as a fluctuating condition, for many years. Howie
et al (1975) defined a group of children as "otitis prone"
on the basis of their having 6 or more episodes of OME before
the age of 6 years. All these children had their first
episode before the age of 18 months. The question posed by
these findings is, how best can the "otitis prone" group of
children be detected and identified. One method clearly
demonstrated by Howie and his colleagues is close observation by dedicated pediatricians. Of considerable value also
would be definition of at risk groups. Some of these are
well known; for example, cleft palate children (Paradise and
Bluestone, 1974); infants in intensive care (Balkony et al,
1978); infants whose mothers have complications pre- or post-
natally (Jaffe et al, 1970); and premature infants (Warren
and Stool, 1971). Other groups may yet need to be identified
and characterized.

Unfortunately, tympanometry employing conventional
equipment has been shown to be unsuited to the examination
of middle ear function up to the age of 6 to 7 months
(Paradise et al, 1976; Balkony and Zarnock, 1978). Beyond
this age, screening tympanometry may be employed (Tos et al,
1979), provided the difficulties of assembling the infants to
a central clinic for examination can be overcome. Elicita-
tion of the acoustic stapedius reflex might prove to be a
simpler and more reliable test for the presence or absence
of OME. A clear reflex response is almost invariably indicative of absent middle ear dysfunction and although absence of

a reflex does not necessarily indicate OME, it would certainly
suggest the need for further investigation. Early studies of
the acoustic reflex in infants (Keith, 1975; Bennett, 1975;
Stream et al, 1977), suggested that the reflex was not elicit-
able in the majority of neonates even in the absence of OME.
However, Allred (1974) indicated that the apparent absence
was probably a function of the probe frequency of the impedance measuring system, rather than being indicative of either
a middle ear condition or the slow maturation of the reflex
response. Weatherby and Bennett (1980) have recently confirmed this conclusion. In their study of 44 neonates aged
from 10 to 169 hours, they employed a detection system with
a variable probe frequency. At 220 Hz, none of the infants
produced reflexes. As the frequency of the probe tone was
progressively increased from 400 to 800 Hz, higher percent-
ages of reflexes were obtained until with probe tones above
800 Hz, all the neonates showed clear reflexes to probe
frequencies up to 1.8 KHz. Much work remains to be done,
however, before this test can be applied as a routine procedure. Weatherby and Bennett comment that even though they
were experienced in evaluating neonates, testing proved
lengthy. This was principally due to the need to obtain,
and the difficulty in obtaining, a complete pressure seal in
the infant meatus.

     In summary, there is a very real need to identify,
diagnose and effectively treat, at the earliest opportunity,
children who are "otitis prone". Only in this way can
irreversible auditory learning disasters be prevented and the
potential of the children maximized. There is a pressing
need to make all those involved in infant care aware of the
potentially damaging nature of OME, and there is an equally
pressing need to seek the most effective form of remediation,
both medical and ecucational.

                          REFERENCES

Balkany, T.J., Berman, S.A., Simmons, M.A. and Jafek, B.W.
     "Middle ear effusion in neonates" Laryngology 88:398 -
     405, 1978.

Bennett, M.J. "Acoustic impedance bridge measurements with the neonate" British Journal of Audiology 9:117 - 124, 1975.

Brooks, D.N. "Impedance bridge studies on normal hearing and hearing impaired children" Acta Oto-rhinolaryngologica Belgium 28:140 - 145, 1974.

Brooks, D.N. "School screening for middle ear effusion" Annals of Otorhinolaryngology Suppl. 25:223 - 228, 1976.

Brooks, N.D. "Possible long-term consequences of middle ear effusion" Annals of Otorhinolaryngology Suppl (in press), 1980.

Brownlee, R.C., DeLoache, R.W., Cowan, C.C. and Jackson, H.P. "Otitis media in children: Incidence, treatment and prognosis in pediatric practice" Journal of Pediatrics 75:636 - 642, 1969.

Dalzell, J. and Owrid, H.L. "Children with conductive deafness. A follow-up study" British Journal of Audiology 10:87 - 90, 1976.

Downs, M.P. "The expanding imperatives of early identification" in Bess, F.H. (ed.) Childhood Deafness (New York: Grune & Stratton), 1977.

Fisher, B. The Social and Emotional Adjustment of Children With Impaired Hearing Attending Ordinary Classes. M.Ed. Dissertation - University of Manchester, 1965.

Glasscock, M.E. "Complications of otitis media" in Glorig, A. and Gerwin, K.S. (eds.) Otitis Media (Springfield, Ill: C.C. Thomas), 1972.

Hamilton, P. and Owrid, H.L. "Comparisons of hearing impairment and socio-cultural disadvantage in relation to verbal retardation" Journal of the Society of Teachers of the Deaf 17:30 - 36, 1974.

Hersher, L. "Minimal brain dysfunction and otitis media" Perceptual and Motor Skills 47:723 - 726, 1978.

Holm, V.A. and Kunze, L.H. "Effects of chronic otitis media on language and speech development" Pediatrics 43:833 – 839, 1969.

Howie, V.M., Ploussard, J.H. and Sloyer, J. "The 'Otitis-prone' condition" American Journal of the Disabled Child 129:676 – 678, 1975.

Jaffe, B.F., Hurtado, F. and Hurtado, E. "Tympanic membrane mobility in the newborn" Laryngology 80:36 – 48, 1970.

Kaplan, G.J., Fleshman, J.K., Bender, T.R., Baum, C. and Clark, P.S. "Long term effects of otitis media: A ten year cohort study of Alaskan Eskimo children" Pediatrics 52:577 – 585, 1973.

Katz, J. "The effects of conductive hearing loss on auditory function" ASHA 20:879 – 886, 1978.

Keith, R.W. "Middle ear function in neonates" Archives of Otolaryngology 101:376 – 379, 1975.

Keith, R.W. and Bench, R.J. "Stapedial reflex in neonates" Scandinavian Audiology 7:187 – 191, 1978.

Lewis, N. "Otitis media and linguistic incompetence" Archives of Otolaryngology 102:387 – 390, 1976.

Ling, D. The Education and General Background of Children With Defective Hearing. Unpublished Ph.D. Thesis, Cambridge University Institute of Education, 1959.

Paradise, J.L. and Bluestone, C.B. "Early treatment of the universal otitis media of infants with cleft palate" Pediatrics 53:48 – 54, 1974.

Paradise, J.L., Smith, C.G. and Bluestone, C.D. "Tympanometric detection of middle ear effusion in infants and children" Pediatrics 58:198 – 210, 1976.

Stream, R., Stream, K., Walker, J. and Breningstall, G., as cited by Keith, R.W. and Bench, R.J. "Stapedial reflex in neonates" Scandinavian Audiology 7:187 – 191, 1978.

Struggles, D.E. Personal Communication (1975).

Tos, M., Poulsen, G. and Hancke, A.B. "Screening tympano-
    metry during the first year of life" Acta Otolaryngologica
    88:388 - 394, 1979.

Warren, W.S. and Stool, S.E. "Otitis media in low birth
    weight infants" Pediatrics 79:740 - 743, 1971.

Weatherby, L.A. and Bennett, M.J. "The neonatal acoustic
    reflex" paper submitted to Scandinavian Audiology, 1980.

Webster, D.B. and Webster, M. "Neonatal sound deprivation
    affects brain stem auditory nuclei" Archives of Otolaryn-
    gology 103:392 - 396, 1977.

Zinkus, P.W., Gottlieb, M.I. and Schapiro, M. "Development
    and psychoeducational sequelae of chronic otitis media"
    American Journal of the Disabled Child 132:1100 - 1104,
    1978.

IMPEDANCE MEASUREMENTS IN INFANTS

Jerry L. Northern
University of Colorado, Denver, Colorado

Introduction

There is significant contradictory evidence in the
literature regarding the merit of performing acoustic
impedance measurements in infants. Margolis (1978) describes
the situation well with his statement that impedance measurements in infants have provided results that are "... both
promising and perplexing." Although early research studies
of the utilization of impedance measures with infants were
favorable, subsequent studies suggested that tympanometry
is invalid in infants less than 7 months of age. Recent
studies have challenged these findings and blamed previous
erroneous conclusions on the singular use of tympanometry
upon which to predict the presence of middle ear effusion.

It is the purpose of this paper to examine in detail the
numerous assorted research studies dealing with clinical
impedance measurements in infants. Broader applications of
impedance measurements used in the prediction of degree of
sensory-neural hearing loss in children, and the application
of impedance techniques to the management of hearing aids is
also discussed. It is not the purpose of this paper to discuss acoustic impedance as a routine screening procedure for
infants, but rather to focus on current clinical applications
and potential utilization of impedance measurements with
infants and other non-verbal children.

Tympanometry/Acoustic Reflex
in Infants

The initial systematic research on impedance testing of
infants was reported by Robert Keith, Ph.D., of the University of Cincinnati Medical Center. In an effort to determine
whether impedance audiometry could be effectively used with
newborns, Keith (1973) tested 40 healthy infants from the
newborn nursery between 36 and 151 hours of age. The babies
were tested on their stomachs with heads turned during sleep.
He found that results with tympanometry did not differ

markedly from results reported by other researchers in older
children. Keith reported normal tympanograms in 33 of the
infants and a "W-shaped" tympanogram in 7 infants.

Keith (1973) also examined stapedial reflex measurements
in these 40 infants with stimulus presentations of 100 dB HTL
at 500 and 2000 Hz. He reported that stapedial reflex responses were often contaminated by behavioural movement of
the infants. In fact, from 160 stimulus presentations, only
33% resulted in clear stapedial reflex responses. No acoustic
reflex response was noted in 26% of the stimulus presentations, and 4 of the 40 infants showed no acoustic reflex in
either ear initially, although all 4 babies were later confirmed to have normal hearing responses.

In a later study, Keith (1975) investigated the middle
ear function of neonates younger than 36 hours of age. Twenty
healthy babies between the ages of 2½ to 20 hours of age were
tested with tympanometry. The tympanometry results were
similar to those reported in his previous study of infants
older than 36 hours of age. Keith concluded that tympanometry
could be used as a simple, reliable measure of middle ear
function in normal neonates. He also concluded that although
impedance measurements were not the answer to mass infant
screening programs, helpful information about the middle ear
function of infants was easily available in the impedance.

Impedance data from 18 infants between the ages of 3 -
11 months were reported by Susan Jerger et al. in 1974. They
reported "successful" impedance results in 40% of the infants
less than 11 months of age, while 20% showed "incomplete"
results, and "no seal" was reported for 10% of the infants.
S. Jerger et al. reported a systematic increase in the number
of acoustic reflexes present with the increasing age of the
infants, a finding consistent with observations reported previously by Robertson et al. (1968). The number of missing
reflexes decreased from 20% at ages 0 - 35 months, to only 5%
at ages 60 - 71 months. S. Jerger et al. also reported that
there is a systematic increase in the incidence of reflexes
at 90 dB HTL (from 7% at ages 0 - 35 months to 33% by ages of
60 - 71 months). The authors offered two explanations for
the absence of acoustic reflexes in very young children:

1) it is possible that the acoustic reflex arc undergoes
    maturation during the early years of childhood; and/or

2)   the reflex arc is complete in the noenate but there may be
     a relatively high incidence of undetected middle ear
     abnormality in very young children.

The authors also concluded that the impedance technique
offered the single most powerful tool for pediatric evaluation. They warned, however, that impedance findings cannot
stand alone, and that impedance should only be interpreted
in combination with some independent assessment of hearing
sensitivity level. Unfortunately, this warning has been
largely unheeded.

    Impedance utilization with infants seemed to be a reason-
ably well accepted clinical tool until the publication of an
article by Paradise, Smith and Bluestone (1976). Their evaluation of 280 children ranging in age from 10 days to 5 years
showed a high positive correlation (86%) between tympanometry
and otoscopy for subjects over 7 months of age. However, poor
correlation was found between the two measures in infants
less than 7 months of age. In fact, from 43 infants less
than 7 months of age, 40 of 81 ears had confirmed middle ear
effusion (determined by myringotomy), yet 24 of the 40
abnormal ears displayed normal tympanograms. The authors concluded that although the use of tympanometry had much to
offer in the diagnosis of middle ear effusion, its use
(tympanometry) was not recommended in infants less than 7
months of age.

    Howie et al. (1976) with outspoken disbelief of the
Paradise et al. findings in infants less than 7 months of
age, quickly set out to replicate the study with his own
comparative evaluation of tympanometry and otoscopy in neonates. Howie and his colleagues found that from 59 ears with
confirmed middle ear effusion (by myringotomy) 26 showed
normal tympanograms and they, thus, emphatically stated that
the results and conclusions of the Paradise group were
accurate and should not be questioned or challenged.

    Zarnoch and Balkany (1978a, 1978b), reported findings of
normal tympanograms in 6 of 7 intensive care unit newborns
with confirmed middle ear effusion. They evaluated 50 normal
newborns less than 24 hours of age, and 35 high risk intensive
care unit neonates under 2 months of age. They found a high
incidence of middle ear effusion (34%) in the ICU babies,
especially in those neonates with nasotracheal orotracheal
intubation. They concluded that "... tympanometry was somewhat cumbersome, time-consuming and often an intrusion to the

busy ICU nursery". In a subsequent published letter, Zarnoch
(1978) commented that re-evaluation of their data might show
the diagnostic accuracy of tympanometry in infants to be 82%
correct, which she indicated reflected well the use of tympanometry in infants.

Although most infant impedance research in the early
1970's was conducted with low frequency probe-tone (220 Hz)
impedance meters, some neonate studies were conducted with
the Grason-Stadler 1720 Otoadmittance Meter which uses a
higher frequency (660 Hz) probe-tone. The results were
again contradictory. Cannon et al. (1974) evaluated 31 normal
neonates and concluded that the use of the otoadmittance
meter was reliable in the assessment of middle ear function.
Shurin and his colleagues (1977) reached the opposite conclusion, that the otoadmittance meter was impractical for the
routine testing of young infants and children because of the
longer test time required and the highly sensitive nature of
the instrument to any subject movement.

Reichert et al. (1978) examined 878 3 month old infants
with otoscopy and tympanometry. All infants were examined
tympanometrically while being held in their mothers' arms
and being comforted with a pacifier or bottle. The authors
concluded that tympanometry produced a low diagnostic specifi-
city (accuracy in identifying non-diseased individuals) with
a high number of false-positive results -- 16 "flat" tympanograms were found in ears that were otoscopically normal. In
their discussion, Reichert et al. recognized that inclusion
of the measurement of the acoustic reflex may have provided
different results than were obtained only with the use of
tympanometry.

Jerger has long cautioned clinicians against the use of
any single impedance measure to reach a diagnostic conclusion. He has repeatedly pointed out that "tympanometry alone
is useful to only a limited degree" in making diagnostic judgments (1970)". Jerger and Hayes (1980) stated that in the
"diagnostic application of impedance audiometry there are no
absolutes; ... the results of any single impedance measurement
are usually ambiguous and have little individual value."

Keith (1978) summarized the situation by stating it is
imperative that tympanometry and stapedial reflex testing
always be done together. To do less, according to Keith,
results in statements that "... tympanometry is neither
accurate nor reliable for use in screening infants". Keith

expressed concern that such a general statement will be
interpreted by some as indicating that the impedance battery
is not valid or reliable for infants under 7 months of age.
This misinterpretation is unfortunate in that it may result
in reluctance to use a valuable diagnostic tool with a population of individuals who are difficult to examine both otoscopically and audiometrically.

Studies published by Orchik et al. (1978a, 1978b) clearly
show that prediction of middle ear effusion on the basis of
tympanometric data alone is difficult at best, unless the
tympanogram is a flat, non-mobile pattern where a 90% occurr-
ance of effusion is present. Orchik's studies proved that
tympanometry with acoustic reflex threshold measurement show
the highest correlation to surgical findings relative to the
presence of middle ear effusion. That is to say, the combination of tympanometry and measurements of acoustic reflex
threshold are superior to the use of either impedance component alone as a predictor of the presence of middle ear
effusion.

Schwartz and Schwartz (1978) also published data which
supported the combined use of tympanometry and acoustic
reflex measurement to identify middle ear effusion. They
examined 85 ears of 46 infants below the age of 7 months.
They found that 16 of 20 ears displayed a normal tympanogram
despite pneumo-otoscopic evidence of effusion. However, the
acoustic reflex was absent in all 20 ears with effusion.
They concluded that while a normal tympanogram cannot be
considered evidence of a mobile tympanic membrane or effusion-
free middle ear, the presence of an acoustic reflex with a
normal tympanogram supports normal middle ear function.
Freyss et al. (1979) also found that the presence of the
acoustic reflex provided a higher sensitivity than tympanometry for separating normal dry middle ears from middle ears
with fluid.

A pilot study by Dedman and Robinette (1973) on the
potential use of the acoustic reflex as a tool for infant
screening showed that consistent acoustic reflex measurements
could be obtained only in neonates older than 72 hours of age.
Abahazi and Greenberg (1977) measured acoustic reflex thresholds in 62 normal infants between 1 month and 12 months of
age. They used pure tones (500, 1000 and 2000 Hz), broadband
noise, low-pass noise and high-pass noise to elicit the
reflex. Only 23 of the 62 infants showed acoustic reflex
responses to all stimuli, while the remaining 39 infants had

acoustic reflexes, but to less than the total number of
stimuli. The findings suggest that as the age of an infant
increases, less stimulus intensity is required for the acoustic reflex threshold. Keith and Bench (1978) showed that the
acoustic reflex is clearly present in all normal infants by
3 weeks of age.

McCandless and Allred (1978) produced an extensive study
of the emergence of the acoustic reflex in 53 infant subjects
tested daily in the hospital nursery and tested weekly following their hospital discharge. These researchers evaluated
two probe-tone frequencies, 220 Hz and 660 Hz, and established
acoustic reflex thresholds with a bracketing procedure for
stimuli of 500, 1000, 2000 and 4000 Hz. The tympanometry
results showed an average middle ear pressure of +26 mm H_2O
from birth to 48 hours of age, which did not resolve to
0 mm H_2O until after the 4th week of life. The infant acoustic reflex thresholds showed a range from 70 dB to 100 dB HTL
with no significant threshold change over the first 6 weeks
of life. The average infant acoustic reflex threshold was 94
dB HTL at birth, with only an average decrease of 3 dB during
the initial 6 weeks of age. McCandless and Allred spoke
highly of the advantages of the 660 Hz probe-tone in measurement of the infant acoustic reflexes. With the 660 Hz
probe-tone and the 500 Hz eliciting stimulis, 89% of the
infants showed acoustic reflexes during the initial 48 hours
of life. The 220 Hz probe-tone with a 500 Hz eliciting
stimulus showed acoustic reflexes in only 4% of the infants
during the same 48 hour period. The acoustic reflex was
noted in some infants as early as 4 hours after birth.
Although the 220 Hz probe-tone was superior for tympanogram
tracings, the 660 Hz probe-tone was clearly better for acoustic reflex measurements in infants. The use of a low-
frequency eliciting reflex stimulus was recommended since
the incidence of infant acoustic reflexes present decreased
as the reflex eliciting stimulus was increased in frequency.

In contrast to the studies which questioned the efficacy
of tympanometry with infants, successful tympanometric
results with 91 infants between 4 weeks and 17 months were
reported by Groothuis et al. (1978, 1979). These clinicians
used otoscopy and tympanometry in 549 evaluations to study
the pathogenesis of acute and chronic otitis media. Normal
tympanograms and normal otoscopy findings correlated highly
in 92% of the evaluations; flat tympanograms and abnormal
otoscopy findings were correlated 93% of the time. However,

the intermediate negative pressure tympanograms and otoscopy
correlated only 59% of the time. Groothuis et al. reported
that the tympanometric examination took about 45 seconds.
Crying infants were given a bottle to suck during the test,
which was relatively unaffected by the sucking behaviour.
Finally, the authors reported that no flat tympanograms were
found in otitis free infants.

The Groothuis studies provide some especially interesting findings:

1) because of the report of Paradise et al. regarding the
    shortcomings of tympanometry in infants less than 7 months
    of age, Groothuis et al. examined their data separately
    for infants older and younger than 7 months. They found
    that the high correlation of tympanometry and otoscopy
    findings were similar in infants above and below 7 months
    of age;

2) when a non-mobile tympanogram appeared in an asymptomatic
    infant in the study who had not previously had otitis
    media, acute otitis media developed within one additional
    month;

3) the resolution of otitis media was often prolonged as
    long as six months in 60% of the infants.

The authors concluded that tympanometry is a most useful tool
and may be utilized for the earlier identification and more
accurate follow-up of acute otitis media in infants.

No aspect of impedance and infants is unassailable. In
regard to tympanometry accompanied by acoustic reflex measurement, Schwartz and Schwartz (1979) reported in 30 children
from 4 months of age with acute otitis media, that tympanometry sensitivity in identifying acute otitis media was only
74.5%, while acoustic reflex measurement was equally discour-
aging with a test sensitivity of 71%. However, the acoustic
reflex was absent in 95% of those ears which exhibited a flat
tympanometric pattern.

More recently, Schwartz and Schwartz (1980) offered
further observations on tympanometric findings in young
infants with middle ear effusions. Their subjects were 28
infants ranging in age from 1 to 5 months. All infants were
diagnosed with strict pneumo-otoscopic criteria to have
middle ear effusion. Of the 40 effusion ears, 30 displayed

the expected flat tympanogram, while 8 effusion ears showed
normal tympanogram. The remaining 2 ears had negative
pressure peaks. Analysis of the 8 false-negative tympanograms
revealed that 6 of the 8 infants were between the ages of 1
and 2 months, and the remaining 2 infants were 3 and 5 months
of age. Hence, the conflicting tympanograms were almost all
from infants within the first 12 weeks of life. The tympanograms from infants older than 3 months were reasonably accurate and in accordance with clinical findings.

The Infant Aberrant Tympanogram

Much discussion has been generated to explain the high
incidence of false-negative findings using tympanometry as a
predictor of middle ear effusion. Initially, Paradise et al.
(1978) concluded that in infants less than 7 months of age,
many of the ears with effusion had "normal" tympanograms,
presumably because external auditory canal walls in infants
tend to be highly distensible. Paradise et al. graded canal
wall distensibility on a scale of 0 to +4, and found that
distensibility indeed varied inversely with age, with the
sharpest drop-off occurring just after 6 months of age.
Similar data on canal wall distensibility were presented by
Schwartz and Schwartz (1978) for 85 infant ears. They also
suggested that "... it is entirely possible that the bimodal
or W-shaped tympanogram... is related to the distensible ear
canal walls of the infant and not to a hyper-mobile tympanic
membrane."

According to Margolis (1978) the explanation for the
"W-shaped" tympanogram is due to the resultant physical interaction among the properties of acoustic reactance, acoustic
resistance, ear canal pressure and probe-tone frequency. Roy
Sullivan, Ph.D., of Adelphi University, suggests that the
hyperdistensible neonatal ear canal walls may act as a shunt
resistance at ambient air pressure, providing an alternative
path for the shunting of acoustic energy from the external
canal, independent of middle ear status. At negative and
positive relative meatal air pressure values, the canal walls
are contracted and expanded respectively, lessening the resistive shunt effect on the total external canal impedance.
Sullivan concludes that with 220 Hz probe-frequency tympanometry, those considerations result in a pseudo-normal tympanogram in an effusion-filled middle ear and a W-shaped tympanogram in fluid-free neonatal ears harboring negative middle ear
pressure. One peak of the W-shape tympanogram will center at,

or near, ambient air pressure due to the loss of sound energy
in the neonatal ear canal through the resistive shunt of the
hyperdistensible canal walls. The more negative of the bio-
modal tympanogram peaks would represent the maximally com-
pliant point of negative middle ear pressure.

Schwartz and Schwartz (1980) argue that one should expect
a monotonically increasing tympanogram if the canal wall distensibility theory is correct. Positive air pressure introduced into the pliable infant external ear canal increases
the canal volume and, thus, decreases the trapped probe-tone
sound energy. The volume of the ear canal should then
decrease with artifically induced negative air pressure,
thereby increasing the probe-tone sound energy. The result
of this action would produce a monotonically increasing
tympanogram as a function of changing relative canal air
pressure from -200 mm H_2O to $+200$ mm H_2O.

Himmelfarb et al. were the most recent authors to publish
information regarding infant tympanogram patterns (1979). They
observed 6 different tympanogram patterns dependent upon the
acoustic impedance property measured and the frequency of the
probe-tone. They concluded that atypical tympanometric
patterns are due to the arithmetic interaction between
acoustic resistance and acoustic reactance. From a clinical
point of view, Howie (1979) suggested that the position of the
infant during the impedance test may provide the answer to the
false-negative tympanogram. Thus, fluid-filled middle ears
may show normal tympanograms if the neonate is in a prone
position with the test ear pointed up, permitting the fluid
to settle toward the medial aspect of the middle ear space
and "freeing" the tympanic membrane to move normally.

At any rate, it is clear that clinicians using tympanometry in young infants should expect some unique patterns.
Misdiagnosis should decrease when tympanometry is accompanied
by acoustic reflex measurement. Because of the numerous
possibilities for error in impedance measurements in infants,
such patients should be tested by clinicians well experienced
with impedance audiometry.

Clinicians using impedance audiometry with infants are
urged to heed several guidelines:

1. Learn to recognize overall patterns in the impedance test
    battery. Do not use any _single_ impedance test to reach
    diagnostic conclusions.

2. Pay little attention to the absolute value, per se, of any
    of the impedance test results. Finicky clinicians may
    overlook the true clinical picture if they become too
    concerned with the absolute numbers of specific impedance
    diagnostic conclusions.

3. Beware of implicit diagnostic conclusions based only on
    impedance measures. No test is infallible; the impedance
    technique is a strong, supplementary tool, but the
    sophisticated clinician bases final decisions on the
    total patient presentation of complaint, history,
    physical examination, audiometry (if possible), behaviour-
    al observations and an impedance test battery.

Hearing Sensitivity Prediction
With the Acoustic Reflex

     Sensory-neural hearing loss can be estimated by use of
the acoustic impedance meter and the Sensitivity Prediction
from the Acoustic Reflex (SPAR) test. Originally developed
by Niemeyer and Sesterhenn in 1974 and revised by Jerger et al.
(1974), the procedure is based on a comparison of acoustic
stimuli. The concept of the SPAR technique is that the presence of sensory-neural hearing loss predictably reduces the
expected acoustic reflex threshold difference between the
pure tone stimuli and the noise signal. Numerous studies
have confirmed the predictive accuracy of the SPAR test in
the identification of sensory-neural hearing loss (Northern
and Downs, 1978).

     Jerger et al. (1978) found that accurate prediction of
sensory-neural hearing loss by the SPAR test is a function of
the patient's chronological age. Fortunately, the predictive
accuracy of the test is most successful in children between
the ages of 0 and 10 years. In the Jerger et al. (1978)
study, 100% of the children predicted to have normal hearing
did, indeed, show normal audiograms. Severe sensory-neural
hearing loss was predicted accurately in children 85% of the
time. Prediction of moderate sensory-neural hearing loss in
children was less accurate (54%) due to the complex interaction of several variables, including degree of hearing loss,
audiometric configuration and type of reflex activating signal.
Unfortunately, minor middle ear disorders, even with normal
audiograms, may have a significant effect on acoustic reflex
measurement -- and thus, influence the predictive accuracy
of the SPAR test results.

Although the SPAR test can be accomplished with children of virtually any age and can be completed in minimal time with standard equipment, no substantive evaluation of SPAR with infants has been reported (Newman et al. 1974). Margolis and Popelka (1975) found that their study group of neonates between 2 and 4 months of age had normal acoustic reflex thresholds, and concluded that the hearing sensitivity prediction procedures used to detect hearing loss in adults should be similarly predictive in the infant population. In fact, they applied the computational procedure of Jerger et al. (1974) to the 10 normal infants used in their study and found that all would be predicted to have normal hearing. Margolis and Popelka did suggest, however, that mild sedation for the infants might be worthwhile to make the acoustic reflex measurement procedure more successful.

There is little question that competent use of the SPAR test would greatly enhance the typical auditory evaluation of children, but additional research is needed to confirm utilization of the SPAR test with infants. An excellent review of all aspects of predicting hearing loss from the acoustic reflex has been published recently by Hall (1980).

Impedance and Hearing Aid
Management in Children

A considerable volume of literature is now available concerning the use of impedance measurements related to hearing aid selection, fitting and management (Northern, 1979). The objective nature of impedance testing suggests that this technique has application with hearing aids and non-verbal patients, particularly children and infants. Madell (1976) emphatically stated that acoustic impedance testing should preceed every hearing aid evaluation session with children. Although the clinical application of impedance techniques is well established and routinely accepted, the use of acoustic impedance as an "objective" hearing aid procedure needs additional research and refinement.

Brooks (1975) pointed out that middle ear disorders generally result in an increase in hearing loss which may have a deleterious effect on hearing aid utilization. If a child's sensory-neural hearing loss is increased by 15 - 25 dB, which is not uncommon in conductive hearing problems, the child will require additional output from the hearing aid.

As the hearing aid is turned up to provide more gain, acoustic
feedback may result, creating distortion and disturbance. In
many hearing aids, increasing the gain to approach the maximum power output of the aid introduces unwanted distortion,
thereby reducing the effectiveness of the hearing aid.
Impedance measures are, of course, extremely sensitive to the
continuing presence of middle ear disorder and should be conducted routinely in the management of the infant or child who
wears a hearing aid.

Studies have also been reported to show the influence of
negative middle ear pressure (identified using tympanometry)
to evaluate hearing thresholds. Cooper, Langley, Meyerhoff
and Gates (1977) examined 1,133 children with negative pressure tympanograms between -150 and -400 mm H_2O and noted their
hearing threshold levels to be elevated by as much as 25 dB.
Norris, Jirsa and Skinner (1977) concluded that audiologists
should expect conductive loss of approximately 8 dB in the
speech frequency range with a middle ear pressure of -100 mm
H_2O, and approximately 20 dB when negative middle ear pressure
reaches -400 mm H_2O. This study points out that the greatest
threshold shift as a consequence of negative middle ear
pressure occurs at the midpoint of the speech frequency range,
a fact which has considerable significance for childhood
hearing aid users with poor Eustachian tube function.

Rubin (1976) cited the importance of impedance measurements with deaf children because of the high incidence of
middle ear pathology in that population. She reported that
in 1 year, 50% of the 16 hearing impaired toddlers and babies
in the Lexington Infant Center demonstrated middle ear pathology. All the infants were given routine impedance testing
during each session of the hearing aid evaluation procedure
and fitting to rule out fluctuant hearing loss. Rubin indicated further that the audiologist must be certain that a
child's middle ears function normally when "real ear" hearing
aid measurements are used as an indication of specific hearing aid performance.

Weber and Northern (1978) described a technique based on
impedance measurements for the selection of children's hearing
aids. They indicated that the aided acoustic reflex is a
reliable method for determining hearing aid gain for non-
verbal children. Weber and Northern suggest putting the
impedance probe in the ear contralateral to the hearing aid
(Figure 1), using a constant sound field input of average

level environmental sounds or conversational speech. The
gain control of the hearing aid is slowly raised until the
acoustic reflex is barely observable on the impedance meter.
Setting the gain just below the acoustic reflex level will be
safely under the patient's loudness discomfort level, thereby
mitigating against the possibility of amplification overfit.
Such "objective" impedance fitting techniques might have
definite beneficial application in infant hearing aid situations, however, considerable research is still needed before
such techniques can become clinical routine.

FIGURE 1:   SCHEMATIC MODEL OF TECHNIQUE FOR SELECTION OF
             CHILDREN'S HEARING AIDS.

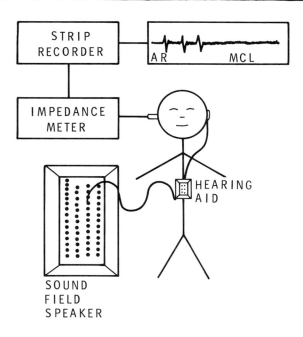

Summary

Utilization of acoustic impedance measurements in infants
have received considerable attention thus far in the literature, but consensus of opinion is varied. Aberrant tympanometric results may be expected with infants, including "W-
shaped" tympanograms as well as pseudo-normal tympanograms
from fluid-filled middle ears. However, impedance results
in infants may provide accurate, valuable information, provided the tests are accomplished by experienced clinicians
who do not depend upon any single test element in the impedance test battery, who use tympanometry accompanied by
acoustic reflex measurement, and who are cautious about making
implicit diagnostic conclusions based solely on impedance
measurements. Impedance techniques with infants can be used
to estimate the presence of sensory-neural loss and to help
guide in the selection, fitting and management of hearing
aids. There is great need, at this time, for additional
research in all aspects of impedance measurements with
infants to help resolve the numerous areas of controversy.

REFERENCES

Abahazi, D.A. and Greenberg, H.J. "Clinical acoustic reflex
    threshold measurement in infants" Journal of Speech and
    Hearing Disorders 62:514 - 519, 1977.

Balkany, T.J. and Zarnoch, J.M. "Impedance tympanometry in
    infants" Audiology & Hearing Education 4:17 - 19, 1978.

Bennett, M. "Acoustic impedance bridge measurements with
    the neonate" British Journal of Audiology 9:117 - 124,
    1975.

Brooks, D.N. "Middle ear effusion in children with severe
    hearing loss" Impedance Newsletter (American Electromedics
    Corp., Acton, Mass.), 4:6 - 7, 1976.

Cannon, S.S., Smith, K.E., Reece, C.A. and Thebo, J.L.
    "Middle ear measurements in neonates: a normative study
    (abstract)" Asha, 16:564, 1975.

Cooper, J.C., Langley, L.R., Meyerhoff, W.L. and Gates, G.A. "The significance of negative middle ear pressure" Laryngoscope 87:92 - 97, 1977.

Dedmon, D.H. and Robinette, M.S. "The acoustic reflex as a tool for neonatal screening" Audecibel 22:202 - 210, 1973.

Elner, A., Ingelstedt, S. and Ivarsson, A. "The elastic properties of the tympanic membrane system" Acta Otolaryngologica 72:397 - 403, 1971.

Freyss, G., Narcy, P., Manac'h, Y. and Toupet, M. "Acoustic reflex as a predictor of middle ear effusion" Proceedings of the 2nd International Symposium on Recent Advances in Otitis Media with Effusion, Annals of Otorhinolaryngology In Press, 1980.

Groothuis, J.R., Altemeier, W.A., Wright, P.F. and Sell, S.H.W. "The evolution and resolution of otitis media in infants: tympanometric findings" in Impedance Screening for Middle Ear Disease in Children, Harford et al. (eds.) (New York: Grune & Stratton), 1978.

Groothuis, J.R., Sell, S.H.W., Wright, P.F., Thompson, R.N., and Altemeier, W.A. "Otitis media in infancy: tympanometric findings" Pediatrics 63:435 - 442, 1979.

Hall, J.W. "Predicting hearing loss from the acoustic reflex" in Clinical Impedance Audiometry, Second Edition, Jerger, J. and Northern, J. (eds.) (Acton, Mass.: American Electromedics Corp.), 1980.

Himelfarb, M. Popelka, G. and Shanon, E. "Tympanometry in normal infants" Journal of Speech and Hearing Research 22:179 - 191, 1979.

Howie, V.M., Grabowski, M.L. and Ploussard, J.H. "Comparison between impedance audiometry and pneumatic otoscopy in the diagnosis of middle ear effusion in the young infant" Presented at the Fourth Annual Meeting of the Society for Ear, Nose and Throat Advances in Children, New Orleans, L.A., November, 1976.

Jerger, J. "Clinical experience with impedance audiometry" Archives of Otolaryngology 91:311 - 324, 1970.

Jerger, J., Burney, P., Mauldin, L. and Crump, B. "Predicting hearing loss from the acoustic reflex" Journal of
Speech and Hearing Disorders 39:11-22, 1974.

Jerger, J., Hayes, D., Anthony, L. and Mauldin, L. "Factors
influencing prediction of hearing level from the acoustic
reflex" Monographs in Contemporary Audiology (Minneapolis:
Maico Hearing Instruments, Inc.), 1:1, 1978.

Jerger, J. and Hayes, D. "Diagnostic applications of impedance audiometry: Middle ear disorder; Sensorineural
disorder" Chapter 6 in Clinical Impedance Audiometry
(Second Edition) Jerger, J. and Northern, J. (eds.)
(Acton, Mass: American Electromedics Corp.), 109 - 127,
1980.

Jerger, S., Jerger, J., Mauldin, L. and Segal, P. "Studies
in impedance audiometry II: Children less than 6 years
old" Archives of Otolaryngology 99:1 - 9, 1974.

Keith, R.W. "Impedance audiometry with neonates" Archives of
Otolaryngology 97:465 - 467, 1973.

Keith, R.W. "Middle ear function in neonates" Archives of
Otolaryngology 101:376 - 379, 1975.

Keith, R.W. "The use of impedance measurements in infant
hearing programs" in Early Identification of Hearing Loss
Mencher, G. (ed.) (Basel: S. Karger), 1976.

Keith, R.W. and Bench, R.J. "Stapedial reflex in neonates"
Accepted for publication in Scandinavian Audiology, 1978.

Madell, J.R. "Hearing aid evaluation procedures with children" in Hearing Aids: Current Developments and Concepts
Rubin, M. (ed.) (Baltimore: University Park Press), 1976.

Margolis, R.H. and Popelka, G.R. "Static and dynamic acoustic
impedance measurements in infant ears" Journal of Speech
and Hearing Research 18:435 - 443, 1975.

Margolis, R.H. "Tympanometry in infants: State-of-the-art"
in Impedance Screening for Middle Ear Disease in Children,
Harford et al. (eds.) (New York: Grune & Stratton), 1978.

McCandless, G.A. and Allred, P.L. "Tympanometry and emergence
    of the acoustic reflex in infants" in Impedance Screening
    for Middle Ear Disease in Children, Harford, et al. (eds.)
    (New York: Grune & Stratton), 1978.

Niemeyer, W. and Sesterhenn, G. "Calculating the hearing
    threshold from the stapedius reflex threshold for different
    sound stimuli" Audiology 13:421 - 427, 1974.

Newman, R.L., Stream, K.S. and Chesnutt, B.C. "Application
    of the Neimeyer method of predicting hearing loss in neo-
    nates and infants" (abstract) Asha 16:564, 1974.

Norris, T., Jirsa, R. and Skinner, B. "The effect of air
    pressure on pure tone thresholds" Read before the annual
    meeting of the American Auditory Society, Miami, Florida,
    1977.

Northern, J.L. "Hearing aids and acoustic impedance measure-
    ments" Monographs of Contemporary Audiology 1:2 (Maico
    Hearing Instruments Corp., Minneapolis, Minn.) 1978.

Northern, J.L. and Downs, M.P. Hearing in Children Second
    Edition (Baltimore: Williams and Wilkins), 1978.

Orchik, D.J., Dunn, J.W. and McNutt, L. "Tympanometry as a
    predictor of middle ear effusion" Archives of Otolaryn-
    gology 104:4 - 6, 1978a.

Orchik, D.J., Morff, R. and Dunn, J.W. "Impedance audiometry
    in serous otitis media" Archives of Otolaryngology 104:409 -
    412, 1978b.

Paradise, J.L., Smith, C. and Bluestone, C.D. "Tympanometric
    detection of middle ear effusion in infants and young
    children" Pediatrics 58:198 - 206, 1976.

Reichert, T.J., Cantekin, E.I., Riding, K.H., Cohn, B.L.
    and Bluestone, C.D. "Diagnosis of middle ear effusion in
    young infants by otoscopy and tympanometry" in Impedance
    Screening for Middle Ear Disease in Children, Harford
    et al (eds.) (New York: Grune & Stratton), 1978.

Robertson, E.D., Peterson, J.L. and Lamb, L.E. "Relative impedance measurements in young children" Archives of Otolaryngology 88:162 - 168, 1968.

Rubin, M. "Hearing aids for infants and toddlers" in Hearing Aids: Current Developments and Concepts Rubin, M. (ed.) (Baltimore: University Park Press), 1976.

Schwartz, D.M. and Schwartz, R.H. "A comparison of tympanometry and acoustic reflex measurements for detecting middle ear effusion in infants below seven months of age" in Impedance Screening for Middle Ear Disease in Children, Harford et al. (eds.) (New York: Grune and Stratton), 1978.

Schwartz, D.M. and Schwartz, R.H. "Acoustic immittance findings in acute otitis media" in press, Proceedings of 2nd International Symposium on Recent Advances in Otitis Media with Effusion" Annals of Otorhinolaryngology, 1980.

Schwartz, D.M. and Schwartz, R.H. "Tympanometric findings in young infants with middle ear effusion: Some further observations" Submitted to International Journal of Pediatric Otolaryngology, 1980.

Shurin, P.A., Pelton, S.I. and Finkelstein, J. "Tympanometry in the diagnosis of middle ear effusion" New England Journal of Medicine 296:412 - 417, 1977.

Sullivan, R. Personal Communication. Adelphi University, New York, 1980.

Tos, M., Poulsen, G. and Hancke, A.B. "Screening tympanometry during the first year of life" Acta Otolaryngologica 88: 388 - 394, 1979.

Weber, H. and Northern, J.L. "The Colorado State Health Program for Selection of Children's Hearing Aids" in Binaural Hearing and Amplification, Volume II, Libby, E. Robert (ed.) (Chicago: Zenetron Corp.), 1980.

Zarnoch, J.M. and Balkany, T.J. "Tympanometric screening of normal and intensive care unit newborns: Validity and reliability" in Impedance Screening for Middle Ear Disease in Children, Harford et al. (eds.) (New York: Grune & Stratton), 1978.

Zarnoch, J.M. "In support of tympanometry with infants"
    Letter to the Editor, <u>Audiology & Hearing Education</u> 4:5,
    1978.

AUDITORY BRAINSTEM RESPONSE: A CONTRIBUTION TO INFANT ASSESSMENT AND MANAGEMENT

John T. Jacobson
Dalhousie University, Halifax, Nova Scotia

Michael R. Seitz
University of Alabama, Birmingham, Alabama

George T. Mencher
Nova Scotia Hearing and Speech Clinic, Halifax, Nova Scotia

Valerie Parrott
Janeway Child Health Centre, St. John's, Newfoundland

Introduction

The concept of early management means many things to many people. Based on one's personal background, education and working relationship with the parents and infant with a hearing impairment, the focus of early management may change dramatically. This concept of diverse input was reflected in the Saskatoon Conference on the Early Diagnosis of Hearing Loss, which recommended that Auditory Brainstem Response (ABR) audiometry be included in the comprehensive evaluation of infants suspected of hearing impairment or found to be at risk for hearing loss. While ABR has been used primarily as a diagnostic technique to assess the integrity of the peripheral auditory system, it also offers a unique input into the necessary long-term management strategy of the hearing impaired child. As stated by Ruben and also Downs elsewhere in this text, evidence suggests that management techniques are inappropriate without ongoing otolaryngological and audiological reassessment. Recognizing then, that successful intervention is only as strong as its weakest link, the contribution of ABR is a logical component in the continuing management process. This paper will:

1)   review the development of ABR audiometry in infants;

2) describe an ongoing high risk hearing screening program
    which utilizes ABR; and,

3) discuss future implications of soundfield ABR audiometry.

     Auditory brainstem response (ABR) audiometry has proven
itself to be a successful procedure in the objective evaluation of the peripheral auditory system. These brainstem
potentials reflect stimulus related electrical activity
generated from the auditory nerve and brainstem nuclei.
Although auditory brainstem activity was initially recorded
by Sohmer and Feinmesser (1967), it was the work of Jewett
and colleagues who accurately reported its origin (Jewett,
1969, 1970; Jewett, Romano, and Williston, 1970; Jewett and
Williston, 1971; Jewett and Romano, 1972). Brainstem onset
responses consist of a series of 7 wavepeak configurations
usually measured within the first 8 to 12 milliseconds (msec)
post-stimulus, using far-field recording techniques. Wave I
is described as a reflection of the compound cochlear-
acoustic nerve action potential and is negative in polarity
(Picton, Hillyard, and Krausz, et al., 1974; Picton and Fitzgerald, 1980). Waves II-VII represent synchronous electrical
activity sequentially derived from the brainstem nuclei and
auditory pathway (Buchwald and Huang, 1975; Goldenberg and
Derbyshire, 1975; Gilroy, et al., 1977; Stockard, Stockard,
and Scarborough, 1977). Each wavepeak is designated by a
Roman numeral (I-VII) and separated in latency by approximately 1 millisecond (Jewett and Williston, 1971). The
specific wavepeak latencies are affected by numerous stimulus
parameters as well as pathological and non-pathological conditions of the auditory system which must be taken into consideration prior to an accurate diagnostic assessment (Picton,
1977; Stockard, Stockard and Scarborough, 1978; Jacobson,
Morehouse and Seitz, 1980).

     Figure 1 displays a series of brainstem response tracings
recorded at a rate of 33.3/sec. from an adult male. Each
replicated tracing represents the sum of 2000 averaged
responses. For clarity, Waves I through VII are labelled at
70 dB normal hearing level (nHL). An inverse relationship
exists for Wave V latency as a function of intensity. That
is, as intensity decreases, Wave V latency increases. Latency
is seen to increase from 6.0 msec at 70 dB to 8.08 msec at
20 dB nHL. In ABR audiometry, the interpretation of Wave V
latency-intensity characteristics has proven to be the most
diagnostically useful in providng accurate estimates of
auditory threshold sensitivity. In addition to an

assessment of hearing acuity, neurological interpretation can
be ascertained by determining interpeak latencies (IPL)
between Waves (I-V). In this manner, an accurate account of
the neural conduction time between peaks and, thus, presumably
transmission time through the auditory system, can be recorded
(Starr and Achor, 1975; Stockard, Stockard and Scarborough,
1978).

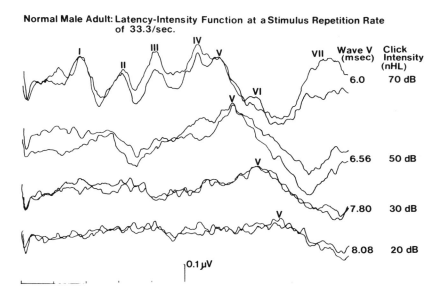

Figure 1. A series of auditory brainstem response tracings recorded at a rate of 33.3/sec from a normal
hearing adult male. Responses are the sum of 2000 averages at 70 dB, 50 dB, 30 dB, and 20 dB nHL.
For clarification, Waves I through VII are labelled at 70 dB nHL. Wave V latencies in milliseconds
(msec) are shown at each intensity.

ABR: Infant Assessment

     The use of ABR audiometry as a tool in the diagnosis of
hearing loss in newborns has been a most recent development.
Hecox and Galambos (1974) and Hecox (1975) were among the
first investigators to report extensive data on the use of
click stimulus ABR techniques with infants. Their studies
dealt primarily with the latency of ABR Wave V in children

three weeks to three years of age. Wave V latencies which
were recorded down to a level of 20 dB HL were demonstrated
to decrease as a function of both stimulus intensity and
maturational age from birth to approximately eighteen months.
The reduction in Wave V latency to age, established the need
for independent norms for various age groups within the
infant population. More importantly, however, the study
demonstrated that ABRs could be successfully obtained from
very young infants, and these procedures were clinically
useful in assessing peripheral auditory function in an age
group that was either too young or unable to respond to
traditional audiological procedures.

     In a follow-up study, Shulman-Galambos and Galambos
(1975) reported Wave V brainstem response latencies obtained
from 24 premature infants initially confined to an Intensive
Care (IC) nursery. The actual ABR testing occurred immediately
prior to discharge from the IC nursery at a time when the
infants were considered medically healthy. Their results
substantiated the earlier work of Hecox and Galambos (1974).
Wave V latencies increased systematically across all intensities tested (60 dB to 30 dB SL) at a rate of approximately
0.4 msec per 10 dB stimulus attenuation. Conversely, 0.3 to
0.5 msec reductions were seen in the Wave V latency as gestational age progressed from 34 to 42 weeks. The significance
of these results is not only in the data, but in the fact
that ABRs can be reliably recorded from non-sedated, premature infants without concern to fatigue, habituation, or
alterations in the sleep state. Under comparable conditions,
similar findings have been reported in adults (Amadeo and
Shaguss, 1973; Picton and Hillyard, 1974; Starr and Achor,
1975; Picton, et al., 1977; Stockard and Jones, 1977).

     Salamy and colleagues (Salamy, McKean and Buda, 1975;
Salamy and McKean, 1976; Salamy and McKean, 1977) have
investigated maturational changes associated with brainstem
responses in newborns and infants. Their results substantiated
the earlier work of Hecox and Galambos (1974) showing a reduction in Wave V latencies as age increased to approximately
twelve months. Their data also suggested that peripheral
transmission (as measured by absolute latency for Wave I) and
central transmission (as measured by the interpeak latency
(IPL) between Waves I and V) mature at different rates. While
the peripheral transmission process (Wave I) approximates
adult Wave I latency by six weeks of age, differences in
central transmission (Wave I-V IPL) did not equate until one
year of age. Salamy and colleagues concluded that

maturational change as measured by peripheral and central
transmission time is a reflection of myelogenesis of the auditory pathway. Salamy, et al, (1978) also described maturational change as a function of presentation rate in 209
subjects ranging in age from birth to three years. At slower
presentation rates (10-40/sec) only the newborn group (n = 45)
produced deviations in recovery of the Wave V and interpeak
latency values when compared to all other subjects tested;
however, at faster rates (50-80/sec) these age related differences were not observed. Alterations in latency values due
to presentation rate have been attributed to neural refractory
change and appear to be fully mature at or near birth.

     In a similar study, Starr, et al, (1977) reported the
effects of maturation on latency in 42 infants ranging from
25 to 44 weeks gestational age. Using click stimuli presented
at 75, 65, 45, and 25 dB SL, absolute latency values for
Waves I, III, IV and V and IPL's for Waves I-III, III-V and
I-V were recorded. Absolute latency values agreed with previous infant studies, thus establishing that reliable ABRs
could be obtained from premature infants as early as the 28th
gestational week, when click stimulus are used at an intensity
level of 65 dB SL. The Starr, et al, data supports the contention that both peripheral (absolute Wave I latency) and
central (IPL) transmission are a function of auditory maturation. In their concluding remarks, the authors offer two
independent mechanisms to account for maturational change.
The decreased latency of Wave I was attributed to improvements
in middle ear impedance, cochlear sensitivity, and VIII trans-
duction. Myelination and synaptic efficiency were offered as
vehicles for the improved neural conduction time recorded.

     Recently, a number of reports have verified earlier ABR
data recorded from both premature and full-term infants (Cone
and Hecox, 1978; Finitzo-Hieber and Hecox, 1978; Ocks and
Markland, 1978; Cox, Hack and Metz, 1978; Diaz, Salomon, and
Mena, 1979; Fabiani, et al, 1979; Hazell, Sheldrake and
Reynolds, 1979; and Kileny, Connelly and Robertson, 1979).
While most findings appear similar in nature, differences in
experimental design, populations and pathological and non-
pathological conditions suggest caution in data interpretation.

Development of Infant Screening Programs

     Over the past decade, procedures for newborn hearing
screening programs have been carefully established. In 1970,

the Joint Committee on Infant Hearing Screening, recognizing
the innate problems associated with universal infant mass
screening, urged further research into behavioural screening
programs but could not, at that time, recommend newborn
screening implementation. Based on longitudinal study, a
supplementary statement was issued by the Joint Committee on
Infant Screening (1972). Those recommendations outlined the
establishment of a five item high risk register which
attempted to identify newborns with hearing impairment. In
addition, the committee suggested that any infant determined
to be at risk should be evaluated audiologically during the
first two months of life.

Since then, testing procedures and screening techniques
have continued to be modified and improved. Two international
conferences (Mencher, 1976; Gerber and Mencher, 1978) have
provided new direction to the implementation of infant hearing identification and diagnosis. Recommendations from the
Nova Scotia Conference (Mencher, 1976) emphasized the early
identification of hearing loss and suggested specific screening techniques which might be used for this purpose. Recall-
ing that the successful treatment of a hearing impaired infant
depends not only on early identification, but also on the
establishment of appropriate follow-up procedures for the
refinement of the initial diagnosis and the establishment of
adequate early habilitation programs, the Saskatoon Conference on Early Diagnosis of Hearing Loss (Gerber and Mencher,
1978) was convened. Dealing primarily with methods and
techniques for the establishment, confirmation and definition
of hearing impairment within the first six months of life,
its recommendations centered on diagnostic procedures which
could be accomplished rapidly, accurately, and economically.

With the exception of the crib-o-gram which has seen
limited use, an objective screening technique has not been
utilized for mass infant testing. However, the development
of auditory brainstem response audiometry, which has provided
an objective (recognizing that the results must be subject-
ively interpreted) and precise technique for monitoring the
peripheral hearing mechanism, appears worthy of future consideration. The procedure was so well recognized by the
participants at the Saskatoon Conference that two specific
recommendations concerning it were presented:

"WHEREAS, electric response audiometry has been demonstrated to be a useful and appropriately sensitive tool in the recognition and diagnosis of hearing loss in newborn children as well as other difficult to test infants;

RESOLVED, DIAGNOSTIC CENTERS IN WHICH QUALIFIED ADMINISTRATION OF THE TEST IS AVAILABLE SHOULD INCLUDE ELECTRIC RESPONSE AUDIOMETRY (ERA) IN THEIR BATTERY OF TESTS FOR THE EVAL-UATION OF CHILDREN WHO ARE SUSPECTED OF HEARING IMPAIRMENT.

WHEREAS, there is a clear evidence that a significant propor-tion of children in the neonatal intensive care unit will have a hearing loss; and

WHEREAS, preliminary evidence suggests auditory brainstem response (ABR) audiometry may be a useful screening-diagnostic tool in the earliest possible evaluation of those children.

RESOLVED, FURTHER RESEARCH FOCUSING ON THE USE OF AUDITORY BRAINSTEM RESPONSE AUDIOMETRY (ABR) IN THE NEWBORN INTENSIVE CARE UNIT IS ENCOURAGED."

In addition to the recommendations, specific procedures for use during "Electric Response Audiometry" were established as a model for the screening and clinical diagnosis of hearing impaired infants. Specifically, the statement urged that audigory brainstem response audiometry be utilized within a test battery and that ABR reports should include:

1. Latency of Wave V response as a function of the clicks;

2. Threshold estimate;

3. Statement of the type of hearing loss found, if any; and,

4. Measurement of the I-to-V interval of the brainstem response.

ABR: As a Newborn Hearing Screening
       Procedure

     As an outgrowth of earlier ABR studies with infants and,
no doubt, due in part to the recommendations of the Saskatoon
Conference, ABR audiometry has gained favor as a screening
procedure, primarily for intensive care nurseries. An ABR
screening program which has been used as a model by hospitals
and clinics has been reported by Galambos and colleagues
(Galambos, 1978; Horning, 1979; Schulman-Galambos, and Galambos,
1979). In the model shown in Figure 2, Galambos (1978) offered
a protocol which stated that any infant suspect of hearing
impairment should be tested by ABR within the first two months
of birth. Based on his earlier work, Galambos suggested the
use of independent ear evaluations, and further, that the
absence of an ABR at 60 dB or 30 dB HL be considered failure
criteria.

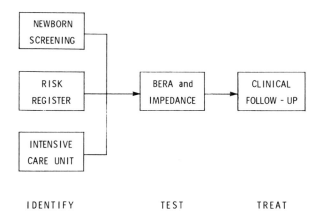

Figure 2.   A scheme proposed to identify neonates with peripheral hearing loss. (Galambos R: Use of
the Auditory Brainstem Response (ABR) in Infant Hearing Testing, in Gerber SE and Mencher GT
(eds): Early Diagnosis of Hearing Loss. New York, Grune & Stratton, 1978, p. 251.)

     In a recent study, Schulman-Galambos and Galambos (1979)
have reported results from their ABR neonatal hearing screening program. They screened 220 normal term infants and 75
newborn infants previously confined to the IC nursery. The
stimulus was a series of 100 micro-second (msec) clicks presented at intensity levels of 60 dB and 30 dB HL independently
to each ear. Infant responses were recorded in a quiet, but
not sound treated testing room.

In the normal group (220 infants) actual ABRs were
derived on a total of 368 ears. Although the variability of
the Wave V latency was judged to be somewhat larger than under
a more controlled testing environment, 85% of all responses
were judged as fair or better. Increased variability was
attributed to equipment noise, patient movement and periodic
personnel interruptions. The results supported the feasibility
of conducting an infant screening program within the confines
of a hospital setting.

Of the total 75 IC nursery infants tested, 21 were "at
risk for hearing loss" based on positive responses from a
high risk questionnaire. From the total number tested by ABR,
four infants (5.3%) were found to be severely hearing impaired.
When these four IC nursery failures were combined with four
other failures from a different high risk follow-up group
(n = 325), the incidence of hearing impairment as identified
by ABR screening was 1 in approximately 50 (2.14%) high risk
infants. This incidence far exceeds the number identified
(1:1000) in a normal newborn population, and supports the
data presented by Simmons (1977) concerning hearing loss and
crib-o-gram failures in the Intensive Care Nursery.

Subsequent studies have shown that the implementation of
ABR audiometry as a screening technique for the identification
of hearing loss in high risk infants appears to be a valid
procedure (Hamilton, Hilding and Mannarelli, 1977; Chisen,
Perlman and Sohmer, 1979; Cox, Hack and Metz, 1979; Horning,
1979; Jacobson, et al, 1980).

An example of the development of ABR as a screening procedure is exemplified in the Infant Hearing Assessment Project
of the Telephone Pioneers of America. This organization
utilizes an ABR system and procedure developed strictly for
"screening" purposes. While experimental results are still
not available, preliminary data from our center and from
others in the United States suggest the system is valid and
reliable, but very time consuming for a screening procedure.
Undoubtedly, more information will be forthcoming on that
program in the future (personal communication, Peltzman, 1980).

ABR: A Clinical Adjunct

The clinical use of ABR audiometry in the assessment of
infant hearing appears limited only by one's imagination.
Numerous studies have been reported which provide pertinent

clinical experiences and suggestions for incorporating ABR
audiometric procedures into existing traditional pediatric
test batteries. For example, Picton (1978) presented an
excellent strategy for evoked potential audiometry with
infants suspected of hearing loss (Figure 3). The strategy
is specifically designed to be utilized with infants who
cannot be assessed accurately with conventional audiometric
techniques. Picton suggests that interpretation of the Wave V
latency–intensity curve function provides diagnostic information about the nature of the hearing loss (conductive vs.
sensory-neural), as well as to its severity. Included in the
diagram is a sequential strategy for the management of an
identified hearing-impaired child.

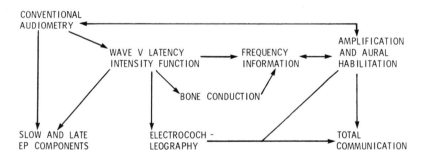

Figure 3.   A tentative strategy for evoked potential audiometry. (Picton TW: The strategy of evoked
potential audiometry, in Gerber SE and Mencher GT (eds): Early Diagnosis of Hearing Loss. New
York, Grune & Stratton, 1978, p. 280.)

Other researchers have used ABR techniques to investigate
specific clinical problems associated with hearing impairment
in children. Mendelson, et al, (1979) reported ABR results
obtained from 63 children ranging in age from 2 to 12 years,
40 of whom were suspected of abnormal middle ear function.
All children were evaluated otoscopically during routine
pediatric examinations. In over 80% of those subjects with
acute supperative otitis media and in 62.5% of those children
with secretory otitis media, Wave I latency was most indicative
of middle ear pathology. Of clinical importance was their
finding which shows a high correlation between aberrant Wave I
latency and abnormal audiometric findings (conductive pathology)
in children who were classified as otoscopically normal.

A group of 82 suspected deaf-blind children were tested using ABR audiometry (Stein, Ozdomar and Daniels, 1979). Of the 79 children from whom ABR data was obtained, approximately 50% failed to respond to click stimuli at intensity presentation levels of 60 dB HL or greater. Thirty-nine per cent of the children who were thought, on the basis of behaviour patterns to be deaf, had near normal peripheral auditory function in at least one ear. Stein, et al, concluded that severely developmentally disabled children can be successfully tested using ABR procedures. Obviously, ABR information can be valuable when planning intervention and treatment strategies for the multiply handicapped child.

Fria and Bartling (1978) reported on the use of ABR audiometry in a clinical setting for 2 years during which 239 children, aged 1 month to 18 years, were evaluated. The majority of those cases (101) were referred based on the results of questionable or unobtainable behavioural testing. Forty-five infants were "at risk for hearing loss", 43 were seen for site-of-lesion determination, 23 exhibited middle ear effusion, 13 infants had meningitis, 8 were suspect of learning disability, and 6 were reported to have had a sudden sensory-neural hearing loss. The data presented in the report indicated the success and usefulness of ABR procedures with a variety of clinical pathologies.

ABR audiometry has also been used successfully with children suspected of autism (Fria, Grundfast and Sabo, 1979; Sohmer and Student, 1978; Student and Sohmer, 1978; Rosenblum et al, 1980) and those with brainstem dysfunction (Nodar, Hahn and Levine, 1979). Additional clinical studies on the use of ABR techniques in pediatric assessment can be found in Davis (1976); Jerger and Hayes (1976); Davis and Hirsh (1977); Mokotoff, et al, (1977); Picton, et al, (1977); Galambos and Hecox (1978); Picton and Smith (1978); Davis and Hirsh (1979); Mainhardt, Davis and Reichert (1979); Weber (1979); Connelly, Kileny and Robertson (1980); and Jerger, Hayes and Jordan (1980).

ABR: An Evaluation Procedure for an
       Infant Screening Program

Health and Welfare Canada, Health Services and Programs Branch, has provided funding for a demonstration/evaluation grant in which all newborns in Halifax are screened for hearing loss at birth. The protocol includes the high risk register, behavioural screening as recommended by the Nova Scotia Conference, and ABR testing of those children who fail the behavioural screening. Two additional groups of infants are also screened and tested as required:

1)   a "special" classification which includes infants from the IC nursery who are not at risk for hearing loss, and any infants for whom there is a request for screening by either a physician or parent; and

2)   a matched number of normal controls. Figure 4 illustrates the flow of the three groups of infants through the screening and evaluation aspects of the program.

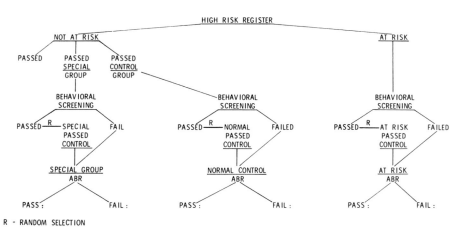

Figure 4.   A flow chart for auditory brainstem response newborn screening. Three categories are shown: (1) at risk for hearing loss; (2) special infant group consisting of parental and physician requests, and intensive care nursery infants not at risk for hearing loss; and (3) normal control group.

Our basic ABR procedure for testing an infant is very simple. Every effort is made to test infants without the use of sedation. That, of course, is highly dependent on the history, age, and status of the infant at the time of testing. However, it has been our experience that children under 4 months of age can be tested without sedation if appropriate measures are taken to insure co-operation. These include sleep deprivation and the scheduling of testing to coincide with feeding. We ask mothers to arrive approximately 20 minutes prior to their scheduled appointment time so they can feed the child at the clinic. Usually, following a minimal waiting period, the majority of infants fall asleep and remain that way throughout the entire test. Electrodes are attached to the baby prior to feeding so that unnecessary movement and contact is kept to a minimum. The parent sits in a reclining chair holding the infant in her arms and with her free hand rests the earphone against the pinna, careful not to occlude or collapse the external auditory canal. Click stimulae are presented monaurally through the earphone and ABR testing techniques are begun. The establishment of ABR threshold sensitivity is based on the replicability of the Wave V component within normal latency limits for the particular gestational age tested. Table I provides the specific testing protocol used for ABR infant screening.

A typical auditory brainstem response from a high risk female infant of 44 weeks gestational age may be seen in Figure 5. For discussion purposes, we have identified Wave latencies I, III, and V and interpeak latencies I-V, I-III, III-V at 60 dB nHL for two presentation rates (10.4/s and 80.4/s). Wave V latencies are also included at 30 dB nHL for each rate. As anticipated, Wave V latencies increased as stimulus intensity decreased at a rate of approximately 0.3 msec per 10 dB stimulus attenuation. These findings are similar to those reported by Hecox and Galambos (1974) and Schulman-Galambos and Galambos (1975). In addition, Wave V latencies are seen to increase as presentation rates increase at 60 dB nHL (10.4/s = 6.88 msec, 80.4/s = 7.36 msec) and 30 dB nHL (10.4/s = 7.56 msec, 80.5/s = 8.44 msec). The increase in Wave V latency as a function of presentation rate substantiates earlier work by Fujikawa and Weber (1977) in infants, and Hyde, Stephens and Thornton (1976), Weber and Fujikawa (1977), and Jacobson, Morehouse and Seitz (1980) in adults.

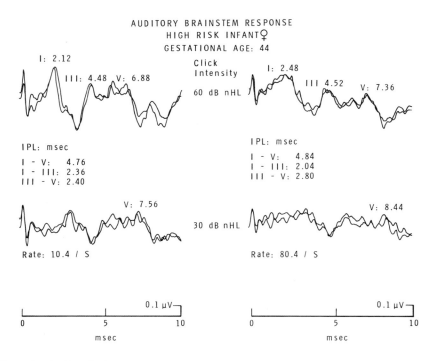

Figure 5.   Auditory brainstem responses recorded from a 44 gestational week old, high risk, newborn female. Responses are shown for one ear at 60 dB and 30 dB nHL at two rates: 10.4/sec and 80.4/sec. Recordings were the result of 2000 averages to an alternating stimulus. The latencies for Waves I, III, and V are given as well as interpeak latencies (I-V, I-III, and III-V) at 60 dB nHL. Wave V latencies are indicated at 30 dB nHL.

We are currently evaluating presentation rate as a function of screening pass-fail criteria. If the identification
and measurement of the Wave V latency were the sole purpose
of ABR screening and, taking into consideration the approximate 2½ minute time difference between a presentation rate of
10.4/s and 80.4/s for 2000 averages, then obviously for
practical purposes, the faster presentation rate would be of
choice. This is particularly true since Wave V resolution is
still maintained at low intensity levels using higher presentation rates. However, if additional wave peak latency
comparisons (IPL) are required for neurological interpretation,
then slower rates which preserve individual wave peak
characteristics must be employed.

Table 1

PROTOCOL FOR NEWBORN ABR SCREENING

1. EQUIPMENT SETTINGS

RATE	10.4/ S, 80.4/ S	SENSITIVITY	10 μV
DURATION	100 μ SEC	BAND PASS	150 - 3000 HZ
SWEEP	10 MSEC	STIMULI	CLICK (ALTERNATE)
REP	2000 MSEC	CHANNELS	1 and 2
DISPLAY GAIN	16		

REAR : ARTIFACT REJECTION : ON; EXTERNAL STIMULUS CONNECTED TO CALIBRATION BOX ; "NORM STIM" X, Y, AND PENLIFT CONNECTED.

2. ELECTRODE PLACEMENT

A + : PZ (FRONTAL) : A- : A_i (EARLOBE) : G : A_C (EARLOBE)

COLLODION TECHNIQUE FOR PZ ELECTRODE

1) CLEAN AREA THOROUGHLY WITH ACETONE ON A GAUZE PAD.
2) PUT ELECTRODE IN PLACE.
3) DROP COLLODION AROUND ELECTRODE.
4) DRY COLLODION WITH COMPRESSED AIR OR HAIR DRYER.
5) INSERT BLUNT NEEDLE SYRINGE THROUGH HOLE IN TOP OF ELECTRODE AND INTRODUCE ELECTRODE PASTE.
6) IMPEDANCE < 5K.
7) IF IMPEDANCE > 5K, SCRAPE SCALP WITH BLUNT SYRINGE INSERTED THROUGH ELECTRODE AND INJECT MORE PASTE. AFTER ELECTRODES HAVE BEEN APPLIED, TAPE WIRES TO CLOTHES AND CONNECT TO AMPLIFIER.
8) CHECK IMPEDANCE ; IF NECESSARY, ABRADE ; SET TO 10^4.
9) FEED BABY AND ALLOW INFANT TO GO TO SLEEP IN MOTHER'S ARMS OR LAYING IN SMALL BASSINET.
10) HAND - HOLD EARPHONE OVER APPROPRIATE EAR - GENTLY SO AS NOT TO COLLAPSE EAR CANALS, MAKING SURE THAT POSITION IS CORRECT.

3. RECORDING PROCEDURE

Q1	60 DB	10.4/ S		Q2	30 DB	10.4/ S
Q3	60 DB	10.4/ S		Q4	30 DB	10.4/ S

RUN EACH QUADRANT SEPARATELY ; RECORD H_1 AND H_2 SUPERIMPOSED. LABEL TRACINGS : NAME, DATE, EAR STIMULUS, INTENSITY RATE.
IF II, IV, VI ARE PRESENT, MEASURE LATENCY.
CALCULATE : I - III LATENCY, I - V , III - V , IV /V : I AMPLITUDE RATIO.

4. RESULTS

IF NORMAL LATENCIES, EAR FINISHED, PROCEED TO CONTRALATERAL EAR.

IF NO RESPONSE AT 60 DB, 10.4/S, INCREASE INTENSITY OUTPUT IN 10 DB INCREMENTS UNTIL WAVE V IS PRESENT. IF QUESTIONABLE OR ABSENT ABR, RE-EXAMINE IN TWO TO FOUR WEEKS USING IDENTICAL PROTOCOL.

Interpeak latencies at 60 dB nHL for rates of 10.4/s and 80.4/s are also provided in Figure 5. When compared to normal adult IPL values (I-V: 4.0 msec, Stockard, et al, 1978), the increased latencies reported in ABR infant literature provides further evidences of maturational change in a newborn population (Salamy and McKean, 1976; Starr, et al, 1977).

Auditory brainstem reponse Wave V mean latencies for 96 newborns are presented in Table II. The infants are classified according to gestational age at the time of testing and condition (at risk, special and normal). Wave V latencies are in response to monaural click stimuli presented at 60 dB and 30 dB nHL at a rate of 10.4/sec. As anticipated, a decrease in Wave V latency occurred as gestational age increased from 40 to 51 weeks in the normal and special categories, but was not apparent in the high risk for hearing loss group (n = 46). These findings would suggest that the auditory maturational process does not appear to be progressing normally in the at risk group under study.

Table 2

AUDITORY BRAINSTEM RESPONSE
WAVE V LATENCY

CLICK STIMULUS :   60 DB NHL   RATE :   10.4/ S

GESTATIONAL AGE : WEEKS	AT RISK	SPECIAL	NORMAL
40 - 43	7.02	7.82	7.10
44 - 47	7.10	7.03	6.88
48 - 51	7.20	6.87	6.70

CLICK STIMULUS :   30 DB NHL   RATE :   10.4/ S

GESTATIONAL AGE : WEEKS	AT RISK	SPECIAL	NORMAL
40 - 43	8.16	8.16	8.01
44 - 47	8.10	7.99	7.36
48 - 51	8.08	7.67	7.27

Table III provides the ABR pass-fail hearing screening
test results from the same 96 newborns. For screening purposes, a failure is considered to be the absence of a replicable Wave V configuration for either ear at the two intensity
levels. There were a total of 12 failures (12.5%), 9 in the
at risk group and 3 in the special group. Of the 12 failures,
8 are still under consideration, 1 has passed on retest, and
3 are confirmed as having a sensory-neural hearing loss.

Table 3

AUDITORY BRAINSTEM RESPONSE
PASS/FAIL HEARING SCREENING BY CATEGORY

	RISK	SPECIAL	NORMAL	TOTAL
Infants Tested	46	37	13	96
Failed	9	3	--	12 (12.5%)
Pass	30	31	7	68 (70.8%)
Incomplete	7	3	6	16 (16.7%)
Retested	5	2	1	8 (8.3%)

The findings of our test results suggest that ABR audiometry is in fact an accurate procedure in monitoring the
peripheral hearing mechanism in newborn infants. Whether ABR
audiometry should be considered a true screening procedure,
however, is a matter of conjecture. If the concept of screening is to provide a reliable procedure which is quick, easy
to administer and interpret, inexpensive and encompasses
large numbers, then ABR audiometry, in its present state of
technological and procedural development, cannot be considered
a suitable tool. Our experience shows that under the best of
conditions (using the procedures described in Table I),

thirty minutes should be considered a minimal time allotted
to test and interpret ABR results from one infant. In the
majority of infants, however, this period will extend to one
hour and in some cases, as long as two hours. In addition,
the cost of commercially available auditory evoked potential
systems is beyond the financial means of all but a few
facilities. Finally, because we are strongly committed to
the fact that the application and interpretation of infant
ABR audiometry should be left in the hands of trained professionals and not to lay individuals, we feel the cost of
ABR screening may be prohibitive.

ABR: A Soundfield Procedure

     The concept of developing an auditory brainstem response
procedure which utilized an open ear (soundfield) technique
evolved while attempting to test an 11 month old baby using
conventional ABR audiometry. The infant had been originally
referred by otology for a complete audiological evaluation.
As a side issue, it has been our policy that, before clinical
ABR audiometry is employed, an otolaryngological and audiological evaluation must be completed. However, after audiometric
testing, which included immittance audiometry, results were
still inconclusive as to the degree of sensory-neural hearing
impairment. It was at this point that ABR audiometry became
an integral part of the total management of this infant.

     Upon arrival, the mother and infant were taken into the
testing booth where electrode placement and feeding took place.
The child fell asleep within a few minutes after feeding. As
the testing was to begin, the child awoke. Although the child
was not overly concerned with the electrode montage, she would
not tolerate placement of the earphone. Every attempt to test
the baby by conventional earphone techniques was thwarted.
Had the parents been local residents, the testing would have
been terminated and rescheduled. Because of the distance
travelled and problems associated with rescheduling, a final
attempt was made to conduct the test using a soundfield
speaker to transduce the click stimuli. While puzzled, the
infant remained quiet, not overly concerned with the new
source of signal stimulation. Apparently the child was more
concerned with the presence of the earphone than the tone
emitted from it. Once the presence of the earphone was
removed, routine testing procedures were carried out in a
soundfield condition. Although the infant did not fall asleep

during the session, reasonable ABR threshold estimates were
recorded. From our testing, we were able to record replicable
wave configurations at 65 dB nHL. While the soundfield procedure removed independent ear assessment, results still provided the clinical audiologist with a threshold estimate
heretofore unobtainable. Subsequent ABR testing under monaural earphone conditions concurred to within 10 dB nHL of
our initial soundfield threshold estimate.

The events of that testing session provided the impetus
for further investigation into the recording of ABRs in a
soundfield environment. Our first intent, therefore, was to
develop normative standards and systematic testing procedures
which could be applied on a routine clinical basis (Parrott,
Jacobson and Seitz, 1980).

Using similar stimulus and recording techniques to those
described in Table I, auditory brainstem responses were
recorded from 30 normal hearing adults under soundfield conditions. A soundfield speaker was placed exactly one meter
from either external auditory canal at zero degrees asimuth
to produce the click stimuli. For comparative purposes,
auditory brainstem responses were recorded under binaural
earphone conditions from the same subjects. Click intensity
differences between conditions were controlled by measuring
perceptual thresholds under both conditions using identical
stimulus parameters as those used to elicit ABRs. A threshold "offset" was incorporated to insure identical intensity
presentation levels under both conditions.

A series of brainstem responses comparing soundfield
and binaural earphone conditions are illustrated in Figure 6.
All responses were recorded from the same individual using
click stimulae presented at a rate of 33.3/sec. Each tracing
is the sum of 2000 averaged responses. Stimulus intensity
which began at 70 dB nHL was decreased in 10 dB steps until
a response could no longer be replicated. A time base of 10
msec was found to be sufficient to analyze binaural earphone
responses whereas a 20 msec window was required for the soundfield condition. All summed responses were replicated, but
for clarity, only one trace is shown.

When brainstem responses were recorded and traced under
each condition (Figure 6), alterations in the waveform were
noted. The earlier waves (I-IV) were not as prominent, showed
a reduction in amplitude, and were not comparable to similar
waves previously described under monaural earphone click

stimulation (Figure 1). Only Waves I, III and V were consistently replicable at higher intensity levels. This reduction
in wave amplitude decreased the probability of accurately
identifying individual wave components. In contrast, Wave V
maintained its stability even at lower intensity levels and
was measured consistently to within 10 dB of admitted high
frequency (2000 Hz - 6000 Hz) behavioural audiometric thresholds. In both conditions, binaural stimulation increased the
amplitude of Wave V while latency remained unchanged. These
findings are similar to those reported by Blegvad (1975) and
Moller and Blegvad (1976).

AUDITORY BRAINSTEM RESPONSES

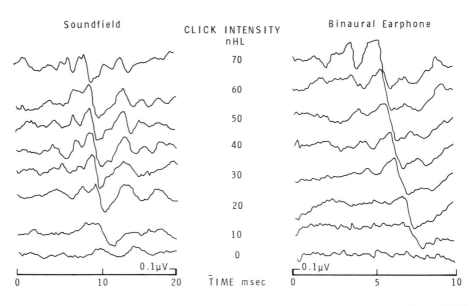

Figure 6. A comparison of auditory brainstem responses under binaural earphone and soundfield
conditions. Click stimuli were presented at a rate of 33.3/sec for each condition. Each tracing (0 dB − 70
dB nHL) represents the sum of 2000 averaged responses recorded from far-field surface electrodes
(vertex-positive, earlobe-negative).

The plotted Wave V latency-intensity curve function for
each condition is displayed in Figure 7. Wave V mean latencies
are seen to increase systematically as intensity decreases
from 70 dB to 5 dB nHL. When quantifying the curve functions,
a steeper slope was derived for the binaural earphone condition. The Wave V latency was reduced 2.85 msec over a 65 dB

range in the earphone condition and 2.06 msec reduction over
the same intensity range for the soundfield presentation.
Wave V produced 3.51 msec longer mean latency difference
when responses were recorded in the soundfield. This increase
in Wave V latency was expected, considering the difference in
distance the stimulus must travel between conditions (1 meter
further). Taking into account the speed and distance the
click stimulus travelled, a 2.91 msec difference was expected.
Parrott, et al, attributed the difference in the expected
latency value (2.91 msec) and the recorded mean latency (3.51
msec) to:

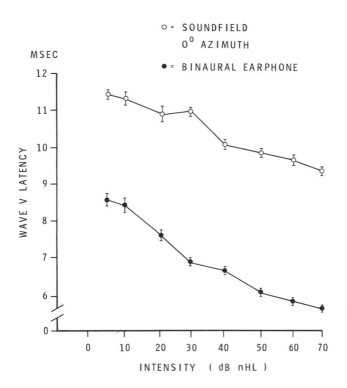

Figure 7.   Plotted mean Wave V latencies and standard deviations for eight ABR intensities (dB nHL).
Two conditions (binaural earlobe and soundfield) are shown for comparison.

1) differences in the frequency response characteristics
   between the TDH-39 earphones and the speaker;

2) differences in the resonance characteristics of the
   occluded and unoccluded auditory canal; and,

3) room reverberation. Although Wave V latency differences
   existed between conditions, the two sets of data were
   significantly correlated and, therefore, highly
   predictive.

ABR: A Hearing Aid Procedure

     The further development of soundfield ABR audiometry may
prove to be advantageous in the long-term management of the
child with a hearing impairment. For example, we have been
experimenting with this technique as a tool for providing
useful information in the determination and appropriate
selection of fitting amplification on infants and children.
The ABR procedure is similar to that previously described for
soundfield testing with the addition of an aided condition.
Figure 8 illustrates a series of brainstem responses recorded
under aided soundfield conditions. Click stimuli were presented through a speaker (zero degrees azimuth) at a rate of
20.4/sec. The subject was an adult female with a mild-to-
moderate, sensory-neural hearing loss. The hearing aid was
fitted on the right ear and appropriate masking was applied
to the contralateral ear. All tracings were based on the
sum of 2000 responses. The brainstem responses were recorded
at a 50 dB nHL intensity level using three gain settings (40
dB SPL, 30 dB SPL, and 20 dB SPL re: ANSI, 1976). The
hearing aid used in this example was a commercially available
post-auricular aid with a high frequency (HF) SSPL of 118 dB,
an HF gain of 57 dB and a wide frequency response curve
characteristic (200 Hz - 5000 Hz).

     The aided ABR patterns seen in Figure 8 are representa-
tive of waveforms recorded under earphone and unaided soundfield conditions. That is, Waves I, III, and V are distinct
and clearly visible at higher intensity/gain settings.
Increases in the Wave V latency are seen to occur as the gain
setting is reduced from 40 dB to 20 dB SPL. With an input of
50 dB nHL, an intensity level which closely approximates the
speech input level used in traditional hearing aid evaluations,
Wave V responses are clearly recognizable at a gain setting
of 20 dB SPL.

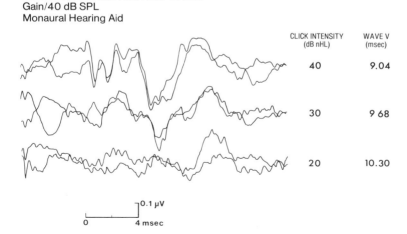

AUDITORY BRAINSTEM RESPONSE:
Click Stimulus 50 dB nHL
Monaural Hearing Aid

	GAIN (dB SPL)	WAVE V (msec)
	40	9.12
	30	9.52
	20	9.68

0.1 μV

0   4 msec

Figure 8.   Auditory brainstem responses recorded under monaural aided soundfield conditions. Three replicated tracings at 40 dB, 30 dB, and 20 dB SPL are displayed. A 50 dB nHL click alternating in polarity was used as stimulus. The stimulus was presented at a rate of 20.4/sec and 2000 averages were analyzed. Wave V latencies for each gain setting are provided in msec.

AUDITORY BRAINSTEM RESPONSE:
Gain/40 dB SPL
Monaural Hearing Aid

	CLICK INTENSITY (dB nHL)	WAVE V (msec)
	40	9.04
	30	9 68
	20	10.30

0.1 μV

0   4 msec

Figure 9.   Auditory brainstem responses recorded under monaural aided soundfield conditions. Three replicated tracings at 40 dB, 30 dB, and 20 dB nHL are shown. Each tracing represents the summed average of 2000 responses presented at 20.4/sec. The hearing aid was maintained at a constant 40 dB SPL gain setting. Wave V latencies (in msec) are shown for each of the three click intensities.

Brainstem responses were analyzed under identical recording parameters with the exception that, in this case, the
hearing aid gain was maintained at a constant 40 dB SPL while
stimulus intensity was reduced from 40 dB to 20 dB nHL
(Figure 9). Consistent with the previous aided series of
responses (Figure 8), the latency of Wave V is seen to
increase as gain setting (and, therefore, total output) is
reduced. It is interesting to note the similarities in Wave
V latency values occurring in Figures 8 and 9. For example,
the Wave V latency in Figure 8 at an output setting of 70 dB
(50 dB nHL click stimulus plus 20 dB SPL hearing aid gain)
produced a latency value of 9.68 msec. This latency is
identical to the Wave V value in Figure 9 at an output of
70 dB; that is, a 30 dB nHL click stimulus plus 40 dB SPL
hearing aid gain. The unaided soundfield ABR Wave V latency
for the same subject was 9.42 msec at 70 dB nHL. The small
difference (0.26 msec) between the monaurally aided and
binaural soundfield conditions may be possibly attributed to
the contribution of the second ear in the unaided condition.

While the soundfield aided auditory brainstem response
procedure is still in a preliminary state, the results
obtained thus far have been promising. Particular caution
is advised in interpreting aided soundfield ABR results. Due
to the possible number of varying combinations of electro-
acoustical hearing aid characteristics, subtle differences
have been noted in the aided response patterns. However,
through further longitudinal study, aided soundfield ABR
audiometry may play an important role in assisting the
audiologist in determining the ear(s) selection and the
appropriate amplification settings required to objectively
fit an infant with a hearing impairment.

Acknowledgments

The intent of this paper has been to provide the reader
with a general over-view of the area of infant auditory
brainstem response audiometry. It should not be assumed that
the studies reported in the text are all-inclusive of the
ongoing research in the field. To those who are currently
involved in infant ABR studies and whom we have not included
in the text, we apologize. To those cited, we hope our
interpretation has been accurate and represents the work

reported. The authors wish to thank Robin Morehouse, M.Sc.,
for his long hours of infant testing, Dr. Terry Picton for
his advice and effort in designing the protocol used in our
infant study, and Donna MacDonald and Barbara Hanson for
their co-operation in manuscript preparation. The infant
screening program described in the text was funded by a
grant from Health and Welfare Canada (#6603-1114-44).

REFERENCES

Amadeo, M. and Shagass, C. "Brief latency click-evoked
   potentials during waking and sleeping in man," Psychophysiology 10:244 - 250, 1973.

Blegvad, B. "Binaural summation of surface-recorded electro-
   cochleographic responses. Normal hearing subjects,"
   Scandinavian Audiology 4:233 - 238, 1975.

Buchwald, J.S. and Huang, C. "Far-field acoustic response:
   Origins in the cat," Science 189:382 - 384, 1975.

Chisen, R., Perlman, M. and Sohmer, H. "Cochlear and brainstem responses in hearing loss following neonatal hyper-
   bilirubinemia," Annals of Otolaryngology 88:352 - 357, 1979.

Cone, B. and Hecox, K. "The brainstem auditory-evoked
   response in neonates," Otorhinolaryngology 86:638, 1978.

Connelly, C., Kileny, P. and Robertson, C. "Audiological
   follow-up in prenatal asphyxia," Paper presented at the
   Canadian Speech and Hearing Association Convention,
   Winnipeg, Manitoba, 1980.

Cox, C., Hack, M. and Metz, D. "Brainstem evoked response
   audiometry in very low birthweight infants," Abstract
   ASHA 21:749, 1979.

Davis, H. "Principles of electric response audiometry,"
   Annals of Otology, Rhinolaryngology and Laryngology
   Supplement 28, Volume 85, 1976.

Davis, H. and Hirsh, S.H. "Brainstem electric response
   audiometry (BSERA)," Acta Otolaryngologica 83:136 - 139,
   1977.

Davis, H. and Hirsh, S.H. "A slow brainstem response for
   low-frequency audiometry," Audiology 18:445 - 461, 1979.

Diaz, L.B., Salamon, R. and Mena, A.M. "Long-term follow-up
   of deaf I.C.U. babies detected by B.S.E.R.," Paper presented at the IERASG Symposium, Santa Barbara, California,
   August, 1979.

Fabiani, M., Sohmer, H., Tait, C., Gafni, M. and Kinarti, R.
   "A functional measure of brain activity: brainstem transmission time," Electroencephalography and Clinical Neurophysiology 47:483 - 491, 1979.

Finitzo-Hieber, T. and Hecox, K. "Clinical applicability of
   the auditory evoked response in neonates," Paper presented
   at the Basic Research Forum American Academy of Ophthalmology and Otolaryngology, Dallas, Texas, October, 1978.

Fria, T.J. and Bartling, V.R. "Brainstem auditory electric
   responses in selected pediatric populations," Paper presented at the American Speech and Hearing Association Convention, San Francisco, California, 1978.

Fria, T.J., Grundfast, K.M. and Sabo, D.L. "Auditory brainstem responses in infants and children," Paper presented
   at the IERASG Symposium, Santa Barbara, California,
   August, 1979.

Fujikawa, S. and Weber, B. "Efforts of increased stimulus
   rate on brainstem electric response (BER) audiometry as a
   function of age," Journal of the American Audiology Society
   3:147 - 150, 1977.

Galambos, R. "Use of the auditory brainstem response (ABR)
   in infant hearing testing," in Gerber and Mencher (eds.)
   Early Diagnosis of Hearing Loss (New York: Grune and
   Stratton), 1978.

Galambos, R. and Hecox, K. "Clinical applications of the
   auditory brainstem response," Otolaryngology Clinics of
   North America 11:709 - 722, 1978.

Gerber, S.E. and Mencher, G.T. (eds.) Early Diagnosis of
   Hearing Loss (New York: Grune and Stratton), 1978.

Gilroy, J., Lynn, G., Ristow, G.E. and Pellerin, R.J.
"Auditory evoked brainstem potentials in a case of "locked-
in" syndrome," Archives of Neurology 34:492 - 495, 1977.

Goldenberg, R.A. and Derbyshire, A.J. "Averaged evoked potentials in cats with lesions of the auditory pathway,"
Journal of Speech and Hearing Research 18:420 - 429, 1975.

Hamilton, L.R., Hilding, D.A. and Mannarelli, R.J. "Screening
hearing in "normal" and "high risk" newborns using brainstem evoked response," Paper presented at the American
Speech and Hearing Association Convention, Chicago,
Illinois, 1977.

Hazel, J., Sheldrake, J. and Reynolds, E. "Auditory evoked
potentials in the newborn," Paper presented at the
Biological Engineering Society International Conference,
September, 1979.

Hecox, K. "Electrophysiological correlates of human auditory
development," in Cohen, L.B. and Salapltik, P. (eds.)
Infant Perception: From Sensation to Cognition (New York:
Academic Press), 1975.

Hecox, K. and Galambos, R. "Brainstem auditory evoked
response in human infants and adults," Archives of Otolaryngology 99:30 - 33, 1974.

Horning, J.K. "High risk registry with brainstem auditory
evoked response follow-up," Hearing Aid Journal 7:32 - 33,
May, 1979.

Hyde, M.L., Stephens, S. and Thornton, A. "Stimulus repetition rate and the early brainstem responses," British
Journal of Audiology 10:41 - 50, 1976.

Jacobson, J., Mencher, G., Morehouse, R. and Seitz, M. "A
neonatal auditory screening program," Paper presented at
the Canadian Speech and Hearing Association Convention,
April, 1980.

Jacobson, J., Morehouse, R. and Seitz, M. "Nonpathological
considerations in the determination of brainstem electric
response activity," Acoustics and Noise Control in Canada
8:22 - 27, 1980.

Jerger, J.F. and Hayes, D. "The cross-check principle in pediatric audiometry," Archives of Otolaryngology 102:614 - 620, 1976.

Jerger, J., Hayes, D. and Jordan, C. "Clinical experience with auditory brainstem response audiometry in pediatric assessment," Ear and Hearing 1:19 - 25, 1980.

Jewett, D.L. "Averaged volume-conducted potentials to auditory stimuli in the cat," Physiologist 12:262, 1969.

Jewett, D.L. "Volume conducted potentials in response to auditory stimuli as detected by averaging in the cat," Electroencephalographic and Clinical Neurophysiology 28:609 - 618, 1970.

Jewett, D.L. and Romano, M.N. "Neonatal development of auditory system potentials averaged from the scalp of the rat and cat," Brain Research 36:101 - 115, 1972.

Jewett, D.L. and Williston, J. "Auditory evoked far-fields averaged from the scalp of humans," Brain 94:681 - 696, 1971.

Jewett, D.L., Romano, M. and Williston, J. "Human auditory evoked potentials: possible brainstem components detected on the scalp," Science 167:1517 - 1518, 1970.

Kileny, P., Connelly, C. and Robertson, C. "Averaged brainstem auditory evoked potentials in asphyxiated neonates," Paper presented at the IERASG Symposium, Santa Barbara, California, August, 1979.

Mainhardt, P., Davis, H. and Reichert, L. "The form of brainstem responses in newborn infants," Paper presented at the American Speech and Hearing Association Convention, Atlanta, Georgia, 1979.

Mencher, G.T. (ed.) Early Identification of Hearing Loss (Basel: Karger), 1976.

Mendelson, T., Salamy, A., Lenoir, M. and McKean, C. "Brainstem evoked potential findings in children with otitis media," Archives of Otolaryngology 105:17 - 20, 1979.

Mokotoff, B., Schulman-Galambos, C. and Galambos, R. "Brainstem auditory evoked responses in children," Archives of
Otolaryngology 103:38 - 43, 1977.

Moller, K. and Blegvad, B. "Brainstem responses in patients
with sensori-neural hearing loss, monaural versus binaural
stimulation. The significance of the audiogram configuration," Scandinavian Audiology 5:115 - 127, 1976.

Nodar, R., Hahn, J. and Levine, H. "Brainstem testing for
site of brainstem gliomas in children," Paper presented
at the American Speech and Hearing Association Convention,
Atlanta, Georgia, 1979.

Ochs, R.F. and Markland, O.N. "Maturational changes of brainstem auditory evoked responses (BAERs) in children and the
effect of increased frequency of stimulation," Neurology
408, April, 1978.

Parrott, V., Jacobson, J. and Seitz, M. "A comparison of
brainstem electric responses obtained under binaural earphone and soundfield conditions," Paper presented at the
Canadian Speech and Hearing Association Convention, April,
1980.

Picton, T.W. "The strategy of evoked potential audiometry,"
in Gerber and Mencher (eds.) Early Diagnosis of Hearing
Loss (New York: Grune and Stratton), 1978.

Picton, T.W. and Fitzgerald, P.G. "A general description of
the human auditory evoked potentials," Personal
Communication.

Picton, T.W. and Hillyard, S.A. "Human auditory evoked
potentials: II. Effects of attenuation," Electroencephalography Clinical Neurophysiology 36:191 - 199, 1974.

Picton, T.W., Hillyard, S.A. and Krausz, H.I. "Human auditory
evoked potentials: I. Evaluation of components,"
Electroencephalography and Clinical Neurophysiology 36:179 -
190, 1974.

Picton, T.W. and Smith, A. "The practice of evoked potential
audiometry," Otolaryngological Clinics of North America
11:263 - 282, 1978.

Picton, T.W., Woods, D., Baribeau-Braun, J. and Healey, T. "Evoked potential audiometry," Journal of Otolaryngology 6:90 - 119, 1977.

Rosenblum, S., Arick, J., Krug, D., Stubbs, E., Young, N. and Pelson, R. "Auditory brainstem responses in autistic children," (In Press). 1980.

Salamy, A. and McKean, C.M. "Post-natal development of human brainstem potentials during the first year of life," Electroencephalography and Clinical Neurophysiology 40: 418 - 426, 1976.

Salamy, A. and McKean, C.M. "Habituation and dishabituation of cortical and brainstem evoked potentials," International Journal of Neuroscience 7:175 - 182, 1977.

Salamy, A., McKean, C. and Buda, F. "Maturational changes in auditory transmission as reflected in human brainstem potentials," Brain Research 96:361 - 366, 1975.

Salamy, A., McKean, C., Pettett, G. and Mendelson, T. "Auditory brainstem recovery processes from birth to adulthood," Psychophysiology 15:214 - 220, 1978.

Schulman-Galambos, C. and Galambos, R. "Brainstem auditory evoked responses in premature infants," Journal of Speech and Hearing Research 18:456 - 465, 1975.

Schulman-Galambos, C. and Galambos, R. "Brainstem evoked response audiometry in newborn hearing screening," Archives of Otolaryngology 105:86 - 90, 1979.

Simmon, F.B. "Automated screening test for newborns: the crib-o-gram," in B.F. Jaffe (ed.) Hearing Loss in Children (Baltimore: University Press), 1977.

Sohmer, H. and Feinmesser, M. "Cochlear action potentials recorded from the external ear in man," Annals of Otology 76:427 - 435, 1967.

Sohmer, H. and Student, M. "Auditory nerve and brainstem evoked responses in normal, autistic, minimal brain dysfunction and psychomotor retarded children," Electroencephalography and Clinical Neurophysiology 44:380 - 388, 1978.

Starr, A. and Achor, L.J. "Auditory brainstem response in neurological disease," Archives of Neurology 32:761 - 768, 1975.

Starr, A., Amlie, R.N., Martin, W.H. and Sanders, S. "Development of auditory function in newborn infants revealed by auditory brainstem potentials," Pediatrics 60:831 - 839, 1977.

Stein, L., Ozdamar, O. and Daniels, M. "Auditory brainstem responses (ABR) with suspected deaf-blind children," Paper presented at the ASHA Convention, Atlanta, Georgia, 1979.

Stockard, J.J. and Jones, T.A. "Central nervous system drugs and the brainstem evoked response," Electroencephalography and Clinical Neurophysiology 43:550, 1977.

Stockard, J.J. and Rossiter, N.S. "Clinical and pathologic correlates of brainstem auditory response abnormalities," Neurology 27:316 - 325, 1977.

Stockard, J.J., Stockard, J.E. and Scarborough, F.W. "Detection and localization of occult lesions and brainstem auditory responses," Mayo Clinic Proceedings 52:761 - 769, 1977.

Stockard, J.J., Stockard, J.E. and Scarborough, F.W. "Nonpathologic factors influencing brainstem auditory evoked potentials," American Journal of EEG Technology 18:177 - 209, 1978.

Student, M. and Sohmer, H. "Evidence from auditory nerve and brainstem evoked responses for an organic brain lesion in children with autistic traits," Journal of Autism and Childhood Schizophrenia 8:13 - 20, 1978.

Weber, B. and Fujikawa, S. "Brainstem evoked response (BER) audiometry at various stimulus presentation rates," Journal of the American Audiology Society 3:59 - 62, 1977.

Weber, B. "Auditory brainstem response audiometry in children," Clinical Pediatrics 18:746 - 749, 1979.

HEARING AIDS FOR INFANTS

Martha Rubin
Lexington School for the Deaf, Jackson Heights, New York

Hearing impairment is a hidden disease, but hearing aids make it visible. Although the baby with a profound congenital hearing loss can be identified early in life and should use amplification as part of a comprehensive program of special education, identification and management usually do not occur until the baby is between 18 and 24 months old (Bergstrom, 1976). The incidence of profoundly hearing-impaired babies in the United States is between 1:1000 and 1:2000 births (Rand, 1974), which makes a deaf baby a rarity in a physician's office and relatively uncommon in a speech and hearing center. One in every 350 births is a hard-of-hearing baby, a child with a loss of 45 decibels or more (Simons, 1978). These babies do not receive early amplification or special services because they are not identified in infancy. In most communities in the United States there is a paucity of neonatal hearing screening programs and follow-up diagnostic services and, thus, hard-of-hearing babies remain invisible and unserved. Both groups of hearing-impaired children need early management programs as soon as possible in order to develop the auditory skills needed for speech and language development. Programs should begin by the third month of life.

Need for Early Management Programs

Babies deprived of acoustic stimulation will develop the acoustic liabilities described by Skinner in 1978, as well as the psycho-social developmental lags which Glenson and her colleagues (1979) traced to early deficits in audition and reciprocal mother-child relationships. Downs (1979) suggested that children with recurrent conductive hearing losses exhibit delays in speech and language similar to those with more severe, sensory-neural hearing losses; although Menyuk (1979) and Needleman (1977) hypothesized that babies with conductive hearing loss may "catch up" in later years. Longitudinal research is needed to prove either hypothesis, but it is known that the short term effects of conductive hearing loss can be devastating.

During the acquisition of language, babies with fluctuant hearing loss cannot develop a stable listening framework. A home in which mother's voice fades in and out can
be frightening to a baby. A valuable illustrative case study
of a 4 month old infant was provided by Beratis and her
associates (1979) in which sleep disturbance, feeding difficulties, and separation anxieties developed as a result of a
bilateral, conductive hearing loss. When this infant
received binaural amplification for a period of three months,
he became more out-going, was willing to nap without the
television set turned on, and subsequently played in a room
without his mother in sight. Both sight and sound were
crucial in helping this infant organize his own affect. This
baby's middle ear disease was limited in time, whereas babies
with sensory-neural hearing losses need extensive remediation
for their handicaps. The usual six to twelve month delay
between the time hearing loss is suspected and the first
fitting of ear molds can easily be cut to a period of no
longer than six weeks. Even if the audiological evaluation
is incomplete by adult standards, hearing aids can be used by
babies at two or three months of age, once a reliable estimate of hearing level has been made (Figure 1.).

Audiological information about hearing impaired babies
is frequently scant. Evaluation must be considered as an
ongoing process during which babies will develop a hierarchy
of auditory skills which can be measured. At birth, infants
are aware of speech rhythms. By three months of age, babies
discriminate consonants, vowels, intonational patterns, duration and intensity. We might expect that a baby with a
sensory-neural hearing loss may possibly experience tinnitus,
sound distortion, recruitment and a limitation in discriminat-
ing signals in the noise of a reverberant room, or a household filled with enthusiastic siblings. Despite the lack of
data about any particular baby's pathological ear, amplification should begin before 3 months of age. Why? The auditory
mode is the most important sensory mode for acquiring speech
and language, and the effects of sensory deprivation during
the critical first year of life may well be irreversible
according to some animal studies (Rubin, 1972; Webster and
Webster, 1977). While it is difficult to generalize from
animal studies to humans, the evidence at hand seems conclus-
ive. It is vital that hearing impaired infants use hearing
aids during this critical time and not at some magical age
determined by cultural, ethnic, medical or audiological mores.
When an estimate of hearing loss is made, a program of

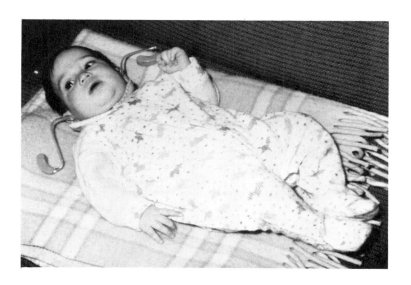

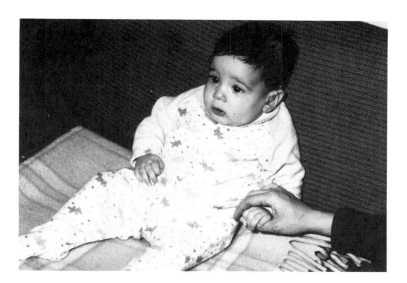

Figure 1.   Three month old baby being fitted with her first ear level hearing aids. In the top photo the long tubing will be cut. In the bottom photo the hearing aids are in place.

habilitation should begin. As Ross (1975) stated, "Hearing
aids are our most valuable rehabilitative tool" and they need
to be a focal point of comprehensive services for special
babies.

Steps in Hearing Aid Use

The first step in the fitting of hearing aids is parental
acceptance of the need for amplification. Recall that hearing
impairment is an invisible handicap, but hearing aids make it
visible. Many of the initial reactions of guilt, anger,
shock and denial surface when parents find it increasingly
difficult to deny the existence of hearing loss. The event
of aiding a baby constitutes an assault on the parents' ego.
The parents' anger is frequently directed at the hearing aid
and the earmold. They question the use of binaural fitting
for their little one because it may block out sound. Their
fundamental assumption is that two hearing aids mean the
baby is deaf, while one hearing aid means their baby is hard-
of-hearing. The mechanisms of denial and displacement need
to be recognized and dealt with during the hearing aid orientation process and, possibly, in a psycho-therapeutic model
nursery (Rubin, 1978A).

Educational information is also shared with parents
during hearing aid orientation. Areas of interest include:

1. rationale for the choice of the hearing aid;

2. description of how an earmold impression will be made;

3. economics of hearing aid use;

4. daily maintenance of the hearing aid; and,

5. realistic expectations about auditory responses of the
   baby.

This information is as new to the family as it is second
nature to the audiologist. The new mother, however, receives
it at a vulnerable time in her life, 3 to 6 months postpartum. The technical aspects need to be shared in a non-
threatening atmosphere. Sound proof chambers and clinical
waiting rooms are to be avoided. White-coated audiologists
may look authoritative, but the non-verbal effect of a white

medical coat is counter-productive to the easy sharing of information. The needs of the young hearing impaired baby and its mother differ from those of the parent and older child who have achieved individuation-separation and who can be helped in a hospital or clinical setting. The mother-infant dyad requires frequent counselling, and should be scheduled weekly when hearing aid use is instituted.

Hearing Aid Selection

Ear level or post-auricular hearing aids are almost universally accepted as the amplification of choice for babies in the United States. These are mainly the linear amplifiers as described by Braida and Durlach (1979). A hearing aid with automatic volume control or a peak clipping limiter should be used for the baby who has a compressed, dynamic range, as revealed by acoustic reflex thresholds for pure tones. The aids fit behind the infants' pinnae and are coupled to the ear mold. Hearing aids are not specifically designed nor produced for young children, a minority con-sumer group, as it would be uneconomical to do so (Sinclair, 1976). Unfortunately, infants are typically limited to per-sonal amplification designed for adults or to carrier wave systems designed for group use (Rubin, 1979).

The design characteristics of presently available commer-cial hearing aids which work well for infants depend on:

1)   ergonomic characteristics;

2)   electroacoustic characteristics; and,

3)   repair capability and cost.

Ergonomic Characteristics

Ergonomic characteristics are the biotechnical proper-ties or design of the hearing aid. Design features critical for infants are length, width, shape vis-a-vis the ear, and location of the microphone. Ear level aids for babies need to conform to the shape and size of the baby's ear. Thick aids tend to distort the helix, and thus aids which accomo-date a battery's thickness rather than an infant's ear should not be selected. A microphone at the pinna picks up leakage around the earmold more easily than a transducer located near

the hook or bow. If feedback becomes a constant annoyance to
the parent, it invariably discourages hearing aid use. A bow
which is molded to the hearing aid in one piece tends to
break easily when dropped, whereas a soft, acrylic bow which
can be screwed on is more robust and is easily replaced. A
soft acrylic bow, however, may slip off easily when the
plastic expands. Audiologists or audio-therapists working
with babies are well advised to have spare bows on hand for
replacement.

Thick wall, or .076 tubing should be used as part of the
coupling mechanism between the hearing aid and the earmold
since thin walled tubing tends to twist on insertion and
break easily. In about 6 months, this tubing will become
hard. Once it loses its flexibility, it can be replaced
easily by the audiologist or audio-therapist. Tubing needs
to be replaced as the baby's ear grows, so that it is always
comfortable and the tubing does not rub or cause irritation.
It may need to be taped across the ear to keep in in place.
The audiologist or audio-therapist should be able to effect
small repairs, to grind down and smoothen rough earmolds,
and to generally alert parents to effective hearing aid use
according to "every day's most quiet needs."

Commercial post-auricular hearing aids contain battery
compartments which are located near the on-off switch,
thereby preventing easy removal of the battery. Battery
compartments are frequently delicate; and, since they are
hinged, they crack.   When this happens, battery contact is
interrupted and the aid's output becomes intermittent.
Parents can learn to identify these problems. For example,
one profoundly deaf, alert parent was able to judge by her
baby's response that the hearing aid output was intermittent,
and she traced the cause to intermittent contact in the
battery compartment. Opening and closing the battery compartment can also unseat the microphone suspension. One otherwise excellent post-auricular aid has the battery compartment housed next to the microphone suspension which is
nudged, moved, and finally either falls off or is pushed
into the hearing aid, resulting in internal oscillation.
Careful handling of the aid and instructions to parents can
result in longer lasting, more functional hearing aid use.

Parents tend to prefer the aid with the best contour,
which is usually the smallest one. Because they dislike
being told, "Push this little dial all the way up and then
back two notches," top priority is awarded to aids with

color coded gain controls or those with numbered gain controls. As the infant's head moves, it is impossible for an
observer to judge whether the volume control is set correctly.
One must check the volume control repeatedly to ascertain
that the setting is appropriate. Hearing aids for infants,
however, cannot be selected solely on ergonomic characteristics, although it is a difficult decision to recommend poorly
designed aids which have excellent electro-acoustic
characteristics.

      Hearing aids worn on the body are still used in many
areas, not because the majority of audiologists feel that
they provide a better signal, but because they are less
likely to be lost and have the potential for easier fitting
and subsequent adjustment. Also, they provide a higher
saturation sound pressure level (SSPL) than post-auricular
hearing aids do when measured in a 2cc coupler. Body worn
hearing aids are robust, and probably should be used for
those infants with multiple handicaps and/or inadequate
mothering. These aids can be enclosed in a small harness and
chosen for ergonomic characteristics such as hidden tone
control settings (which cannot move easily), and separate
battery compartments which fit well and tend not to crack
as easily as flip top battery compartments. Aids need to be
engineered for infants who dribble, wet, and wear layers of
clothing in cool climates. To date, the three major defects
of body aid design for babies are flip top battery compartments, movable switches, and poor engineering design.

Electroacoustic Characteristics

      The electroacoustic characteristics of hearing aids are
measured according to American National Standards Institute
S3.26 specifications in a 2cc coupler or with a Kemar Maniken
which more closely approximates the adult ear (Figure 2).
When Saturation Sound Pressure Level (SSPL) and frequency
response of a hearing aid are measured with a Kemar Maniken
and a Zwislocki coupler, the results are different in the
reference plane, the area behind the earmold simulator. This
reference plane (Figure 3) was denoted as Volume 3 by
Lybarger (1978). Since impedance is inversely proportional
to volume, the SSPL measurements obtained with a 2cc coupler
or with a Kemar Maniken are too low for most of the frequency
range when measured in an infant ear. The physical volume
of an infant's ear is small. The 2cc coupler underestimates
SSPL by almost 5 dB below 1000 Hz and by 20 dB in the area

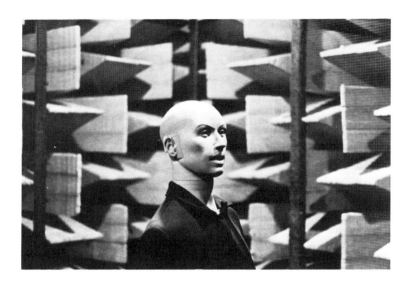

Figure 2.   Kemar Mannikin in Anechoic Chamber at Lexington School for the Deaf.

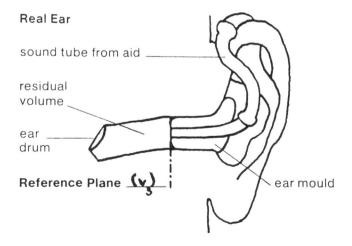

Figure 3.   Sectional view of internal earphone system. (Courtesy of Oticon Corp.)

between 2000 and 2500 Hz (Figure 4). Every time the cavity
volume is halved, there is a 6 dB increase in SSPL. The low
frequency response of the system is affected also by the
hold or bore of the occluding earmold. The bore is usually
made with a .039 inch tool for infants and for adults. Thus,
the volume of air beyond the tip of the earmold cavity and
the impedance of the eardrum influence the frequency response
and SSPL: the smaller the volume the higher the SSPL.

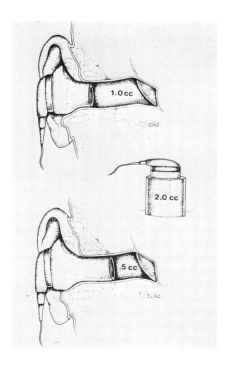

Figure 4.   Comparison of volume of adult ear canal (1.0 cc), child's ear canal (.5 cc) and acoustic
coupler normally used in calibration (2.0 cc). Every time the cavity is halved there is a 6 dB increase in
SSPL. (Illustration courtesy of J. Northern.)

    Amplification used for infants, therefore, needs to be
selected carefully with regard to SSPL-90. While coupler
measurements on high gain instruments show outputs of 128 dB
SPL, it seems reasonable to assume that an SPL of over 140 dB
may be generated based on the physical volume of the infant's
ear. In an effort to adjust the SSPL of hearing aid settings,
an acoustic reflex technique was investigated by McCandless
and Miller (1973), Rappaport and Tait (1975), and Keith (1979).
Keith compared the contralateral speech acoustic reflex
threshold (ART) with the most comfortable loudness level (MCL)

and threshold of discomfort (TD). Results indicated that
speech ART was at the same level as speech MCL and at lower
levels than TD. Further investigation indicated that subjects with speech ART's equal to or less than 90 dB had
their aids adjusted comfortably to the aided speech ART,
while subjects with ART's of 91 dB or above had their aids
adjusted for MCL below the aided ART for speech. Keith's
technique appears to be promising for infant hearing aid
adjustment for speech MCL.

Another method of achieving greater comfort in hearing
aid use was suggested by French-St. George and Barr-Hamilton
(1978) who believed that all earmolds should be vented to
relieve the occluded ear sensation. They recommended the
use of sintered filters which may be valuable for infants –
especially those who pull out aids and demonstrate that the
hand is quicker than the eye at the ear. Although infant's
earmolds are small, diagonal vents with filters can be used.
The size of infants' earmolds precludes the use of parallel
vents. An earmold needs to be remade approximately every
three months to insure a good continuing acoustic seal.

The frequency response of the hearing aid and its effect
on speech discrimination has been researched in older children (Ling, 1978). If an infant has residual hearing in the
speech frequencies, linear amplification is used with a
Kemar response starting at 300 Hz. For the profoundly
impaired infant with a corner audiogram, low frequency
enhancement is desirable. Equalization aids could be a
real breakthorugh were they available commercially. More
often than not, binaural hearing aids are used. Dichotic
release from masking (Rand, 1976) and better discrimination
in noise have been shown as advantages (Ross, 1978). It is
prudent to begin with a monaural fitting until a parent
accepts the aiding process. Thereafter, binaural fittings
are used unless the baby rejects one aid consistently in one
ear while accepting a second aid in the other ear. In that
event, monaural use is recommended until the cause for
rejection is discovered.

In sum, using 2cc coupler measurements or Kemar measurement for babies is misleading. Although precise measurements
are currently as lacking for infants as they are for adults,
it is good practice to choose an instrument with a use gain
of approximately 50% of the pure tone average measured in
the sound field, and then to measure functional gain in the
same mode. Threshold measurements for pure tones, speech,

and for Ling's Five Sound Test (Ling, 1978) can be approxi-
mated using behavioural observation audiometry, brainstem
electric response audiometry, or visual reinforcement audiometry. Real ear aided measurements should be made using the
same audiological technique. Valid observations on the use
of the aid, which are provided by the parent and audio-
therapist, can then be compared with the real ear aided
measurements. The aid which provides a flat response curve,
extended high frequency response, and the best ergonomic
characteristics should be recommended for purchase.

Repair Capability and Cost

It is important to state that, before a hearing aid is
purchased, the baby with residual hearing should experience
amplification and accept it for daily use. During this
time, adjustments can be made on one unit or several models
can be tried until an aid is selected that provides the best
amplification. While this may be costly in terms of "loaner
hearing aids," it appears to be the only way to choose
amplification based on the rapid growth and development of
the child during the first year of life (Rubin, 1980).

In the United States, the recommendation for purchase of
an aid should take into account the availability of insurance
against loss and damage, which several companies offer.
Babies are curious creatures who mouth aids, feed them to
the dog, and cheerfully dismantle them while strapped in an
auto seat. To guard against the loss of a post-auricular
aid in a shopping center, for example, one parent tied a
thread from the tubing of the aid to a pin on the baby's
shoulder. This array resembled the old body worn hearing
aid with one significant difference: the microphone of the
hearing aid was at the ear and, thus, the signal was
received without the effects of body baffle and with a more
optimal signal/noise ratio than the signal received through
a body worn hearing aid. The spectre of a lost hearing aid
in the United States looms large for young parents who
cannot afford the replacement cost.

Factors in Hearing Aid Selection

Middle Ear Infection

A significant factor in hearing aid use for the hearing
impaired infant is susceptibility to middle ear infection.

Rubin (1978B) showed that 65% of the babies enrolled in the
Infant Center of the Lexington School for the Deaf had one
or more episodes of serous otitis media during the first 3
years of life. Implications for hearing aid use for these
children were that electro-acoustic parameters had to be
modified until middle ear infection resolved (Rubin, 1979).
All too frequently, young children are fitted with inappropriate hearing aids during the course of middle ear effusion.
The SSPL and the frequency response which seemed appropriate
to a child with a 100 dB hearing loss is grossly inappropriate
for the same child with a 60 dB hearing level. These babies
subsequently reject their aids and become inconsistent hearing aid users, thereby cutting off the auditory pathway to
information.

    Multiple Handicaps

    The additional handicapping conditions which place these
babies in one or more high risk categories fortunately lead
to early identification of their hearing losses. Despite
early recognition, however, diagnosis and habilitation suffer
severe delays for several reasons. First, many of these
children are served by two agencies. It is not uncommon in
our area, for example, for a baby with Downs Syndrome to be
enrolled for therapy in an Association for Downs Syndrome
school, and for auditory management in a hearing and speech
center. This dual service complicates the fitting and
selection of hearing aids because of the time constraints
placed on the mother. Secondly, it is rare that there is
appropriately trained professional staff to serve the needs
of the multiply handicapped infant. McDermott and Goldblatt
(1979) questioned 211 programs in the United States serving
hearing impaired infants (birth to 3) and reported that 43%
stated that they needed more in-service training on working
with the multiply handicapped. Possibly the transdisciplinary
approach outlined by Conner (1978) may help. A third reason
for delay in habilitation is that many of these babies have
one or more hospitalizations for reconstructive surgery
during which time hearing aids are temporarily abandoned.
When habilitation resumes, regressive tendencies are
evident. Vocalization once begun, may have stopped. One
baby with Weir's Syndrome was hospitalized six times during
a two year period and at age 2.8, she has just begun to say
"mama", to the enormous delight of her mother. Multiply
handicapped babies present the greatest challenge, but they
need an auditory connection to the world around them at the

the earliest possible time.

Summary

It must be stressed that hearing aid fitting and use for
infants is only one aspect of an habilitative program. The
kinds of comprehensive services needed are described elsewhere (Rubin, 1976), but certainly educational services and
continuing diagnostic procedures need to be available on a
weekly basis at a minimum. The degree to which a parent or
parent-surrogate can participate in the early management program is vital to its success.

Hearing impaired infants need early management programs
which include the fitting of hearing aids within the first
six months of life. Hearing aid recommendation should follow
a long trial basis during which time the audiologist can
validate measurement techniques. The selection of hearing
aids depends on ergonomic characteristics, electro-acoustic
parameters, and repair capability vis-a-vis the hearing
impaired baby and its needs.

DISCUSSION

DOCTOR MENCHER
We received a questionnaire at the Nova Scotia Hearing
and Speech Clinic asking if we knew of any recorded incidents
of young babies swallowing batteries and then becoming ill or
dying. In our centre, we have not seen any incidents of that
nature. What do you know about that?

DOCTOR RUBEN
I'd like to mention two related points. First, we have
little rubber hearing aids for our babies to chew on, which
they delight in chewing on if they really want to mouth
hearing aids. Secondly, babies will feed hearing aids to
dogs very easily. I brought that to the attention of the
Federal Drug Administration, but the hearing aid manufactur-
ers indicated that there was nothing, absolutely nothing, in
the hearing aid that attracts dogs. We have not had a
battery eating problem, although when we have children who
are really severely disturbed, we watch them very carefully.

Frankly, I think children prefer earmolds to batteries.

DOCTOR ROBERT RUBEN
     The problem is with the ingestion of the hearing aid
battery. It will sometimes rest in the esophageous and cause
a corrosive esophagitis. To make a long story short, nobody
should die from it, really, but you will have a stricture of
the esophageous. We run into these things every now and
then. I don't have any (in my case load), but I know of
some people who have had hearing aid or similar batteries
swallowed, causing corrosive esophagitis in children; so
this is not a potential problem but a real problem. If a
child does swallow a battery, you want to get them to burp
it up pretty quickly, if you can. Certainly, don't wait
before you get them proper medical help.

REFERENCES

Beratis, S., Rubin, M., Miller, R.T., Galenson, E. and
     Rothstein, A. "Developmental aspects of an infant with
     transient moderate to severe hearing impairment" Pediatrics
     63:153 - 155, 1979.

Bergstrom, L.B. "Congenital deafness" Northern, J. (ed.)
     Hearing Disorders (Boston: Little, Brown and Co.), 1976.

Braida, L.D.,Durlach, N.I., Lippman, R.P., Hicki, B.L.,
     Rabinowitz, W.M. and Reed, C.M. Hearing Aids (ASHA
     Monographs, Rockville, Md.), 1979.

Connor, F.P.,Williamson, G.G. and Sipee, J.M. Program Guide
     for Infants and Toddlers with Neuromotor and Other
     Developmental Disabilities (New York: Teachers College
     Press), 1978.

Downs, M. "Minimal auditory deficiency syndrome" Audiology,
     An Audio Journal for Continuing Education (New York:
     Grune & Stratton), 1979.

French-St. George, M. and Barr-Hamilton, R.M. "Relief of the
     occluded ear sensation to improve earmold comfort" Journal
     of American Audiological Society 4:30 - 35, 1978.

Galenson, E., Miller, R., Kaplan, E. and Rothstein, A. "Assessment of development in the deaf child" Journal of American Academy of Child Psychiatry 18:128 - 142, 1979.

Keith, R.W. "An acoustic reflex technique of establishing hearing aid settings" Journal of American Audiological Society 5:71 - 75, 1979.

Ling, D. "Auditory Coding and recoding" in Ross, M. and Giolas, T. (eds.) Auditory Management of Hearing-Impaired Children (Baltimore: University Park), 1978.

Lybarger, S.F. "Earmolds" in Katz, J. (ed.) Handbook of Clinical Audiology (Baltimore: Williams and Wilkins), 1978.

McCandless, G. and Miller, D. "Loudness discomfort and hearing aids" National Hearing Aid Journal 7:28 - 32, 1972.

McDermott, S. and Goldblatt, B. New Preparation Program for Teachers/Supervisors of Infant Programs for the Hearing-Impaired, B.E.H. Grant 451 AG 60422, 1979.

Manyuk, P. "Development in children with chronic otitis media: design factors in the assessment of language" Annals of Otology, Rhinology and Laryngology Supp 80, 2:78 - 88, 1979.

Needlemen, H. "Effects of hearing loss from early recurrent otitis media on speech and language development" in Jaffee, B.F. (ed.) Hearing Loss in Children (Baltimore: University Park), 1977.

Rand Corporation Improving Services to Handicapped Children (The Rand Corporation, Santa Monica, California), 1974.

Rand, T.C. "Dichotic release from masking" Journal of Acoustical Society of America 55:678 - 680, 1974.

Rappaport, B. and Tait, C.A. "Acoustic reflex threshold measurement hearing aid selection" Archives of Otology 102:129 - 132, 1976.

Ross, Mark "Hearing aid selection for the preverbal hearing-impaired child" in Pollack (ed.) Amplification for the Hearing-Impaired (New York: Grune and Stratton), 1975.

Ross, M. "Classroom acoustics" in Katz, J. (ed.) Handbook of Clinical Audiology (Baltimore: Williams and Wilkins), 1978.

Rubin, M. "Auditory deprivation in infants" Journal of Communication Disorders 5:195 - 204, 1972.

Rubin, M. "Amplification for infants and young children" Audiology, an Audio Journal for Continuing Education (New York: Grune and Stratton), 1975.

Rubin, M. "The Lexington program for infants" in Gerber, S.E. and Mencher, G.T. (eds.) Early Diagnosis of Hearing Loss (New York: Grune and Stratton), 1978a.

Rubin, M. "Serous otitis media in severely to profoundly hearing-impaired children, ages 0 - 6" Volta Review 80:81 - 85, 1978b.

Rubin, M. "The relation between impedance findings and hearing aid selection for deaf infants" Volta Review 81:436 - 441, 1979.

Rubin, M. "Meeting the needs of hearing-impaired infants" Pediatric Annals 9, 1980.

Simmons, F.B. "Identification of hearing loss in infants and young children" Otolaryngology Clinics of North America, Vol 11, 1978.

Sinclair, J. "Electroacoustics standards" in Rubin, M. (ed.) Hearing Aids: Current Developments and Concepts (Baltimore: University Park), 1976.

Skinner, M.W. "The hearing of speech during language acquisition" Otolaryngology Clinics of North America Vol 11, 1978.

Webster, D. and Webster, M. "Neonatal sound deprivation affects brainstem auditory nuclei" Archives of Otology 13:392 - 396, 1977.

AMPLIFICATION IN THE HABILITATION OF THE YOUNG DEAF CHILD

Marion P. Downs
University of Colorado, Denver, Colorado

One of the greatest miracles that we will ever see is
the incomparable feat accomplished by the plastic brain of
the young hearing impaired infant in making order out of the
cacophony of sound that comes to him through a hearing aid.
The fact that the infant brain, in its early language learn--
ing, can utilize this sound has occasioned the long-term,
prodigious effort to identify hearing impaired infants at an
early age and to apply appropriate amplification to them.
As Mark Ross (1977) has said, "the early, appropriate, and
supervised use of hearing aids is probably the single most
important therapeutic tool we have to assist the hearing
impaired child".

Because these things are so, the placing of hearing aids
on children is a task that must be approached with grave
care. Unfortunately, infants and young children cannot give
us the kind of responses that allow us to make hearing aid
selections for hearing impaired adults. Therefore, present
theory would have us extrapolate what we know about hearing
aid fittings for adults, who can give us the desired responses
and project that knowledge to hearing aid fittings for the
young infant. This idea seems to make it all very simple,
but the fact is, of course, that we do not have adequate
knowledge about many facets of hearing aid fitting. We do
not have realistic expectations for the possible benefits
of hearing aids on adults, nor do we understand all the
variables involved in fitting hearing aids on adults. We are
not even certain that we understand the best method of performing real ear measurements of hearing aid function on
adults. Therefore, the extrapolation of knowledge of an
adult's hearing aid fitting to a child's hearing aid fitting
is going to be a tenuous proposition at best. The validity
of such extrapolation is also questionable because, in the
case of adults, we are dealing with a fully developed central
auditory nervous system that has utilized and assimilated
acoustic material for a lifetime and has developed all of the
necessary strategies for interpreting language through the
auditory channel. In the infant, on the other hand, we are
presenting acoustic input to a brain that has never heard
auditory signals and has developed neither functioning

199

auditory pathways nor cortical interpretation of sound. The
only thing the infant has going for it is the plasticity of
its brain during the first years of life, something which
facilitates the process whereby auditory input develops meaning, and it is limited only by the extent to which the
acoustic signal is complete or partially complete. The fact
that this signal must be the best possible one for the
individual child places a frightfully heavy responsibility
on the shoulders of the audiologist making the hearing aid
recommendation. There will never be any way to know whether
we have done the right thing in a given case. So, we must
simply forge ahead and combine our clinical insight with our
pragmatic knowledge of how hearing aids function.

    Five aspects of amplification seem to be relevant to
the selection of hearing aids for the younger child:

1. expectation of benefit;

2. general type of hearing aid;

3. upper limits of amplification;

4. lower limits; and,

5. frequency selection.

Expectations for Benefit

    Many years ago, in desperation to find a formula that
would predict success or failure in hearing aid use, I
attempted to compile a "deafness management quotient" which
would allow such a prediction. It included the degree of
residual hearing, the extent of central intactness, the state
of intellectual factors, the conditions of the family con-
stellation, and the impact of socio-economic factors. In
general, this formula has held up fairly well when applied
retrospectively to hearing impaired populations. However, it
has become apparent that other parameters should be added to
such a quotient -- parameters which may not be measurable,
but which could possibly be within the purview of the physio-
logically oriented otologist to predict.

    Such factors have been looked at by McCandless and
Parkin (1978), who surveyed 140 hearing aid users and related
the success or failure of hearing aid use to the site of

of lesion involved. They utilized differential diagnostic
auditory tests as the criteria for categorizing the site of
lesion in their adult hearing impaired population. There
are, of course, questions about the validity of auditory
tests in determining a specific site of lesion, but certainly
when combined with adequate diagnosis, there is some reason
to feel confident that a reasonable estimate might be made.
McCandless and Parkin determined in their survey whether or
not hearing aids were being worn successfully as a function
of the amount of time the aids were worn. The results of
their survey are as follows:

N = 140	Site of Lesion	Successful Use
	Conductive	94%
	Cochlear	84%
	Neural	30%
	Central	6%

In all, only 55% of the aids were found to be worn the
majority of time; nearly 30% were partially or totally
rejected.

What McCandless and Parkin are saying has far-reaching
implications. Histopathologists have reported for many years
that neural lesions due to neural presbycusis, syphilis, or
VIIIth nerve tumors, have markedly low discrimination;
whereas, sensory lesions, in the presence of sufficient
residual hearing, can be expected to have fairly good discrimination. This fact controverts the theory of phonemic
regression which assumes that the low discrimination scores
of many presbycusic losses are due to "central problem" - a
concept difficult to demonstrate. McCandless' and Parkins'
category of central problems was compiled from actual known
traumatic or other adventitious brain damage.

Although site-of-lesion audiometric tests cannot be
done on infants and young children, an otologic diagnosis
can serve to give some clue as to the possible site of lesion
in the case of a hearing impaired infant or young child. One
can relate the classical temporal bone pathology types to
the etiology, and develop some gross types of classification,
as per Black et al (1971).

1) Michel type: agnesis of the inner ear

There is total absence of the inner ear and auditory
nerves so there is no possibility of hearing of any sort.

2) Mondini type: bony and membraneous labyrinthine dys-
    genesis

Although there may be malformation of the bony labyrinth,
the hearing loss will be due to cochlear lesions, while the
spiral ganglion cells and higher auditory pathways will be
normal. Where residual hearing is found, the prognosis for
hearing aid use should be excellent. It should be noted
that there is a possibility of progression of the hearing
loss in a case with a Mondini ear.

3) Scheibe type: cochleo-saccular degeneration

The hearing loss is due to Organ of Corti degeneration,
and good discrimination can be expected to be present in
proportion to the amount of hearing that is present. This
pattern is found in many genetic hearing losses and is also
present in viral endolabyrinthitis caused by measles, mumps
or rubella. It has been our observation that cases of
rubella have excellent prospects for developing good discrimination when wearing a hearing aid, if the hearing loss
is identified early.

Michel and Mondini pathologies can be identified by
polytomography, but in the living child, the Scheibe type
can only be inferred from the etiology.

There are also other clinical entitles which are
associated with known temporal bone pathologies, such as
hearing loss due to an infection of bacterial meningitis.
Where meningitis affects the inner ear, it most probably
destroys not only the Organ of Corti, but the cochlear
neurons as well. Therefore, where profound deafness is
found following meningitis, the prognosis for hearing aid
use is very poor. Another clinical entity which has very
poor prognosis for hearing aid use is a congenital syphilitic
infection in which there is \a loss of spiral ganglion cells
and the cochlear and neural cells have become atrophied.
Poor hearing function and limited use of hearing aids can be
expected because of the neural atrophy.

The above listing represents only a small number of the
possible pathologies whose site of lesion can, at this time,
only be based on speculation. A large-scale collaborative

study between otologists and audiologists is necessary in order to provide for better and more accurate prediction of successful hearing aid use by these groups.

General Type of Hearing Aid

The initial consideration of a hearing aid must include decisions as to whether to fit air conduction or bone conduction aids, ear level or body-worn hearing aids, and binaural or monaural modes.

Bone Conduction Versus Air Conduction

The only time that a bone conduction hearing aid should be placed on a child is when it is physically impossible to wear air conduction or when it is medically hazardous. In cases of total atresia, there is no other means of amplification than bone conduction, and in life-threatening ear disease where an earmold would exacerbate the disease, air conduction aids are contraindicated. But only in such extreme cases of ear disease should bone conduction hearing aids be allowed. It has been our experience, after fitting hundreds of children with bone conduction hearing aids within the first 3 or 4 months of life, that none have developed language skills up to their potential abilities.

In the past, it has been felt that bone conduction aids are as effective as air conduction for the child with a conductive hearing loss. As a consequence, such aids have been recommended with only minimal concomitant speech and hearing therapy. What has not been recognized is that the signal transmitted by the bone conduction receiver is very much like that which would be received by a mild sensory-neural hearing loss. That is, the high frequency sounds are distorted or not heard as clearly through bone conduction as through air conduction. The problem has been that we are not able to measure a bone conducted signal as accurately as an air conducted signal, so we do not really know what kind of speech energy is actually reaching the ear via bone conduction. It has only been through sad experience that we have realized that a child who is given a bone conduction hearing aid in the early months of life should be considered a child with a sensory-neural hearing loss, and speech, language and hearing therapy should be as intensive as that given to a child with a congenital sensory-neural hearing loss.

Ear Level Versus Body Worn Aids

At the present time, the electroacoustic characteristics of ear level aids are almost equal to those of body type aids. Therefore, there is no reason to recommend body type aids except in the following instances:

1. Where bone conduction aids are indicated. Even then, there are instruments now made that can be placed completely on the head and held on a headband. Here, one has the advantage of having the sound source on the head where head turning can accomodate the head shadow effect.

2. Where feedback from the earmold cannot be eliminated at high volumes. This is really the most stringent limitation of ear level aids, for it is sometimes difficult to obtain an earmold that has adequate seal and, thus, will prevent feedback. However, heroic efforts should be made to obtain a well-sealing earmold before resorting to a body type aid. One possibility is a CROS-type fitting, which permits a farther distance between the microphone and the ear.

3. Where there is a very severe mixed hearing loss. If, for example, a child has a sensory-neural loss around 60 dB and an additional conductive loss of 60 dB, he would need a total output of at least 140 - 150 dB, which can be obtained only with a body-type hearing aid. With this type of hearing loss, there is almost no limit to the saturation output that can be tolerated and the dynamic range will be almost as large as in the normal ear.

The advantages of ear level aids include:

1) elimination of clothing noise and muffling from clothing placed over the aid unit microphone;

2) enabling of the head to play a role in the spatial separation of sound sources;

3) the ability to use directional microphones which give an advantage in noise.

In other words, the use of ear level aids permits true binaural hearing in every sense of the word which, as we will see, is the recommended mode.

Binaural Versus Monaural

A true binaural hearing aid fitting is the fitting of choice in 99% of the cases. The only two exceptions are:

1)   when it is absolutely certain that one ear has no usable hearing whatsoever; and,

2)   if it becomes apparent after an adequate trial of two aids that the child does better with one than with two. In our experience, only one child has been found to fit this category.

As Ross (1977) has stated, "With properly fitted binaural hearing aids the brain is able to correlate the time, frequency and intensity differences of the sound reaching each ear." This results in:

1)   improved abilities to localize sound sources;

2)   loudness summation (less intensity is required for the two ears than one ear to reach an equal loudness sensation);

3)   improved foreground-background differentiation, which improves the hearing of the speech signal in noise; and,

4)   enhancement of the head shadow effect (with one aid the speech coming from the other side is attenuated by 6 dB before reaching the aided ear).

With a monaural fitting or a Y-cord fitting, the above advantages do not occur. Therefore, we can state unequivocally at this time, that binaural fitting is the most advantageous for practically every hearing impaired child. A new two-volume series, edited by E. R. Libby and entitled Binaural Hearing and Amplification (Zenetron, Chicago, 1980), has just become available. With this publication, the agrument on binaural aids is ended, once and for all. It may, indeed, be over-kill.

Upper Limits of Amplification

Here we are really dealing with two questions:

1. Are there hearing losses so profound that a hearing aid
    need not be recommended?

2. Can a case be made for the need to limit the saturation
    output of hearing aids more than is presently prescribed
    for young children?

The first question concerns itself with the fact that
there may be cases where there is no possibility of any
remaining hearing that will respond to amplification. Such
a situation might occur in the classic Michel pathology, or
in those cases of meningitis where the neural structures are
completely destroyed. There also may be other instances
where the residual hearing is so slight as to be practically
non-functional. The general rule to follow in the case of
young infants and children is always to fit a hearing aid,
unless there is definitive evidence that no usable hearing
exists. And even where the latter situation holds, it is
our policy to apply hearing aids, either air conduction or
bone conduction, in the hope that some vibratory response
will be useful in separating the presence of sound from the
absence of sound.

The second question is open to a great deal more argument. What are the limits of saturation outputs for hearing
aids for young children? Several studies have been reported
which point to the possibility that some losses may be
exacerbated by improper upper limits. None of the studies
meets the rigorous requirements of scientific inquiry,
however, and the only evidence that has been supplied is
anecdotal in nature. That is not to decry anecdotal evidence;
as a matter of fact, one of the most telling reports was made
by Heffernan and Simons (1979) (see Figure 1). There is no
question that this child did receive a temporary threshold
shift from wearing the hearing aid that had been fitted.
And if one accepts the theory that temporary threshold shift
after noise exposure presages permanent threshold shift, then
this child's hearing was indeed in danger of progression as
a result of the type of amplification that had been given to
him. Such a concept requires closer scrutiny.

The theory of temporary threshold shift as a precursor
of permanent threshold shift has been applied only to normal
hearing ears, so any attempt to extrapolate it to an already
damaged ear or one with a congenital hearing loss is specula-
tive at best. Nonetheless, all of us have seen similar
instances that have taken the same course that Heffernan and

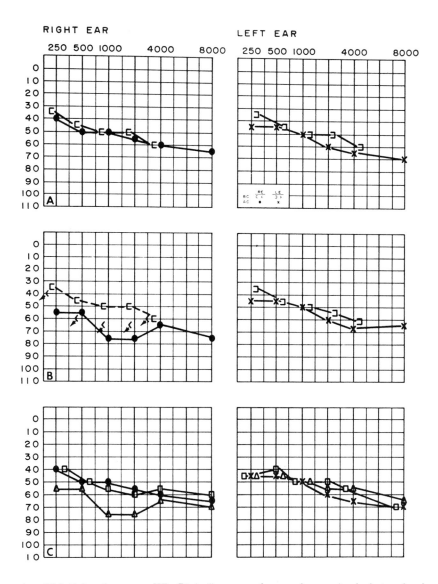

Figure 1. (A) Initial audiogram on HT. (B) Audiogram performeα after wearing body-type hearing aid for 7 months on right ear. Note the absence of responses to bone conducted stimuli on that side. (C) Serial audiograms contrasting air conduction thresholds over an 8 month period. ●-●- Initial test; Δ-Δ- After wearing aid for 7 months in the right ear; □-□ After 14 days of "auditory rest." (This material provided through the courtesy of P. Heffernan and M. Simons, and is taken from their article: "Temporary increases in sensorineural hearing loss with hearing aid use," *Annals of Otology, Rhinology and Laryngology* 88:86−91, 1979.)

Simon's case did, and we too have reduced the saturation
level of the hearing aid.

   None of the studies in this area has come to grips with
the fact that a certain number of congenital hearing losses
will be progressive, whether a hearing aid is worn or not.
There has been a recent flurry of interest by otolaryngologists about congenital progressive hearing loss. It is
thought that where progression occurs, a Mondini bony cochlear
malformation is responsible. There have been verbal reports
which speculate that the progression in such cases is due to
enlarged endolymphatic ducts, and if the endolymphatic sac is
shunted, the progression will be halted. A large number of
such procedures have been reported, with no further progression of hearing loss evident over the period of time that
these procedures have been done. From a scientific point of
view, it will be difficult to prove or disprove the efficacy
of this kind of surgery as there is no way to establish
controls for a rigidly researched study.

   The fact that some otologists are now placing the blame
for the progression of some hearing losses on the physical
features of the congenital ear, illustrates the uncertainty
regarding what causes progressive hearing losses. Like the
surgery for the Mondini ear, there is simply no way that a
scientific investigation can do a controlled study of this
problem. The only evidence we have is individual and anecdotal, as whatever large surveys have been recorded have been
done without benefit of any controls, either inter- or intra-
subject (Kinney, 1961; McCrae and Farrant, 1965; McCrae,
1968a, 1968b). A comprehensive review of the literature by
Mills (1975) covered the studies to that date. Since then,
it seems that anecdotal reports are more prevalent, as
illustrated by the Heffernan and Simons report.

   Anecdotal reportage is a game any number can play and
we, too, have contributed our experiences in reports that we
have made on "Catastrophic Inner Ear Symptoms" (Downs,
Bergstrom and Wood, 1980). One report concerns a series of
12 children and adults with congenital hearing losses of
varying degrees, who have experienced temporary or permanent
progressive hearing loss accompanied by vertigo (Tullio
effect), tinnitus, and reduced discrimination. The onset is
always sudden and is always related to some sort of acoustic
experience while a hearing aid is being worn. That is, the
subjects report a sudden loud noise through the hearing aid

and an immediate onset of tinnitus, vertigo, discrimination
loss, and apparent reduction in hearing. In some cases, the
hearing has progressed to a permanently lower level, and in
others it has returned to its previous level following rest
or heroic medical intervention. The latter has included
stellate ganglion block, heparin, nicotinic acid and antihis-
tamine. The fact that the symptoms always begin with an
acoustic experience has led us to reduce the SSPL of the hearing aids worn and also to recommend split frequency band
fittings (see below) on the theory that less amplitude reaching a cochlea will best benefit a particularly susceptible
ear. This type of "sudden-onset" problem has been found in
isolated recessive deafnesses, in maternal rubella syndrome
deafness, in dominant syndromes such as Stickler's syndrome,
and in unknown causes. The question, of course, remains
whether the "acoustic experience" is caused by an inner
acoustic experience or whether the aid has transmitted a
loud sound in the environment that has impinged on a sensitive ear.

    The jury is still out on the question of injury to the
ear from hearing aids. A table describing the studies reporting pro and con statements has been produced by Markides
(1980). It is reproduced here as Table I. It can be seen
that there is extreme polarization in the two sides of this
question. Two statements can be made with fair certainty:

1. Just as in the normal population, there will be some
ears that have unusual susceptibility to noise exposure, and
almost any levels of constant noise will cause progression
of hearing loss. The number of such ears probably ranges
from 1 - 5%, so we are faced with the same dilemma that OSHA
(Occupational Safety and Health Administration) has; namely,
that there is no single criterion that can be established
that will protect all the ears in a population (Ward, 1969).
Like OSHA, we will have to arrive at some sort of trade-off
principle in this regard.

2. One hundred and twenty dB should be the absolute upper
limit for hearing aids for sensory-neural hearing losses.
Danaher and Pickett (1975) noted that, in subjects with very
profound hearing loss, the loudness discomfort level was 128
dB SPL which is close to 115 dB hearing level. The most
comfortable hearing level was around 125 dB SPL, which,
again, may be closer to 105 - 110 dB hearing level. Hood
and Poole (1966) stated that 90% of their cochlear-impaired

TABLE I: DO HEARING AIDS DAMAGE THE USER'S RESIDUAL HEARING?

Author	No. of persons in sample	No. of persons affected	Stated Max. acoustic output of hearing aids in dB SPL	Amount of deterioration observed in dB
YES				
Kinney (1953)	8,800	16	?	?
Moller & Rojskaer (1960)	390	9	120	?
Kinney (1961)	178	41	146?	10-25
Sataloff (1961)	1	1	?	20 (TTS)
Ross & Truex (1965)	2	2	139	25-35 (PTS)
Macrae & Farrant (1965)	87	?	121-126	906 1102
Ross & Lerman (1967)	18	9	130	102 904
Macrae (1967, 1968)	4	4	130	4-5 (ETS)
Macrae (1968)	32	?	115-117	402
	40	?	117-119	309
	38	?	120-124	801
	24	?	125-130	806
Ballantyne (1970)	1	1	140	20-30 (PTS)
NO				
Holmgren (1940)	?		?	
Murray (1951)	?		130	
Naunton (1957)	120		126	
Brockman (1959)	9		?	
Whetnell	?		?	
Barr & Wedenberg (1965)	84		130	
World Health Organization (1967)	?		?	
Bellefluer & Van Dyke (1968)	58		?	
Roberts (1970)	278		?	
Hine & Furness (1975)	21	125-136?		
Derbyshire (1976)	100		100+	
Markides (1976)	100		116-136	
Markides & Aryee (1978)	55		116-136	
UNDECIDED				
Harford & Markle (1955)	1		?	

subjects had loudness discomfort levels between 95 and 105 dB
SPL. The normal ear probably begins to distort at 115 - 120
dB SPL. It is logical to assume, therefore, that the pathological ear, which at those levels uses the same hair cells as
the normal ear does, will also distort the speech signal at
that point. Thus, we have many reasons for not recommending
hearing aids with more than 115 dB SSPL for cases of pure
sensory-neural hearing loss. When a mixed loss occurs, the
limits will be increased by the amount of the conductive
hearing loss.

Lower Limits of Amplification

     As short a time as 5 years ago, it was generally con-
sidered that hearing aids should not be recommended for
children unless hearing loss averaged 25 - 30 dB or more.
Since that time, a large number of reports in the literature
have combined to convince us that in many instances, hearing
losses as low as 15 dB or even less may be significantly
handicapping to the very young child and, therefore, consideration should be given to a hearing aid trial for such
losses. Slight losses accompany serous otitis media - that
insidious, asymptomatic disease of early childhood which has
now been demonstrated to be devastating to some children's
later language development. As a matter of fact, even
fluctuating hearing losses of this sort - where as much as
half the time the hearing may be normal - can be handicapping
to the child's auditory language learning development.

     A number of studies have accumulated to give us this
new picture of the harmful effects of serous otitis on the
child's functioning. For example, a series of retrospective
studies of children with histories of recurrent otitis media
beginning in the first year of life demonstrated that their
auditory language learning skills are significantly lower
than those of normal controls (Kessler and Randolph, 1979;
Needleman, 1977; Lewis, 1976; Holm and Kunze, 1969; Howie,
1978). Results of another series of studies indicated that
when children in special classes for language learning problems are examined, a significant proportion of them have
been shown to have had histories of recurrent otitis beginning in the first year of life (Zinkus et al, 1979; Katz,
1976; Masters and March, 1978).

     Animal studies have confirmed the fact that there are
central nervous system correlates to conductive hearing

losses which occur early in the animal's life. Webster and
Webster (1979) gave newborn mice conductive hearing losses
for 45 days, then sacrificed the animals and compared their
central auditory pathways with those of normal controls.
The conductive loss group was found to be deficient in the
size and number of neurons in the cochlear nuclei cells of
the superior olivary complex and in the trapezoid body. In
a further experiment, Webster and Webster restored the hearing of a similar experimental group of mice. After 45 days
of deprivation, the experimentors allowed the mice to hear
normally until 90 days, at which time the animals were
sacrificed and neuronal examination made. It was found that
there was no restitution of neuronal size or numbers in the
affected areas of the auditory pathways. Thus, it appears
that when deprivation occurs during critical periods in the
development of central auditory processing, permanent damage
results.

Why should such mild conductive hearing losses produce
damage quite out of proportion to their severity? The reason
lies in both the nature of conductive loss and that of speech
energy. Normal speech has been shown to range from around
30 dB SPL to 75 dB SPL (Skinner, 1978). The difficulty is
that when we speak of the total amount of energy in a speech
stimulus, it does not mean that the total speech content is
heard well enough for learning purposes. The unvoiced consonant parts of speech may be 20 - 30 dB softer than the
vowel sounds that contain most of the energy. In fact, some
of these unvoiced consonant sounds may not be heard at all in
rapid speech, but most of us have learned so well the strategies that are necessary to fill in for these missing sounds
that we may not even notice that they are not present. But,
an infant or young child who is learning speech and language
cannot do that. He must hear every part of the speech signal
very thoroughly in order to learn language well.

Skinner (1978) has stated that "Even a mild hearing loss
will cause the short, unstressed words (e.g., it, if, is) and
the less intense speech sounds (voiceless stops and fricatives) to be inaudible. This loss of cues results in a delay
in normal acquisition of language. The acoustic cues of
speech that are audible will be perceived differently by a
child with a conductive impairment compared to one with a
sensory-neural impairment". These conclusions of Skinner
have recently been corroborated by a very nice study by
Dobie and Berlin (1979). These researchers prepared a 10
second speech utterance by recording it through "correcting
filters which shape the signal as if it were processed through

an ear at about the 40 phon level". They then digitized the
selection in a computer and displayed it oscillographically.
After this, they attenuated the display to simulate the way
a 20 dB hearing loss would hear the speech. They compared
this display with unattenuated oscillographs. Spectro-
analyses of each 600 milliseconds of speech were compared.
The oscillographs were read independently by a number of
readers who segmented, marked and located the onset of the
various phonetic utterances. When this synthesis of a 20 dB
hearing loss was inspected, the authors found precisely what
Skinner had predicted: "A potential loss of transitional
information, especially plural endings, and related final-
position fricatives was highly likely ... Very brief utterances or high frequency information could be either distorted
or degraded if signal noise conditions were less than satisfactory." Dobie and Berlin felt this degradation would
reduce information from the acoustic signal in these ways:

1)   morphological markers might be lost or sporadically mis-
      understood;

2)   very short words which are elided often in connected
      speech will lose considerable loudness;

3)   inflections or markers carrying subtle nuances such as
      questioning and related intonation contouring can, at
      the very best, be expected to come through inconsistently.

Thus, Skinner's predictions were confirmed by an ingenious
study which is certainly a landmark report.

     In addition to confirming Skinner's predictions, Dobie
and Berlin also presented some data which may allow us to
extrapolate from Webster and Webster's study on mice to the
human condition. BSER readings were done on a child who had
had a long history of early and recurrent serous otitis, but
who at a later age had perfectly normal hearing. This child
was subjected to a two-click interactive BSER and results
were compared with responses from a normal child. The otitis
media child showed inconsistency in her two ear interactions,
and a different polarity and latency for the so-called
interactive responses. The authors feel that they may,
indeed, be describing a measurable physiological correlate
to the effects of long standing but resolved conductive
hearing loss similar to the anatomical studies of Webster
and Webster.

These recent studies have now substantiated that language is adversely affected by early fluctuating hearing loss
from serous otitis, however mild it may be. We have found
that infants with fluctuating hearing losses can successfully
wear very mild hearing aids. The aids we have selected have
the following characteristics:

1. Small size. There are a few aids available that are
small enough to be accommodated easily by the infant ear.
Although larger aids can be worn, it is more appropriate
to utilize the smaller size when possible.

2. SSPL level lower than 90 dB. These aids should, preferably, be set at approximately 80 dB SSPL, a level which can
be tolerated by the normal ear for long periods of time
without discomfort or injury.

3. Gain of around 20 dB. The amount of gain is, of course,
limited by the reduced output, but no more than 20 - 25 dB
is an acceptable level.

Although there is no question that these hearing aids
can be worn successfully by young infants, the fact is that
it taxes all the ingenuity of the audiologist and hearing
therapist to see that such a hearing aid is worn. A mandatory concomitant of the hearing aid is a home language stimulation program which should be recommended whether or not a
hearing aid is tried. Successful hearing aid use requires a
great deal of co-operation, understanding, and dedication by
both parents to keep the hearing aid on the child, and equal
dedication by the managing physician, audiologist and hearing
therapist. Perhaps no more than 50% of the children we
consider for hearing aids will have successful hearing aid
use.

Our indications for this kind of educational treatment
(home language stimulation program plus trial with hearing
aids) are as follows:

I. Three months duration of serous otitis media:

    A) Condition:
        (1) Constant serous otitis media, or
        (2) Failure of tubes, or
        (3) Recurrent bouts.

B) Action:
    (1) Speech and language evaluation,
    (2) Immediate home language stimulation program if
         the evaluation shows weakness,
    (3) Watchful waiting if evaluation is normal.

II. Six months duration of serous otitis media:

A) Condition:
    (1) Constant SOM, or
    (2) Failure of tubes, or
    (3) Recurrent bouts.

B) Action:
    Complete aural rehabilitation program, including
    home language stimulation program and consideration
    of, or trial with, hearing aid.

Frequency Selection

       Ever since the famous (or infamous) Harvard report of
1947 (Nichols, 1947), the controversy has raged regarding
"selective" frequency response. Generally, audiologists
have tended to "mirror" the audiogram, which in adults, most
often produces better results on articulation tests utilizing PB word lists. Theoretically, the fitting with high
frequency emphasis would eliminate the "upward spread of
masking". This means that the low frequency representation
produced by moderate levels of environmental noise, when
amplified through a hearing aid, may produce a masking effect
on the higher frequencies, making speech intelligibility
difficult. A dilemma arises because it is now apparent that
low frequency energy may be more important than we had
thought, as many of the supra-segmental aspects of speech
are carried in the low frequencies (Franklin, 1975). High
frequency emphasis would leave out these aspects. A fitting
which appears to circumvent both of these problems has been
suggested originally by Franklin (1975) and by Weber and
Northern (1980). They propose that if high frequency signals
are presented to the right ear and low frequencies to the
left, the brain will fuse the speech signal and eliminate the
upper spread of masking while offering the requisite low
frequency signals to one ear. The basis of this proposal
rests on studies by Dirks (1964), Shankweiler and Studdart-
Kennedy (1970), Nagafuchi (1970), Ling (1971), and Franklin
(1975). Briefly, these studies indicate that:

1) in the dichotic state (where different auditory signals
   arrive simultaneously at the right ear and at the left
   ear) the right ear recognizes consonant–vowel nonsense
   syllables significantly better than the left ear.

2) in this state, monosyllabic word discrimination is
   superior in the right ear over the left ear.

3) in the dichotic state, predominance of the right ear is
   evident as early as age 3, suggesting that the left
   hemisphere of the brain is dominant for speech by age 3.

     Thus far there is only anecdotal reportage on the bene-
fits of split frequency band amplification. However, those
who have used it over several years' time have felt confident
that it provides many advantages over the standard binaural
fitting. Not only do we see improved speech discrimination
in almost every instance, but the fitting allows us to use
binaural amplification split frequency bands on hearing
losses that are widely asymmetrical. We follow the practice
of the Colorado Department of Health (Audiology Department)
in:

1) placing emphasis on the use of limited power output aids
   (less than 115 dB SPL) as well as the use of compression
   circuits on all aids in excess of 105 dB SPL;

2) in objective technique to determine specific gain settings; and,

3) special consideration for binaural fittings, including
   dichotic, for children.

     Following is the procedure (from Weber and Northern,
1980):

1. The acoustic system for a very young child is selected
on the basis of the patient's audiometric configuration
which may be determined as awareness threshold levels using
speech, narrow band noise, and/or pure tone signals. The
system can be tuned more finely as the child matures to a
level when reliable objective/subjective information is
forthcoming.

(a)   A child demonstrating an audiometric configuration
      of normal/near normal hearing levels extending
      upward through 500 Hz, with high frequency hearing
      loss bilaterally, should be tested in the binaural
      state using open earmolds, coupled with high fre-
      quency emphasis hearing aids. If acoustic feedback
      prevails, hearing aids with broader frequency res-
      ponse patterns will be utilized.

(b)   A child demonstrating bilateral profound hearing
      loss with a "corner audiogram" of hearing levels
      measurable only at 125 Hz, 250 Hz and/or 500 Hz at
      high intensity levels should be tested in the bi-
      naural state, with hearing aid producing low fre-
      quency energy extending downward to at least 100 Hz
      (and preferably lower). A standard earmold should
      be utilized. The principles of maximum power
      selection and gain selection described earlier in
      this manuscript should be rigidly enforced.*

2. A child demonstrating any other bilateral, sensory-neural
hearing loss should be tested in the dichotic state with a
hearing aid in the right ear set for high frequency amplification and a hearing aid in the left ear set with a low frequency setting. Standard earmolds should be utilized.

When feasible, special considerations will be made to
provide additional auditory signal differences between the
hearing aids fitted in the dichotic state, such as:

(a)   providing a directional microphone hearing aid for
      the right ear and an omni-directional microphone
      hearing aid for the left ear. Directional micro-
      phone hearing aids also tend to supply higher fre-
      quency ranges than do their own omni-directional
      counterparts.

---

* As previously described, Ling's study (1975) disclosed
   that no child performed worse with binaural fitting than
   with monaural fitting. However, the reverse was not true,
   particularly where the hearing aid was not worn in the
   dominant ear. Although the right ear appears to be the
   dominant ear for speech/language processing in most people,
   the exception does exist. Therefore, unless the patient
   can objectively/subjectively demonstrate monaural advantage,
   the binaural state will be selected).

(b)   providing the two hearing aids 180° out of phase
       with each other. The phase shift is available upon
       request through the hearing aid dealer or manufact-
       urer at minimal or no additional cost. Phase shift
       of 180° is achieved by reversing the receiver leads
       or microphone leads to the amplifier of one of the
       hearing aids.

   Split frequency band fittings may be suspect because
they appear to offer the utopian ideal of a universal fitting
for all types of hearing loss. Nonetheless, it behooves all
audiologists to prove to themselves whether the claims made
for this type of fitting are accurate or not.

Summary

   We live in the best of all worlds and times for hearing
aid fittings. Scientific investigation is beginning to
clarify the relationship between successful hearing aid use
and site of lesion. We have options available to use that
allow free choice of any type of hearing aid, whether it is
the body worn or ear level, air conduction or bone conduction,
large, small, or medium sized. We can successfully limit the
amount of sound that goes into an ear where necessary, or we
can produce enormous volumes where needed. We can place
hearing aids on ears that may be normal part of the time and
have very mild losses the rest of the time, without damaging
the ear in any way. We have available a variety of options
for frequency selection that may eventually solve the fitting
dilemmas of the past. What is most gratifying is that,
through conferences such as these Canadian meetings, we have
established acceptable screening procedures for identifying
at an early age, all hearing losses that need amplification.
If we utilize effectively all the knowledge that is presently at our disposal, we cannot fail to achieve the best
welfare of the hearing impaired child.

DISCUSSION

DOCTOR JACOBSON
   It has been observed that the threshold of discomfort
in an impaired ear is usually somewhere about the same place
it is for normal ears. The hydrodynamics of the basiler

membrane do not change, whether we have a pathological or
non-pathological auditory system. Sandwin and Krantz
reported in 1975 that the threshold of discomfort in the
impaired ear is 112 dB. McCann, in 1975 and 1976, said you
shouldn't use an aid with an MPO of more than 170 dB. On the
other hand, we know that we are sometimes dealing with profoundly impaired children who, even if you give an aid with
an MPO of 170, are not going to hear anything at all. I
would like us to deal with the ethics of that issue. I don't
know which way to go. Do we forgo the aid? Or, do we say,
let's take the chance of acoustic trauma. - It's better than
not hearing. Two other issues I find fascinating. One is
split band amplification, and the other, of course, amplification of mild conductive losses, which I might bring to
your attention, was one of the recommendations from the
Saskatoon conference.

REFERENCES

Ballantyne, J. "Iatrogenic deafness" The 16th James Yearsley
    Memorial Lecture Journal of Laryngology and Otology
    84:967 - 1000, 1970.

Barr, B. and Wedenberg, E. "Prognosis of perceptive hearing
    loss in children with respect to genesis and use of hear-
    ing aids" Acta Otolaryngologica 59:464 - 474, 1965.

Bellefleur, P.A. and Van Dyke, R.C. "The effects of high
    gain amplification on children in a residential school
    for the deaf" Journal of Speech and Hearing Research
    11:343 - 347, 1968.

Black, F.O., Bergstrom, L., Downs, M. and Hemenway, W.
    Congenital Deafness (Boulder: Colorado University Press),
    1971.

Brockman, S.J. "An exploratory investigation of delayed
    progressive neural hypacusis in children" Archives of
    Otolaryngology 70:340, 1959.

Danaher, E.M. and Picket, J.M. "Some masking effects pro-
    duced by low frequency vowel formants in persons with
    sensorineural hearing loss" Journal of Speech and Hearing
    Research 18:261 - 271, 1975.

Darbyshire, J.O. "A study of the use of high power hearing
   aids by children with marked degrees of deafness and the
   possibility of deterioration in auditory acuity" British
   Journal of Audiology 10:74 - 82, 1976.

Dirks, D. "Perception of dichotic and monaural verbal material and cerebral dominance for speech" Acta Otolaryngologica 58:73 - 80, 1964.

Dobie, R.A. and Berlin, C.I. "Influence of otitis media on
   hearing and development" Otitis Media and Child Development, Suppl. 60 Annals of Otology, Rhinology and Laryngology 88:1 - 111, 1979.

Downs, M.P., Bergstrom, L. and Wood, R.P. Unpublished
   research, University of Colorado Health Sciences Centre,
   1958.

Franklin, B. "The effect of combining low and high frequency
   passbands on consonant recognition in the hearing impaired"
   Journal of Speech and Hearing Research 18:719 - 727, 1975.

Harford, E.R. and Markle, D.M. "The atypical effect of a
   hearing aid on one patient with congenital deafness"
   Laryngoscope 65:970 - 972, 1955.

Heffernan, P. and Simons, M. "Temporary increases in sensorineural hearing loss with hearing aid use" Annals of
   Otology, Rhinology and Laryngology 88:86 - 91, 1979.

Hine, W.D. and Furness, H.J.S. "Does wearing a hearing aid
   damage residual hearing?" The Teacher of the Deaf 73:261 -
   271, 1975.

Holme, V.A. and Kunze, L.H. "Effect of chronic otitis media
   on language and speech development" Pediatrics 43:833 -
   838, 1969.

Holmgren, L. "Can hearing be damaged by a hearing aid"
   Acta Otolaryngologica (Stockh) 42:539, 1940.

Hood, J. and Poole, J. "Tolerable limit of loudness: Its
   clinical and physiological significance" Journal of the
   Acoustical Society of America 40:47 - 53, 1966.

Howie, V.M. "Acute and recurrent acute otitis media" in
Hearing Loss in Children, Jaffee, B.F. (ed.) (Baltimore:
University Park Press), 1978.

Katz, J. "The effects of conductive hearing loss on auditory
function" ASHA 20:879 - 886, 1978.

Kessler, M.E. and Randolph, K. "The effects of early middle
ear disease on the auditory abilities of third grade
children" Journal of the Academy of Rehabilitative
Audiology 12-2:6 - 20, 1979.

Kinney, C.E. "Hearing impairment in children" Laryngoscope
63:220 - 226, 1953.

Kinney, C.E. "The further destruction of partially deafened
children's hearing by use of powerful hearing aids"
Annals of Otology, Rhinology and Laryngology 70:828 - 835,
1961.

Ling, A. "Dichotic listening in hearing impaired children"
Journal of Speech and Hearing Research 14:793 - 803, 1975.

Lewis, N. "Otitis media and linguistic imcompetence"
Archives of Otolaryngology 102:387 - 390, 1976.

Macrae, J.H. and Farrant, R.H. "The effect of hearing aid
use on the residual hearing of children with sensorineural
deafness" Annals of Otolaryngology 74:409 - 419, 1965.

Macrae, J.H. "TTS and recovery from TTS after use of powerful hearing aids" Journal of the Acoustical Society of
America 43:1445 - 1446, 1967.

Macrae, J.H. "Recovery from TTS in children with sensorineural deafness" Journal of the Acoustical Society of
America 44:1451, 1968a.

Macrae, J.H. "Deterioration of the residual hearing of
children with sensorineural deafness" Acta Otolaryngologica
66:33 - 39, 1968b.

Markides, A. "The effect of hearing aid use on the user's
residual hearing" Scandinavian Audiology 5:205 - 219,
1976.

Markides, A. and Aryee, D.T.K. "The effect of hearing aid use on the user's residual hearing – A follow-up study" Scandinavian Audiology 7:19 – 23, 1978.

Markides, A. "The effect of hearing aid amplification on the user's residual hearing" in Binaural Hearing and Amplification, Vol II, Libby, E.R. (ed.) (Chicago: Zenetron Corp.), 1980.

Masters, L. and March, G.E. "Middle ear pathology as a factor in learning disabilities" Journal of Learning Disabilities 11:103 – 106, 1978.

McCandless, G.A. and Parkin, J.L. "Hearing aid performance relative to site of lesion" Otolaryngology 86:181, 1978.

Mills, J.H., Gengel, R.W., Watson, C.S. and Miller, J.D. "Temporary changes of the auditory system due to exposure to noise for one or two days" Journal of the Acoustical Society of America 48:524 – 530, 1970.

Moller, T.T. and Rojkaer, C. "Injury to hearing through hearing aid treatment (Acoustic trauma)" paper presented at the Fifth Congress of International Society of Audiology Bonn, Germany, 1960.

Murray, N.E. "Hearing aids and classification of deaf children" Report CAL-IR-Z Commonwealth Acoustic Laboratories, Sydney (cited by Macrae and Farrant), 1951.

Nagafuchi, M. "Development of dichotic and monaural hearing abilities in young children" Acta Otolaryngologica 69:409 – 414, 1970.

Naunton, R.F. "The effect of hearing aid use upon the user's residual hearing" Laryngoscope 67:569 – 576, 1957.

Needleman, H. "Effects of hearing loss from early recurrent otitis media on speech and language development" in Hearing Loss in Children, Jaffe, B. (ed.) (Baltimore: University Park Press), 1977.

Nichols, R.H., Jr. "Physical characteristics of hearing aids" Laryngoscope 57:31 – 40, 1947.

Roberts, C.   "Can hearing aids damage hearing" Acta Otolaryn-
     gologica 69:123 - 125, 1970.

Ross, M. and Truex, H.   "Protecting residual hearing in
     hearing aid users" Archives of Otolaryngology 82:615 - 617,
     1965.

Ross, M. and Lerman, J.   "Hearing aid usage and its effect
     on residual hearing: A review of the literature and an
     investigation" Archives of Otolaryngology 86:639 - 644,
     1967.

Ross, M.   "Hearing aids" in Hearing Loss in Children, Jaffe,
     B. (ed.) (Baltimore: University Park Press), 1977.

Sataloff, J.   "Pitfalls in routine hearing testing" Archives
     of Otolaryngology 73:717 - 726, 1961.

Shankweiler, D. and Studdert-Kennedy, M.   "Hemispheric
     specialization for speech perception" Journal of the
     Acoustical Society of America 48:579 - 594, 1970.

Skinner, M.W.   "The hearing of speech during language
     acquisition" Otolaryngological Clinics of North America
     11:631 - 650, 1978.

Ward, W.D.   "Effects of noise on hearing thresholds" Proceed-
     ings of the Conference on Noise as a Public Health
     Hazard. American Speech and Hearing Association,
     Monograph, 40 - 48, 1969.

Weber, H.J. and Northern, J.L.   "Selection of children's
     hearing aids: Colorado Department of Health Program"
     in Binaural Hearing and Amplification, Libby, E.R. (ed.)
     (Chicago: Zenetron Corp.), 1980.

Webster, D.B. and Webster, M.   "Neonatal sound deprivation
     affects brain stem auditory nuclei" Archives of Otolaryn-
     gology 103:392 - 396, 1977.

Whetnall, E. and Fry, D.B.   The Deaf Child (London:
     William Heinemann Medical Books, Ltd.), 1964.

World Health Organization. <u>The Early Detection and Treatment Of Handicapping Defects In Young Children</u>, Special Report, distributed by Regional Office for Europe, Copenhagen, 1967.

Zinkus, P.W., Gottlieb, M.L. and Schapiro, M. "Developmental and psychoeducational sequelae of chronic otitis media" <u>American Journal of Disabled Children</u> 132:1100 - 1104, 1978.

EARLY HABILITATION: A BLEND OF COUNSELLING AND GUIDANCE

Agnes H. Ling Phillips
Dalhousie University, Halifax, Nova Scotia

Hearing impairment, especially when severe or profound, drastically reduces the possibility for children to develop intelligible speech, good linguistic skills, and educational standards commensurate with their intellectual abilities. Where hearing loss is not detected in infancy and/or where there has been no intervention, abnormal patterns of mother-child communication tend to emerge (Goss, 1970; Ling and Ling, 1976). There is markedly less verbalization on the part of the mother and less vocalization on the part of the child. In fact, both the quantity and quality of vocalization from hearing impaired children have been reported as poorer than normal quite early in life (Lenneberg, 1967; Mavilya, 1969; Manolson, 1972).

Follow-up studies on children who participated in early intervention programs beginning prior to age three have demonstrated significant improvement in speech skills (Lach, Ling, Ling and Ship, 1971), in personal-social, hearing and speech, and performance skills (Ling, 1971) and in mother-child communication (Greenstein, Greenstein, McConville and Stellini, 1976; Ling and Ling, 1976). Near-normal achievement has been reported in spoken language (McConnell and Liff, 1975; Leckie, 1975), social skills (Kennedy and Bruininks, 1974), academic skills (Rister, 1975; McClure, 1977), reading (Doehring, Bonnycastle and Ling, 1978), and in speech (Ling and Milne, 1979).

The early intervention programs which have been successful in preparing severely and profoundly hearing impaired children to function well at an early age in regular classes appear to have many features in common. These include active involvement of staff members in detection, diagnosis and management; the provision of counselling, guidance and education for parents; parents who accept a primary role in habilitation; careful and frequent audiological and otological monitoring to ensure maximum utilization of residual hearing; the development of communication by spoken language; a strong and lasting personal interest in the families on the part of the professionals; systematic evaluation of progress; and professionals who are also engaged in research and/or teaching.

Parent-centered programs do not reach a large portion of the population, nor are they successful with all families who enroll. Some parents lack the stamina to cope with the special needs of a hearing impaired child in addition to their other family commitments. Sometimes there is a lack of compatibility between parents and professionals, sometimes parents transfer to child-centered programs, and sometimes professionals lack the essential technical or counselling skills. Parent-centered programs may be criticized for being elitist, as it is only those who do not have to work outside the home who are able to devote the necessary time and energy required to raise a family which includes a hearing impaired child. The type of close working relationship which facilitates habilitation is most readily achieved when parents and professionals share common educational, social and cultural backgrounds, and have similar aspirations for the child.

The positive results reported from parent-centered programs contrast with those of studies reviewed by Moores (1978) where intervention did not begin until about three years of age and where programs were child, rather than parent, centered. Temporary gains also typified the outcome of child-oriented programs for disadvantaged children. In his review, Bronfenbrenner (1975) reported that enduring gains were obtained by children whose parents were viewed as the primary agents of intervention, and where the focus was on assisting mothers to interact verbally with their children while engaged in some joint activity.

More recent studies confirm the long-term benefits of programs which foster the development of strong mother-infant communication (Levenstein, 1979; Shipman, 1979).

Communication Development in
the First Six Months

Between birth and three or four years of age, the normal hearing child develops the ability to converse fluently in the language spoken by the family. Such communication involves the integration of auditory, vocal, cognitive, linguistic, and interpersonal skills. Of these, audition is the only one which is already highly developed at birth.

The infant's ability to perceive minute differences between speech sounds provides a powerful avenue for acquiring spoken language. On the other hand, the baby's vocalizations are sparse and undifferentiated. Smiles and coos from appreciative adults reinforce rudimentary efforts and lead to exploration of vocal capacities. Listening both to self and others, the infant develops increasing control over the speech musculature so that by about 9 months of age, the child is capable of imitating a wide range of intonated babble patterns. Such skill will be of great value as he begins to unravel the language he hears around him and attempts to approximate words and phrases.

Interpersonal skills can be seen to emerge very soon after birth. When a mother holds her baby and visually absorbs his physical appearance, the infant reacts in some way, perhaps moving his arms or legs, gazing at her face, or crying. In interacting with their tiny infants, mothers provide stimulation through all sense modalities. The infants hear their mother's voices, see their facial expressions, and feel their touch. Infants return their mother's gaze, move in response to their touch, and vocalize in response to their mother's voice. Such turn-taking behaviour is a prominent feature of mother-infant communication (see Anderson, 1979; Kretschmer and Kretschmer, 1979; for reviews and discussion).

Beyond the age of 6 months, cognitive and linguistic skills converge with auditory, vocal and interpersonal skills and out of this intricate background, spoken language emerges. The interaction of parent and infant becomes increasingly verbal until by age 3, about half of each partner's communication is verbal, while the other half is composed of non-verbal aspects (Ling and Ling, 1974).

A growing appreciation of the relevance of parent-infant interaction to the development of communication is likely to foster the drive towards identification of hearing impairment in newborn infants. Furthermore, increased sophistication of testing techniques is helping to make such identification a reality. However, such very early diagnosis creates problems as well as promises.

Problems Relating to Diagnosis
in Newborns

    Parental reactions to being informed of suspected or
confirmed hearing loss can be expected to vary according to
whether there was awareness that the infant might be born
with an impairment, whether the infant is a firstborn child,
and whether the infant has multiple anomalies and/or is
receiving intensive care. Parental reactions are also likely
to vary according to the prior life experience, general
approach to life, educational, socio-economic, cultural and
religious backgrounds and, of course, to personalities.

    When hearing loss has not been expected, parents may
suffer extreme shock when they are informed that their infant
does not respond normally to sound. They may refuse to
believe the diagnosis, especially when there is no visible
evidence. Alternatively, they may argue that hearing impairment is not a serious problem, that modern medical science
will provide a cure, or that a "bionic" ear can compensate
entirely for the problem. When the permanence of the loss
and the need for long-term habilitation are stated, some
parents may become quite hostile to the professionals who
have diagnosed the impairment, yet cannot effect a cure.
Other parents may be very practical and accepting, and ready
to take whatever habilitative steps are recommended. Such
action may, however, be a cover for feelings that they dare
not admit but which will surface in due course.

    In cases where parents have been prepared for the possi-
bility that their infant might be hearing impaired, the
shock of discovery is not so great, though the pain and
grief may be just as strong. They have usually hoped for a
"normal" child. Parents who are themselves deaf may also be
upset at the diagnosis as they, too, may have hoped for a
normal hearing child.

Firstborn Infants

    The diagnosis of hearing impairment in a newborn infant
who is a firstborn child creates special problems. The parents have not yet had a chance to adapt to their new role as
parents. They may consider this child as evidence of their
failure as a couple. They are denied the joy and pride of
showing off their baby for all to admire. When the diagnosis

is announced in the first week or so of life, before the
parents have had time to become strongly attached or bonded
to their infant (Klaus, 1976), they may reject him, at least
temporarily, and normal patterns of parent-infant interaction
may be disrupted. They may handle the baby mechanically and
as little as possible, rarely smiling or playing with him.

Multihandicapped Infants

        At the present time, since most screening programs are
directed at the at-risk population, hearing impairment is most
likely to be detected in newborns with additional problems.
Consequently, with the exception of those at risk because of
family history, infants diagnosed as hearing impaired may be
babies whose very survival is in question. Parents of such
infants may not be able to cope with yet another problem and,
thus, may resist habilitative procedures.

        In summary, the major problems relating to the diagnosis
of hearing impairment in newborn infants would seem to be:

1) extreme shock leading to the possible disruption of the
    normal parent-infant bonding process, especially with
    firstborn infants; and,

2) the difficulty of convincing parents of the serious conse-
    quences of hearing impairment, the benefits of an early
    start to habilitation, and the major role which they, as
    parents, should play in the habilitative program.

Such parental reactions pose problems for the clinician who is
eager to initiate habilitation. In contrast, when a child is
approaching 2 years of age, is not responding to sound, not
understanding speech, not beginning to talk, and is becoming
a behaviour problem, the need for habilitation is usually
quite evident to the parents and their behaviour less extreme.

        The foregoing discussion should not be construed as a
rejection of the value of early detection. Rather, it is
intended to stress the need for parent counselling, and to
warn clinicians against arousing false expectations. Early
identification, even when combined with an immediate start to
habilitation, should not be expected to prevent all the usual
consequences of profound prelingual hearing impairment. A
successful outcome will not be achieved simply by fitting

appropriate hearing aids, giving some advice on their use, and providing a few counselling sessions. The more severe the loss, the more detailed the guidance will have to be, and the more counselling the parents will require if they are to persist in helping their child over the long term. However, where early detection is linked with a comprehensive program of habilitation geared to the needs of the individual infants and their families, there is a greater chance of the child reaching maximum potential.

HABILITATION

A comprehensive habilitation program is one which responds to the needs of infants and their families. Examples of such programs are described in the literature (McConnell, 1968, Northcott, 1971; Elwood, Johnson and Mandell, 1976; Ling and Ling, 1978; Simmons-Martin, 1978).

Infant Needs

Parents may need to be assured that the needs of their hearing impaired infants are largely the same as those of other infants. In order to thrive, the infant needs to be loved and cherished, as well as being fed, bathed, and diapered. Because an infant requires the comfort of physical contact, it should not be left unattended for long periods. Babies are attentive to facial expression and should be encouraged to smile and vocalize. The hearing impaired infant's particular need is to develop effective communication with those in the immediate family. To this end, the child should be fitted with appropriate amplification to facilitate the development of residual hearing, the expansion of vocal repertoire, and the acquisition of spoken language. Full use of sensory modalities should be encouraged. Where appropriate, alternate systems of communication should be utilized. Such a decision should be based on the child's assessment by a team of professionals and in consultation with the parents.

Family Needs

The parents will require psychological support (counselling) to facilitate their adjustment to having an infant with
special problems and needs; factual information relating to
their child's impairment, together with extended discussions
of its implications; and guidance as to techniques which can
be utilized to help overcome some of the special problems.
The parents may also require help to balance the special
needs of the hearing impaired infant with those of other
family members (Luterman, 1979; Murphy, 1979). The parents'
personal needs should not be overlooked.

From Diagnosis to Habilitation

In a sense, habilitation begins during the course of
diagnosis as the several professionals involved interpret
test findings. In particular, the audiologist has a considerable role to play at this juncture (Northern and Downs, 1974;
Rubin, 1978; Stream and Stream, 1978). The ability to interact sensitively with parents may well set the tone for their
acceptance of the diagnosis and their willingness to consider
taking the first steps in the habilitative program.

A smooth transition from the diagnostic to the habilitative setting is important, especially where different personnel or agencies are involved. This can be achieved either
by one of the members of the diagnostic team accepting responsibility for habilitation, or by the habilitationist being
invited to observe and/or participate in some of the audiological assessment sessions.

Role Clarification

Clarification of the respective roles of the parents
and professionals is essential. It is evident that the parents are the best persons to provide direct help to the baby
since the development of communication skills is essentially
a full-time project depending on one-to-one relationships
available on a day-in, day-out basis. The clinician can
achieve very little in weekly sessions. Therefore, the
parents have to be helped to accept a primary role in their
child's habilitation. However, the professional should be
careful not to lay the entire responsibility on the parents,

especially in the very early stages when they are still in a
state of shock. The clinician should explain his/her role
(and that of other members of the management team) in undertaking an ongoing assessment of the child's abilities and
needs; interpreting test results to parents; providing background information about hearing, speech, language and
communication; planning an individual program (jointly with
the parents); and demonstrating techniques for the appropriate use of hearing aids and the development of communication.
The clinician also should be prepared to provide considerable
psychological support for the parents, either personally or
by referral to another professional.

Counselling and Guidance

     While the parents' need for counselling is generally
acknowledged, different programs have chosen to fill this
need in different ways. Some utilize a team approach with a
psychiatrist, psychologist, or social worker providing counselling for parents individually and/or in groups, and a
teacher/clinician/parent adviser undertaking guidance with
respect to technical and practical aspects. Alternatively,
the habilitationist may take on the dual role of clinician/
counsellor for most families, consulting with or referring
to a psychiatrist or psychologist when necessary. The
greater availability of information on parent counselling
makes such an approach more feasible than it formerly was
(Stream and Stream, 1978; Luterman, 1979; Murphy, 1979).

     The provision of counselling and guidance concurrently
can be especially helpful during the initial phases of habilitation. Counselling responds to parents' personal needs to
work through the stages of mourning (see Moses and Wulatin,
chapter in this text), while guidance related to the management of the hearing loss enables them to respond to their
child's needs and may alleviate feelings of helplessness.

     Parents can be encouraged to talk directly into their
baby's ear so that there may be a chance to hear the voice
and feel the breath stream. Parents can be asked to discover what provokes gurgles, coos and smiles, while holding
the baby face-to-face. The clinician/counsellor can demonstrate techniques relating to the use of hearing aids and the
stimulation of vocalization. Parents can also be asked to
observe and record their infant's responses to the sounds of

his/her own vocalizations (Ling, 1977). Evidence of progress
will usually create hope and lead to a reduction of pain and
anxiety about the child's future. The proportion of counselling versus guidance is likely to vary in relation to
individual needs, and from one session to another.

Guidance is not a matter of telling the parents what to
do and how to do it, but rather consists of explaining the
nature of the problem and working with them to find solutions
which seem appropriate for their particular infant and family
situation. When specific procedures are considered essential
to the child's habilitation, these should be explained
carefully.

Parents whose firstborn is a hearing impaired infant
may require more extensive counselling and guidance than
experienced parents. As new parents, they are likely to
feel insecure about many aspects of their child's development
and their ability to respond to basic, let alone, special
needs. The clinician/counsellor should avoid taking the role
of expert, but should aim to develop the parents' confidence
in their ability to help their infant. Because of their
daily experience with the baby, they will know how he likes
to be held, what makes him smile, when he is ready to sleep,
what position he is most comfortable in, and so forth.
Parents should be encouraged to respond to their infant as
an individual, and to be aware that some babies are quiet
and contented, while others are active and need lots of
stimulation. Most parents (and clinicians) will enjoy
Brazelton's (1969) book on this topic.

In the case of the multihandicapped infant, the
clinician/counsellor may have to help the parents to get
delight from the baby, and to see that he/she is cute and
lovable. The clinician should show interest in the infant's
daily development, empathize with feeding or sleeping problems, point out new achievements (e.g., holding up head well,
showing curiosity in new visual environments, grasping
objects, etc). The parents may need to be reinforced for
smiling, talking to and playing with their baby. Parents of
multihandicapped children will be especially appreciative of
frequent contact with professionals, either in person, by
telephone, or by letter.

The clinician/counsellor who becomes involved in the
habilitation of a multihandicapped infant and his parents
must be prepared for the eventuality that the infant might

die, and for the ensuing feeling of loss experienced by both
the counsellor and the infant's parents. Elisabeth Kubler-
Ross' (1969) book <u>Death and Dying</u> may be helpful. The person
undertaking habilitation has to be prepared to share the
sorrows and the joys experienced by the family. The counselling relationship involves caring and should not be
attempted by someone who wishes to remain detached.

The Young Clinician

     The young clinician may initially feel more comfortable
with technical and informational aspects of habilitation, but
insecure when faced with parents who are distressed at the
discovery that they have a hearing impaired baby. Little
progress is likely to be made, however, if the clinician is
not able to respond to the parents' emotional state. In my
view, habilitation depends on the development of a close
working relationship between the parents and the person providing guidance relating to the everyday management of the
hearing impaired infant. Moving outside the technical area
involves taking risks. In a counselling relationship, one
is offering oneself and consequently, there is the fear that
one might be rejected. The counselling relationship will
develop gradually as the young professional shows concern,
by both word and action, for the infant and the family.
Parents will respond to someone who shows a willingness to
listen when they are ready to talk about how they feel, who
is ready to share their problems, accept their grieving, and
respect their viewpoints. Considerable satisfaction is
obtained as the parents gradually come to accept the reality
of the hearing impaired and become able to take constructive
steps towards more active participation in their child's
program.

Continuity of the Habilitation
Program

     The long-term nature of the habilitation program should
be acknowledged by both professionals and parents from the
outset. An early start to habilitation does not cure hearing
impairment. To make the most of their potential, hearing
impaired children (even those with moderate losses) will
require special intervention throughout their school life.
The nature and amount of support services required can be

expected to vary from time to time and from child to child.
Parents, too, should continue to have access to counselling
and guidance services. In addition, parents have a continuing need to increase their knowledge in the areas which
relate to their child's hearing impairment.

Parent Education

        The concept of a spiral curriculum (Bruner, Goodnow and
Austin, 1967) has been utilized in the education of hearing
impaired children by Blackwell and his colleagues (1978) and
could be applied to parent education too. In the early
stages, parents can be introduced to basic information about
the ear and hearing, the nature and extent of their baby's
hearing loss, and the early stages in the development of
speech, language and communication. As the parents adjust
to their child's impairment, the clinician/counsellor can
help them extend their knowledge in such areas as audiological assessment, hearing aid technology, behaviour management
and/or whatever topics are of importance. The learning
process may involve reading, discussion, films, seminars,
and conferences. Informed parents are less vulnerable to
the loss of a particular professional and can contribute more
to their child's habilitation on a long-term basis.

Conclusion

        The drastic consequences of prelingual hearing impair-
ment and an increasing awareness of the important nature of
the infant's early experience have helped researchers persist
in their effort to diagnose hearing impairment in newborn
infants. Because parents tend to react to such early diagnosis with strong feelings of loss, which may interfere with
the development of normal parent-infant interaction, counselling is viewed as an integral and continuing part of the
habilitation program. To play an effective role, parents
also need guidance. A clinician/counsellor can help parents
in establishing rich patterns of interaction with their
infants and demonstrate techniques in maximizing the use of
residual hearing and expansion of vocal repertoire. In order
to foster enduring gains from early intervention, parents
should also be provided with opportunities to increase
their knowledge in areas related to hearing impairment. The
day-to-day needs of the family with a hearing impaired child

are being seen as being best met by a professional who is
able to offer a blend of counselling and guidance.

ACKNOWLEDGMENTS

This chapter is dedicated to the 1980 graduating class of
audiology, School of Human Communication Disorders, Dalhousie
University, Halifax, Nova Scotia.

DISCUSSION

DR. SUSAN MATTINGLY
    Many of us are in the position of working with children
much older than the 1 to 2 month age group. This is, unfortunately, I think, a process of diagnostic facility. Is it
your feeling, now that you've had the experience, that it's
any less difficult for a parent to accept a hearing loss with
these very very young infants from the very beginning, or is
it more difficult for them because they have not established
good maternal bonding?

DOCTOR PHILLIPS
    Well, I think it's rather hard to say that the parents
accept it more readily at one time than another. I think
that once the child has reached 2 years of age, there is no
doubt in the parents' mind that the child really requires
habilitation. However, they will still have to go through
the grieving process, even then. If you begin directly at
birth when the infant is only a few weeks old, then I think
you're in serious trouble because you may well break up the
initial building of a parent-infant relationship. Fortunately, I think, the diagnostic process doesn't work fast
enough. This does, in fact, give the parents and the infant
opportunity to get to know one another a little bit before
someone starts interfering and saying "you've got to do this;
you've got to do that."

DR. ANDREE SMITH
Because of the emphasis on counselling, and obviously, counselling goes beyond an interpretation of the results and how hearing aid works, I was wondering if you felt that we should include more formal training in counselling in our training programs in speech and audiology?

DOCTOR PHILLIPS
This is something about which I'm really very much concerned. I had to learn the hard way, on the job, and I know that when I started out as a teacher of hearing-impaired children, I was quite happy to dispense advice to parents about what they should do and how they should bring up their children. That was true until I had children of my own and discovered it wasn't so easy. But now there really is a lot of information available about counselling. I have recently taught a course in counselling to second year audiology students and, in fact, have dedicated my paper to them. I've found it quite helpful to encourage students to read quite widely in the area of human development, to read Elisabeth Kubler-Ross' book "On Death and Dying" and to make comparisons between that book and, say, David Luterman's "Counseling Parents of Hearing-Impaired Children. I do that as a means of trying to help students develop some kind of feeling, some kind of understanding for what parents experience. If the audiologist, in particular, does have or does develop real sensitivity, I believe that will make a fantastic contribution to the habilitation of the child and the parents.

DOREEN POLLACK
With reference to your comment about the problem in bonding in the early weeks, I had a rather quick feeling of anxiety last night when Doctor Mencher showed the results of the neonatal screening and there were over 100 babies who were brought back for retesting and a very small number were diagnosed as deaf. As a mother of children myself, I began to wonder - and I have wondered for a long time in my own neonatal screening - how I would have felt to be kept "on the hook" for several weeks with a newborn baby, wondering whether that baby had a hearing loss or not?

DR. GEORGE MENCHER
    Actually, of those 100, many were retested before the
parents were even involved. Our procedure is screening in
the newborn nursery, and failures go directly over to the
audiology center as a part of the routine hospital procedure.
So, most times the parents are not even involved at that
stage of the game, because we don't want to alarm them. Our
neonatologists have been very concerned about that. Our
parents are notified after failure in the audiology center.
Further, we do, throughout the entire screening, tell the
mothers that this is a screening procedure which does turn
up a lot of false positives. We also emphasize throughout
the entire program that there's no reason for parents to be
concerned until we get concerned. Nevertheless, your point
is well made. I have the same fears myself.

DR. PHILLIPS
    I think this is one of the big advantages of techniques
such as brainstem audiometry, which allow a firm diagnosis
to be made in newborn infants. When we undertook mass screening of newborns in the '60's, follow-up behavioural testing
was carried out at 1 month and often we were still unable
to confirm or deny a hearing loss. We certainly saw a lot
of agitated parents, and the pediatricians really became
very concerned. That was one of the reasons why we discon-
tinued screening of the entire population of newborn infants.
It just created too much anxiety.

REFERENCES

Anderson, B.J. "Parents' strategies for achieving conversa-
    tional interactions with their young hearing-impaired
    children" in A. Simmons-Martin and D.R. Calvert (eds.)
    Parent-Infant Intervention: Communication Disorders
    (New York: Grune & Stratton), 1979.

Blackwell, P., Engen, E., Fischgrund, J.E. and Zarcadoolas,
    C. Sentences and Other Systems: A Language and Learning
    Curriculum for Hearing-Impaired Children (Washington, D.C.:
    Alexander Graham Bell Association), 1978.

Brazelton, T.B. Infants and Mothers (New York: Dell Publishing Co.), 1969.

Bronfenbrenner, U. "Is early intervention effective?" in B.Z. Friedlander, G.M. Sterritt and G.E. Kirk (eds.) Exceptional Infant, Volume 3, Assessment and Intervention (New York: Brunner/Mazel), 1975.

Bruner, J.S., Goodnow, J. and Austin, G. A Study of Thinking (New York: Science Editions, Inc.), 1967.

Doehring, D.G., Bonnycastle, D. and Ling, A.H. "Rapid reading skills of integrated hearing-impaired children" Volta Review 80:339 - 409, 1978.

Elwood, P., Johnson, W. and Mandell, J. (eds.) Parent-Centered Programs for Young Hearing-Impaired Children (Upper Marlboro MD: Prince George's County Public Schools), 1976.

Goss, R.N. "Language used by mothers of deaf children and mothers of hearing children" American Annals of the Deaf 115:93 - 96, 1970.

Greenstein, J.M., Greenstein, B.B., McConville, K. and Stellini, L. Mother-infant Communication and Language Acquisition in Deaf Infants (New York: Lexington School for the Deaf), 1976.

Kennedy, P. and Bruininks, R.H. "Social status of hearing impaired children in regular classrooms" Exceptional Child 40:336 - 342, 1974.

Klaus, M.H. Maternal-Infant Bonding (St. Louis: C.V. Mosby), 1976.

Kretschmer, R.R. and Kretschmer, L.W. "The acquisition of linguistic and communicative competence: parent-child interactions" in A.T. Murphy (ed.) The Families of Hearing-Impaired Children. Volta Review 81, 1979, (Monograph issue).

Kubler-Ross, E. On Death and Dying (New York: MacMillan), 1969.

Lach, R., Ling, D., Ling, A.H. and Ship, N. "Early speech
    development in deaf infants" American Annals of the Deaf
    115:522 - 526, 1970.

Leckie, D. Language Skills in Hearing-Impaired Children.
    Unpublished M.Sc. thesis, McGill University, Montreal,
    1975.

Lenneberg, E.H. Biological Foundations of Language (New
    York: John Wiley and Sons, Inc.), 1967.

Levenstein, P. "The parent-child network" in A. Simmons-
    Martin and D.R. Calvert (eds.) Parent-Infant Intervention:
    Communication Disorders (New York: Grune & Stratton),
    1979.

Ling, A.H. "Changes in the abilities of deaf infants with
    training" Journal of Communication Disorders 3:267 - 279,
    1971.

Ling, A.H. Schedules of Development in Audition, Speech,
    Language, Communication for Hearing-Impaired Infants and
    their Parents (Washington, D.C.: Alexander Graham Bell
    Association), 1977.

Ling, A.H. and Ling, D. "Communication development of normal
    and hearing-impaired infants and their mothers" in Z.S.
    Jastrzembska (ed.) The Effects of Blindness and Other
    Impairments on Early Development (New York: The American
    Foundation for the Blind), 1976.

Ling, D. and Ling, A.H. "Communication development in the
    first three years of life" Journal of Speech and Hearing
    Research 17:146 - 159, 1974.

Ling, D. and Ling, A.H. Aural Habilitation: The Foundation
    of Verbal Learning in Hearing-Impaired Children (Washing-
    ton, D.C.: Alexander Graham Bell Association for the Deaf),
    1978.

Ling, D. and Milne, M. "The development of speech in hearing-
    impaired children" in F. Bess (ed.) Proceedings of the
    International Symposium on Amplification in Education
    (Washington, D.C.: Alexander Graham Bell Association),
    in press.

Ling-Phillips, A. "Habilitation of hearing-impaired children" in R.W. Keith (ed.) Audiology for the Physician (Baltimore: Williams and Wilkins), 1980.

Luterman, D. Counseling Parents of Hearing-Impaired Children (Boston: Little, Brown & Co.), 1979.

Manolson, A. "Comparative study of intonation patterns in normal-hearing and hearing-impaired children" in A. Rigault and R. Charbonneau (eds.) Proceedings of the 7th International Congress of Phonetic Sciences (The Hague: Mouton), 1972.

Mavilya, M.P. Spontaneous Vocalization and Babbling in Hearing-impaired Children. Unpublished Ed.D. dissertation, Teachers College, Columbia University, New York, 1969.

McClure, A.T. "Academic achievement of mainstreamed hearing-impaired children with congenital rubella syndrome" Volta Review 79:379 - 385, 1977.

McConnell, F. Proceedings Of The Conference On Current Practices In The Management Of Deaf Infants (0 - 3 years) (Nashville: Bill Wilkerson Hearing and Speech Centre), 1968.

McConnell, F. and Liff, S. "The rationale for early identification and intervention" The Otolaryngologic Clinics of North America 8:77 - 87, 1975.

Moores, D.F. Educating the Deaf (Boston: Houghton Mifflin Co.), 1978.

Murphy, A.T. (ed.) The Families of Hearing-Impaired Children Volta Review 81, 1979 (Monograph issue).

Northcott, W.H. "Infant education and home training" in L.E. Connor (ed.) Speech for the Deaf Child: Knowledge and Use (Washington, D.C.: Alexander Graham Bell Association), 1971.

Northern, J.L. and Downs, M.P. Hearing in Children (Baltimore: Williams and Wilkins Co.), 1974.

Rister, A. "Deaf children in mainstream education" Volta Review 77:279 - 290, 1975.

Rubin, M. "The Lexington program for infants" in S.E. Gerber and G.T. Mencher (eds.) Early Diagnosis of Hearing Loss (New York: Grune & Stratton), 1978.

Shipman, V. "Maintaining and enhancing early intervention gains" in A. Simmons-Martin and D.R. Calvert (eds.) Parent-Infant Intervention: Communication Disorders (New York: Grune & Stratton), 1979.

Simmons-Martin, A. "Early management procedures for the hearing-impaired child" in F.N. Martin (ed.) Pediatric Audiology (Englewood Cliffs, N.J.: Prentice-Hall), 1978.

Stream, R.W. and Stream, K.S. "Counseling the parents of the hearing-impaired child" in F.N. Martin (ed.) Pediatric Audiology (Englewood Cliffs, N.J.: Prentice-Hall), 1978.

THE SOCIO-EMOTIONAL IMPACT OF INFANT DEAFNESS: A COUNSELLING MODEL

Kenneth L. Moses
Evanston, Illinois

Madeleine Van Hecke-Wulatin
North Central College

Introduction

The hearing impaired infant has socio-emotional needs which can profoundly affect the development of language and cognition. These children face the same challenges to develop socially and emotionally as the hearing infant. Development in these areas is, however, less assured because of the effects of the impairment upon both infant and parent. A major difficulty experienced by parents is in providing the positive caregiving needed by their impaired infants, while struggling with the grief they feel as a result of having an impaired child. This paper focuses on how professionals can facilitate the grief process in parents, and so ultimately increase the parents' personal growth and ability to cope effectively with the challenge of parenting a deaf child.

The Social-Emotional Development of the Child

The newborn infant is, in many ways, in a primitive state. He has yet to learn that the cries he hears are, in fact, his; that the fingers which find their way into his mouth are fundamentally different from the breast or bottle he receives. The discovery of where his body ends, and the rest of the world begins, is yet to be made. His own basic needs -- to sleep, to be fed, to be held, to be warm -- are probably experienced as undifferentiated discomfort, just as being cared for is felt as being filled and satiated in a simple, total fashion.

The newborn infant seemingly has no expectations from our world. Somehow, from these rudimentary sensations and experiences, the neonate forms a conception of the world and the people surrounding him. The first task is to develop a sense of trust in that world, a feeling of security that one

is loved and will be taken care of (Erikson, 1963). The
establishment of this sense of basic trust is the primary
emotional task of infancy.

In addition, the infant will form its first affectionate,
meaningful relationship with another human being. The infant
will come to distinguish that person from others, to prefer,
to feel safe with, and to use that person as a secure base
from which to explore the world (Ainsworth, Bell and Stayton,
1974; Bowlby, 1969). The establishment of this close attachment to another person is the major social task of infancy.
The processes of developing trust and developing attachment
are entwined; both require similar kinds of interaction
between the infant and the caregiver, and both are partially
mediated by developing cognitive and perceptual abilities.

The Establishment of Trust

Erik Erikson (1963) describes the process that seems
crucial if the infant is to develop a basic sense of trust.
Erikson believes that the infant defines itself as lovable
through sensitive caregiving which occurs predictably. He
writes:

Mothers create a sense of trust in their children
by that kind of administration which in its quality
combines sensitive care of the baby's individual
needs and a firm sense of personal trustworthiness
within the trusted framework of their culture's life
style. This forms the basis in the child for a
sense of identify which will later combine a sense
of being oneself, and of becoming what other people
trust one will become.

Erikson hints at the cognitive changes necessary for the
infant to develop this sort of trust in the mother, and to
experience her caregiving as predictable and dependable. The
infant needs to develop "the recognition that there is an
inner population of remembered and anticipated sensations and
images which are firmly correlated with the outer population
of familiar and predictable things and people" to allow the
mother to become "an inner certainty as well as an outer
predictability."

Schlesinger (1972; 1978) writes on the impact of infant deafness and the development of this sense of trust. Such trust requires a "mutual regulation" between infant and care-giver which is predictable, and largely positive. On the part of the infant, this means the ability to link one's own behaviour to responses made by the caregiver. The infant needs to recognize that cries of pain lead to relief, cries of hunger to food intake, clinging to cuddling, and smiles to a reciprocal social response. Early infant deafness may make it more difficult for the infant to recognize this connection between self behaviour and that of the caregiver (Liben, 1978; Schlesinger, 1972). The hearing infant may perceive the warmth and nurturance of the mother earlier by hearing her voice and the sound of her approach. In contrast, the deaf infant may find it more difficult to see the relationship between expressions of distress and the caregiver's response. Moreover, deafness may lead the hearing impaired infant to organize perceptual input differently, making it more diffi-cult to perceive and retain patterns of stimulus change (Liben, 1978; Schlesinger, 1972).

In addition to those characteristics of the infant which might impair the development of trust, the mother's response to deafness in her child may impede her ability to provide the kind of positive mutual interaction necessary for trust. Mothers must resolve this crisis of parenthood to establish positive relationships with their children (Schlesinger, 1972). This entails a strong sense of self-esteem, yet the birth of an impaired child often has devastating effects upon parental self-esteem (Gordeuk, 1976; Meadow, 1975). Mothers resolve the crisis of pregnancy partly by anticipating positive interactions with the child after birth. The belief that the impairment will diminish such positive interactions generates grief and disappointment which may undermine the parents' ability to be emotionally available to that child. The parents of unimpaired children need cultural and familial support to cope with the demands of parenting. The demands of the deaf child are greater, and parents depend heavily upon professionals who are often perceived as not providing adequate support.

In sum, the infant's limitation and the caregiver's reactions to having a deaf child may impede the development of trust. These same factors may also disrupt the process of attachment.

The Attachment Process

Attachment may be defined as a "focused relationship of
one person to another that includes strong affection and a
mutual regulation of one another" (Yussen and Santrock, 1978).
Attachment requires, first of all, that the infant recognize
that the mother exists even when she is not present, and the
ability to distinguish her from others. The concept that the
mother is a permanent rather than transient part of the
environment has been termed "person permanence", and is akin
to Paiget's (1952) notion of "object permanence", in which
the infant gradually becomes aware that objects exist in the
environment even when they are not physically present.
According to Paiget, the development of object permanence
requires the repeated experience of the loss and reappearance
of objects. The deaf infant may experience difficulty in the
development of person permanence because of a primary reliance on vision, and is thus bound to the immediate environment (Liben, 1978). In contrast, the hearing infant who
recognizes the sound of the approaching mother before she
appears may have an advantage in forming the concept that
she exists, even when she is not in sight.

Similarly, the hearing impaired infant may have more
difficulty perceiving the mother as a distinct individual.
The infant learns to recognize and respond differently to
mother's voice, compared to other voices (Wolff, 1966). This
suggests that the hearing infant recognizes the mother as a
separate individual based on a composite of cues: her
physical appearance, voice, smell, etc. The deaf infant is,
in effect, deprived of one of the cues available to the
hearing infant, thus, possibly delaying the attachment process.

In addition to requiring that the infant be capable of
distinguishing a caregiver from others, secure attachment
also requires that the infant and caregiver experience their
relationship as reciprocal. It seems important that the
infant not only respond to the caregiver, but recognize that
she responds to the infant's crying, vocalizing, smiling and
eye contact (Bell, 1974; Lewis and Freedle, 1973; Lewis and
Rosenblum, 1974; Lewis, Weinraub and Ban, 1973). Playful
interaction with the infant has been found to be a powerful
determinant of attachment. Infants attach to those adults
who respond positively to their signals for attention, and
who engage in reciprocal play with them. Much of this playful
interaction involves early and frequent patterns of alternating vocalizations by the infant and the caregiver (Schaffer

and Emerson, 1964).

Similarly, the mother needs to be aware that the infant responds positively to her interactions. Changes in the maturing infant seem to facilitate the attachment of the mother to the unimpaired infant. Playful social interactions tend to increase as the infant matures, partly because the infant's demands for physical care diminish in intensity to allow more social responses from the caregiver. The new behaviours exhibited by the maturing infant probably elicit increased interaction. For example, by the third week of life, the unimpaired infant becomes attentive to the sound of the mother's voice and smiles in response to it. This, in turn, evokes a social interaction from the mother (Bell, 1974).

There are several implications for the deaf infant. Clearly, it is less able to perceive and respond to the auditory dimension of the infant-caregiver relationship. The infant's difficulty in recognizing the predictable patterns of response may also result in less awareness of the important reciprocal aspect of interactions with the caregiver. Moreover, the hearing impaired child may be less capable of eliciting playful interactions from the caregiver. Demands may not decline in intensity to the same extent or at the same pace as the unimpaired infant, and the child is certainly less capable of exhibiting novel behaviours in response to the caregiver's auditory messages. The parents of the hearing impaired infant may be so intent on using all verbal interactions as a training ground for language development, that they destroy the potentially playful quality of such interactions (Schlesinger, 1972).

On her part, the impaired infant's mother or caregiver may be less able to engage in the reciprocity which is the cornerstone of attachment. Her own emotional reactions to having an impaired child may make it difficult for her to respond as positively or playfully to the infant as she might otherwise. She may less frequently experience her interactions as having an effect on the child, interfering with her ability to experience the relationship as reciprocal.

The possibility that lack of infant responsiveness may disturb the mother's attachment to her infant is suggested by observations of the attachment process in unimpaired infants. Mothers whose tempermental infants were difficult to comfort, experienced a disturbed attachment to their infants (Robson and Moss, 1970). Mothers of hearing infants interpreted nonresponsiveness in their babies as intentional, and reacted negatively to the lack of responsiveness as though it had personal meaning (Brazelton, Koslowski and Main, 1974).

Implicitly, mothers may experience their deaf infants as being nonresponsive, thereby disrupting maternal attachment. The distress of even very young infants can be soothed by the sound of a human voice (Hetherington and Parke, 1975). Similarly, human tonal patterns and "speechlike behaviour" are extremely effective in eliciting reactions from hearing infants (Eisenberg, 1970). Mothers of children who had "talked" to them less at one year of age were more rejecting and less responsive to their babies' signs of distress during the second year of life (Clarke-Stewart, 1973).

Thus, many of the deaf infant's characteristics which interfere with an attachment to a caregiver may also interfere with the caregiver's attachment to the infant. Mothers of deaf infants appear to experience great frustration and feelings of incompetence as a result of the infant's unresponsiveness (Schlesinger, 1978). Thus, deaf children may be "limited or atypical participants in the social exchange with the parent" (Harris, 1978), leading to a disruption of attachment long before diagnosis occurs. In this regard, it is interesting to note that deaf children of deaf parents often seem to fare better than deaf children with hearing parents (Meadow, 1975), possibly because they are better able to establish the necessary mutuality.

In sum, the deaf child is challenged with the task of becoming "a part of life without hearing the sound-patterns of living" (Levine, 1970). It seems probable that this limitation on the part of the infant, and the repercussions it has on the caregiver, make the development of trust and attachment more difficult for both. These findings imply that the habilitation of the deaf infant needs to consider the infant-caregiver relationship and focus on parental reactions to infant deafness.

Holistic Intervention and Parent Counselling

Over the last ten or fifteen years, many habilitation and rehabilitation professions concerning themselves with children have become aware that one cannot treat a child's sense, function, or limbs in isolation (Friedlander, Sterritt and Kirk, 1975). Indeed, the concepts of the holistic approach have been generally accepted as the only way to successfully habilitate or rehabilitate children. The concept of working with a child's ears, ignoring the rest of that child's functions or developmental struggles, almost seems absurd at this time. Professionals have come to recognize the interrelationship between locomotion, vision, hearing, cognition, and social-emotional development in such a fashion as to understand that children, not functions, develop and grow. Such a conceptualization has had two effects upon the fields: to create interdisciplinary diagnostic and habilitation settings, and to broaden the scope of the training of professionals working with hearing impaired children. Such thinking has been the impetus behind both research and clinical application of the early intervention concept with hearing impaired children. Earlier intervention increases the involvement between professionals and the parents of deaf children.

Unfortunately, not all settings have yet incorporated holistic concepts of how a child develops and what is needed for a child's total habilitation. Professionals have quickly discovered that the necessary cooperation, as well as the attainment of such broad knowledge, does not come easily. Specifically, one of the areas of repeated concern is related to parent counselling; that is, the interactions between parents and those professionals who are primarily trained to work with their children. Generally, a primary stumbling block for the professional is the emotional states that many parents manifest while trying to deal with the impact of having a deaf child. Such emotional states are often a manifestation .of grieving (Buscaglia, 1975; Gordon, 1975; Kubler-Ross, 1969; Moses, 1977, 1979; Stewart, 1978; and Webster, 1976).

Hearing Impairment, Parenting and Grief

In the course of anticipating the birth of a child, parents generate dreams, fantasies, and projections into the future of who or what that child is to be for them. Such dreams are often of an extremely personal nature and hold much promise for the parents' future. The experience of anticipating the birth of a child is a primitive one that stirs people deeply. Unfulfilled needs, yearnings into the

future, wishes to have deficiencies corrected, and desires
to have fantasies maintained are often attached to who or
what that parent needs that yet-to-be-born child to be.
Parents are generally deeply attached to these dreams.

Grief is that process whereby an individual can separate
from someone or something significant that has been lost.
Grieving stimulates a re-evaluation of one's social, emotional and philosophic environment. Such shifts often lead to
positive values and attitudes. Grieving facilitates growth.
Without the ability to grieve, a person cannot separate from
a lost person or "object" and, thereby, in essence, "dies"
with whatever or whomever is lost. These people lose a
present and future orientation and focus only on the past;
that is, only on the "good old days" before they sustained
the loss. Grieving, therefore, is the catalyst of growth,
for with all growth, there is loss, and continuous growth
requires successful grieving.

Grieving is a primarily affective or emotional process.
The affective states are not epigenetic; that is, they have
no specific order; one is not a prerequisite for another,
and indeed, some can be felt simultaneously. Grieving starts
spontaneously and appears to require no learning. The effective states seem to be intrinsic, cross-cultural, and even
evidenced in some animals (Lewis and Rosenblum, 1974).

Most parents find disability to be the great spoiler of
their dreams and fantasies around who or what their impaired
child was to be for them. Most dreams require an unimpaired
child. Therefore, the initial diagnosis oftentimes marks the
point when a cherished and significant dream has been
shattered for the parent. It is that dream that must be
grieved. Unfortunately, the loss of the dream is such a
personal and illusive loss that few people concerned with
the parent of a deaf child understand the nature of the loss
sustained. Indeed, the parent oftentimes does not understand
that it is a dream that he has lost, and therefore, he is
frequently confused by the grief process that follows.

Successful grieving seems dependent upon significant
human interactions; that is, one cannot grieve alone. The
support that the parent of an impaired child needs to successfully grieve ofttimes can come from the professional who is
working with her child, as well as from her spouse, friends,
religious group, community, and/or parent organizations.

Unfortunately, many of the prevalent cultural injunctions evidenced in Western society are contrary to the spontaneous grieving process. The affective states associated with this process are often difficult to accept by both the grieving individual and by those offering support. Ironically, often the people that bereaved individuals need to facilitate grief, discourage it instead. Rather than accepting the denial, guilt, depression, anger and anxiety which are a natural part of the grieving process, those closest to the bereaved individual may view these affective states as psycho-pathological. They may respond with diagnostic labels, expressions of rejection, or behaviour connoting fear. Those wishing to offer support may fail to recognize that each of these affective states serves a specific function which allows the parent to separate from the shattered and cherished dream. The separation then permits the generation of new dreams which incorporate the hearing impairment, and then stimulates the emergence of the coping process. Understanding the value of the emotional states associated with grieving is crucial to offering parents the acceptance they need in order to grieve successfully.

(a) Denial

Denial is perhaps the first affective state seen in the process of greiving. Parents of deaf children deny in a number of different ways. They may reject the diagnosis itself, the permanence of the diagnosis, or the impact of the diagnosis. The parent who has difficulty accepting the diagnosis itself ofttimes argues with the professional diagnostician. This is the parent who refuses to accept what the diagnostician offers, thereby creating an atmosphere that can either prompt the diagnostician to feel insecurity around the accuracy of the diagnosis, or to feel some anger toward the parent. In either case, an adversary relationship may be the end result. The more polite parent, of course, does not confront the professional with denial, but rather simply does not follow through on recommendations or cooperate with attempts to habilitate the child.

Other parents who are denying the impact of the handicap rather than the diagnosis per se, might seem like ideal parents. Such people, in essence, say that they do not understand all the to-do about having a deaf child because "what's the big deal?" They might state that they know that special education has come a long way, that cultural

attitudes have shifted, and that, further, federal legislation has been enacted that offers support for parents of
impaired children and insures equal rights for handicapped
people. Professionals concerned with the field are quite
aware that deafness is, indeed, a "big deal" and that these
parents are likely denying its impact.

Perhaps the process of denial is the most frustrating
one for professionals in the communication disorder field,
because all evidence points to the efficacy of early intervention for child habilitation. To the professional, denying
parents might appear to be in a nonproductive, passive state,
which serves no positive function and often interferes with
parental cooperation in early intervention.

Denial is neither a random, purposeless state, nor a
passive nonproductive one. Denial serves a distinct and
important purpose. For individuals to function within an
environment fraught with danger, each person must establish
a mechanism that keeps him from believing that he is in any
real jeopardy. We cannot live day to day with the fear of
cancer, or death, or dismemberment, or with the fear of having an impaired child. Such fears would keep human beings
from functioning spontaneously. Therefore, most people have
within them a mechanism that makes them feel special and
invulnerable to the actual dangers about them. As a consequence, when something ghastly occurs, and many parents of
deaf children see having an impaired child as a ghastly event,
they are wholly unprepared to deal with such an occurrence.
Parents of impaired children need time to constructively
incorporate what has occurred.

That the denial process is not a stagnant state which
freezes parents into purposeless immobility, is evident when
one compares two parents, one whose child was born unimpaired
and one whose child was born deaf. The parent denying the
deafness would differ emotionally from the parent of the
unimpaired child. Denying parents feel distressed and
agitated (to the point often of experiencing sleep difficulties). They are commonly guarded in their interactions with
others. These behaviours are a sign that the denial process,
far from being passive, is an active process in which much is
occurring underneath the surface on both the preconscious and
conscious levels. The parent is accumulating information and
searching for inner strength, even while consciously fending
off the reality of what has occurred.

Parents of impaired children use denial to buy the time needed to find the inner (ego) strength and the external mechanisms to deal with what has occurred. External mechanisms might include acquiring information, skills and support from family, friends, organizations and professionals. If the denial process was assaulted, and the parent of an impaired child was somehow forced to understand the impact of what had occurred before having the inner strength and the outer mechanisms, that parent would collapse emotionally.

For early intervention to employ a holistic approach, the child must be seen within the context of a family unit (which includes the parents). To exclude the parents in the child's habilitation is like ignoring the influence of the child's auditory functioning on his cognitive development. Professionals working in early intervention, therefore, must be skilled in recognizing and facilitating the grieving process in parents. In particular, they must find ways to not merely tolerate, but to accept parental denial while still offering, to the best of their abilities, those services needed directly by the child.

Parents who are denying are not suffering from a logical deficiency, nor are they usually unable to understand what is being presented to them. An early intervention clinician can rest assured that there are many people telling the parent that he is stupid, destructive, inappropriate or shirking responsibility by denying. Instead, the parent needs someone whose attitude conveys an acceptance that embraces the validity of denial. Implied in the management or counselling of such parents is an avoidance of countless repetitions of the professional's opinion which leaves the parent feeling foolish, ignorant, illogical, or stupid. There are few people who are able to give denying parents what they most need: recognition that the individual is likely a loving parent who, for good reason, cannot currently engage actively in his own child's habilitation.

A case comes to mind of a parent who brought her 5 year old child for an initial assessment to a multi-disciplinary audiology center. With the support of other professionals, the audiologist determined that this child was profoundly deaf. Upon presenting this information to the mother, the audiologist met with strong resistance. The mother repeatedly claimed that the child could hear her name whispered behind her back. The audiologist decided to have the mother

demonstrate this seemingly impossible feat. The clinic was
in an old building with wood slatted floors. The mother
placed her child on that floor and then stood behind her, and
with one stamp of her foot, whispered "Mary". Responding
most adequately to the vibration in the floor, the child
crisply turned around to her mother with a smile. No explanation of how the floor vibrated to stimulate such a response
convinced the mother at that moment that her judgment was
incorrect. It indeed turned out to be a most frustrating
experience for clinician and parent alike, until the battle
was relinquished and the clinician could turn to the mother
and say:

> "It must be most frustrating for you to hear me
> presenting something contrary to what you believe.
> The idea of Mary being deaf seems almost imposs-
> ible for you to accept. Can you tell me a little
> bit about what it would mean to you if, somehow,
> my assessment were correct?"

Although the audiologist's manner of relating did not reverse
the denial, it did precipitate a long-standing, positive
parent/professional relationship. It is such a relationship
that.is as much a cornerstone of a child's habilitation as
are the actual "hands on" early intervention techniques.

    Since denial affords the parent the opportunity to find
the inner strength and the external mechanisms to deal with
having a deaf child, it ultimately ceases when the parent
attains such strengths. At that point, the mechanism of
denial will have served its purpose.

    (b) Guilt

    Guilt, as an affective state associated with grieving,
is generally the most disconcerting of the grief states for
both the parent and the professional confronting it. Parents
of deaf children might manifest guilt in any one of three
general ways. The first is evidenced through parents who
have actual stories documenting that they indeed caused their
child's handicap. Such stories often involve the taking of
drugs during pregnancy, the hiding of known genetic disorders
in the family, the contraction of an avoidable disease, or
other such occurrences that the parents felt were in their
control. This first manifestation of guilt is the most
logical, and the least common. Because of its logical

nature, it seems the least difficult to accept by the professional, although it still is disconcerting. The second
way that parents of hearing impaired children might manifest
guilt appears less logical. It is reflected through the
parents' belief that the impaired child is just or fair
punishment for some specific and awful action that they have
committed in the past. There need not be any logical connection between the nature of the past "transgression" and the
nature of the impairment. The third manifestation of guilt
common in parents of deaf children is of a de facto philosophic nature. This is reflected in the parent who basically
states, "good things happen to good people; and, therefore,
bad things happen to bad people". Such a general belief
leaves the parent feeling guilty simply because the impairment exists.

It is hard for many professionals to accept that so
painful and debilitating an affective state can have any
positive, growth facilitating elements. In the context of
grief, guilt is the vehicle that allows parents to re-
evaluate their existential beliefs. Seemingly each person
holds within himself a personal belief system that acknow-
ledges control over certain events, while allowing other
occurrences to be comfortably attributed to the whims of
chance. How and when one defines certain events as "his
fault" while attributing other occurrences to fate, is an
individual and internal process. The goal is to develop a
system that allows one to be comfortable with classifying
events as within one's own jurisdiction of control, or outside of it. It permits, in effect, avoidance of the absurdity
of assuming full responsibility for all life events, and the
equally absurd position of disclaiming any responsibility.
The guilt which parents of deaf children experience precipi-
tates their re-evaluating the parameters of their
accountability.

The case of a young couple exemplifies the professional
issue concerning guilt. Both spouses in this couple worked.
When their first baby was conceived, the husband encouraged
his wife to stop working. He argued that she was in strenuous
work with children who often times become ill. He went on to
say that women in his family never worked when pregnant. His
wife argued that she felt fine and saw no reason to discon-
tinue her work, especially since her work tenure and her
pregnancy term coincided.

She continued to work and was unfortunate enough to be one of the mothers who contracted rubella during the epidemic. When telling her story, she would plaintively present the idea that she had caused her child's handicap. Her child, indeed, was born deaf and brain damaged as a result of maternal rubella.

It is most tempting for professionals to try to explain to such a mother that her exposure to rubella was unpredictable, that she could have as easily contracted rubella from her next door neighbor's child as from the children with whom she worked. But logic is as ineffectual with guilt as it is with denial. Professionals in early intervention need to be aware that guilt does not yield to argument, cajoling, coercing, or even irrefutable scientific evidence. This mother's logical system was as viable as that of the professional, but within a different context. She might well have countered that her husband had accurately predicted what would happen if she continued working.

For guilt to be effective in helping the individual sort out why she has an impaired child, she must be able to share those feelings with an empathic, significant other. The professional who fulfills such a role might do so by offering acceptance through an attitudinal framework exemplified by the following possible response: "If you truly believe that you caused your child's hearing impairment, no wonder you feel so badly. Tell me more about it." The prevalent temptation on the part of most professionals is to try to take away the guilt. Indeed, parents will have many other people attempting to argue with them and "fix" the unfixable feeling. It will be the very exceptional person who is able to validate the legitimacy of the parent's feeling without seeming to confirm his judgment of fault. To offer such a relationship is to offer a unique opportunity that facilitates the growth.

Nothing will make guilt run its course more quickly than it needs to move. There are events, however, that can perpetrate this difficult phase. It is a significant other person that can make the difference. If the professional can accept guilt as part of a normal, necessary and facilitative process of grief, the parent will detect that and likely engage in a more substantial and ultimately constructive relationship with the professional. In contrast, the professional who views guilt as psychopathology, or who has a condescending view towards parents who manifest guilt, will impair the relationship between the parent and the professional. As guilt successfully offers the vehicle for the re-examination of the parent's existential values, it will cease on its own.

Incidentally, the manner in which the parent manifests the guilt often reflects the nature of the particilar handicap. Many parents of deaf children feel that their child's disability is a specific punishment in the area of communication (Mindel and Vernon, 1971). Again, it is the empathic professional who can offer the most to a parent presenting such a feeling. There is nothing to be cured or fixed. There is only an affective state to be facilitated.

(c)   Depression

Depression, interestingly in Western culture, is almost always seen as psychopathological. Although it is one of the affective states most commonly identified with grief, most professionals attitudinally relate to a depressed individual as being one who must be treated with special deference and care. Unfortunately, such attitudes are usually contradictory to what is needed by the parent who is depressed through grieving precipitated by the impact of having a deaf child.

For the purposes of understanding the processes of depression in grief, depression is defined as being anger turned inward; that is, anger toward oneself. This simple definition has general clinical accpetance, although the etiologies, dynamics, and characteristics of various depressions are obviously far more complex than such a definition might convey. Nonetheless, this definition is useful in understanding the dynamics of depression as a grief state. For what reason are parents of hearing impaired children angry with themselves, one might ask? The answer to such a question leads one into the area that depression serves; that is, the area of potency versus impotence or competency versus incompetence.

Parents can view their potency as existing somewhere between two extreme vantage points. One can feel that they were impotent to prevent whatever occurred to their child and feel anger toward themselves for their "useless impotent state"; or they can feel that they were always potent enough to have prevented what occurred, and, therefore, are self-enraged that they did not act before it was too late.

In the face of a negative and permanent occurrence,
adults in this culture are forced to re-evaluate the nature
of their potency and competence. Their personal definitions
concerning self-value and productivity become threatened.
Depression offers the vehicle that encourages this re-
evaluation. Depressed people assume the vantage point that
they are impotent, incompetent, incapable, and of little
value, given that they can have no impact on something so
close to them -- something that they want so very much to
change.

A woman who dramatically exemplified the dynamics of
depression was one who had always been the mainstay and
strength of her family. She had been through many struggles,
and had emerged as the support of everyone around her. She
was widowed fairly early in life, and left to raise her only
son. At age eight, that son became seriously ill with a
kidney disease that required the risky use of a potentially
ototoxic drug. Unfortunately, he was deafened overnight.
Months after this occurrence, this woman was feeling severe
depression. As it was an uncommon affective state for her
to manifest, the family became alarmed and alerted the professionals who were connected with her son. Upon interview,
she stated that she felt broken, that there was nothing left
within her, and that she was impotent to heal the affliction
that she found in the most significant person in her life.
She felt incompetent and incapable. The temptation on the
part of the professional to argue against such feelings is
powerful. One often wishes to point out to the parent how
much she can do for her child, that indeed she is the mainstay and center of her child's habilitation. Although such
statements may be true, they do not fit her perception of
this occurrence. To feel capable, potent, and competent,
this parent needed to feel that she could make her child
"normal" once again. This, evidently, was impossible and,
therefore, she saw herself as a failure.

It often takes special strength within the professional
to sit down with a parent who feels such depression and invite
her to share, in detail, the ways in which she feels incompetent. The professional might create this facilitative atmosphere by sharing an attitude exemplified by the following
statement: "Could you tell me more about the impossible
demand that you feel imposed upon you?" Indeed, the mother
described above found that such an atmosphere enabled her to
reassess her family image of being "the strong one", and to

see how that image only increased the pressure she felt.
From that vantage point, she was able to reassess her capabilities and also the attitudes of significant people around
her. Indeed, the feelings of depression became feelings
which facilitated personal growth.

It is at that point that the input from the professional
made a difference. Depressed people do not need cheering up.
They do not need someone to implicitly deny them the right to
feel depression. Instead, they need someone who will allow
them to feel the legitimate depression that they experience
and further, to be available to talk with them about how
impotent they feel. Unfortunately, most of us were taught to
relate to depressed people in ways which inadvertently leave
them feeling misunderstood, stupid, crazy, inappropriate,
and/or destructive, in addition to feeling depressed.
Depression is part of a normal, necessary and self-sufficient
process of grieving that allows parents to separate from the
dreams and fantasies that they have generated around their
child, and the loss that they have sustained around the
impairment. There is, indeed, value in "wallowing in self-
pity", and "crying over spilled milk". Since what constitutes
reality for each individual is reality as he perceives it,
life truly is "as bad as he thinks it is."

As parents are permitted to experience depression within
an environment of acceptance, they will likely re-evaluate
how they define competency. Such re-definition permits self-
acceptance in spite of not being able to "fix their child".
Again, it is the significant other than can offer the atmosphere facilitating this facet of grief.

(d) Anger

Anger (or rage) is an integral part of grieving. Each
person has an internalized concept of justice that permits
him to move within society and the laws of nature without
undue anxiety or fear of being mistreated. Such a conception
is flexible and changes with maturity. An unpredictable
event, such as having an impaired child, threatens the feelings of security around such a belief system. Whenever one's
sensibilities about order and fairness are disrupted, one
feels frustrated. Frustration, agitation, aggravation,
irritation, annoyance, etc., are all words that parents of
impaired children find on their lips at one time or another,
along with anger and rage. Long ago, psychologists noted that

frustration leads to aggressive feelings. Parents who are
frustrated by the birth of an impaired child, feel anger
towards the deaf child who has intruded upon their lives and
disrupted it in many realms. It is expensive, embarrassing,
time consuming, energy consuming, exposing, and shattering to
have a hearing impaired child in your family. On a more
psychologically primitive level, most parents feel that all
this disruption and pain has emanated from the child.

Since anger toward their child is considered heinous by
most parents, they often displace these angry feelings upon
others; most commonly, spouses, the deaf child's siblings,
and, of course, professionals. Such displacement of anger is
most unfortunate since parents are ofttimes in need of support
from the very people whom they may be alienating through their
anger. As an alternative, parents may direct their anger and
feelings of injustice toward God, science, or "the general
order of things". They may also find solace in directing
their anger into fertile areas concerned with methodological
controversies (e.g., oral/aural versus total communication).
This type of displacement can usually elicit empathic understanding more easily from the people around them. Yet, it
too, prevents the parents from confronting the real root of
their anger, which is the feelings towards the deaf child.

A note of caution here. Professionals are ordinary
human beings and, therefore, liable to make errors. Indeed,
there are some professionals in the habilitation fields whose
own personal motives prompt them to often behave insensitively.
Parental anger generated under such circumstances seems most
apropos and seems to have little to do with the anger that is
part of the process of grieving. Thus, not all anger represents displacement. It is parental anger that seems to have
no basis in reality and/or the prolonged maintenance of a
feeling of anger associated with a justified circumstance
that prompts one to become suspicious of anger associated
with grieving.

The function of anger within the grieving process is that
it allows the parent to reassess and reconstruct the internal
conception of justice which has been disrupted by the birth of
a deaf infant. The parent needs to maintain an internalized
sense of justice in the face of this traumatic occurrence.
Anger, like the other affective states of grieving, serves a
positive role in the growth of the parent. The development of
an internal sense of justice changes with maturity. Consider,

for example, what a teenager sees as being fair, compared to the more flexible and complex view of justice often held by a 40 year old. The parent of an impaired child who is able to incorporate the seemingly unfair circumstance of "having an impaired child without just cause", will have generated a new internal sense of justice which will allow him to cope competently with any future losses. Crisis and its concomitant disruption (in this case anger re: injustice), is the impetus for attitudinal changes that foster competency. The more reality-based one's inner sense of justice, the more competently one encounters life's unpredictable occurrences.

It is crucial for parents to recognize and deal with the anger they feel towards their impaired child. Professionals can help by accepting and relating to that anger when it is presented to them. That is difficult. Parents who are manifesting feelings of injustice in a general fashion are usually more easily accepted by professionals than parents who express feelings of anger toward their children. Professionals have often chosen the habilitation fields because of their sensitivities and their humanitarian attitudes toward people with special problems. Many professionals become quite attached to the children they work with and, indeed, recognize the illogical nature of parents being angry at their deaf children for having disrupted their lives. Nonetheless, this anger appears to be both a common feeling, and one that facilitates the grief process. Professionals who offer parents the opportunity to talk openly about their angry feelings towards their children are providing a kind of support which the parent rarely encounters.

Unfortunately, professionals are typically affected most profoundly by an angry parent, and may act in ways which do not aid the grieving process. The reaction of each professional often depends upon his own self-confidence. The more confident professional may become annoyed with the angry parent, sometimes countering with his own anger. In contrast, the less secure professional can become quite easily frightened by the angry parent. Such professionals are often thrown into an anxious questioning of their own competency, since the parent appears so dissatisfied and, indeed, might be vociferously questioning the professional's capabilities. In either case, the professional is unable to provide the sort of response to parental anger which would facilitate the grief process.

A description of a particular parent can serve as a good example of the anger engendered through grieving. This particular father was a technician in the electronics field, who himself, suffered from a moderate handicap (not related to audition). He knew the suffering that it had caused both him and his parents. As fate might have it, he fathered two children who had hearing impairments that required numerous interventions from professions (surgeries, therapies, special education, and prostheses). The etiology of the impairment was genetic in nature. This father held as a primary value (along with his wife) having a large family. It was very clear to him that the financial pressures he was already suffering, because of the services required by his first two children, prohibited his considering more children. He knew the blunt financial reality -- if he had another hearing impaired child, he would be bankrupt -- a very disagreeable prospect for this proud, competent man. As he saw it, life had dealt him a triple-headed blow: by giving him a handicap, by giving him "bad" genes that caused him to have handicapped children, and therefore, by depriving him of having the family of which he had dreamed.

He had become irrascible, critical, demanding, and generally resistive toward "habilitation" professionals. The school personnel feared him, and medical professionals fought with him. The status quo of parent/professional communications that included this man were strained at very best. In a group experience (that he had reluctantly decided to attend) he began to actively criticize and attack the group facilitator (after having passively resisted any and all issues for the first half of the process). He detailed all the ways that he saw such a group to be useless, and further, all the ways that he saw the facilitator to be a person who could offer very little. He went on to say that he resented participating in an "obvious waste of time", and that he, for one, was going to file a complaint to the administration that was responsible for the professional conducting the group. When the group leader invited him to share more of his feelings by asking him if he felt cheated and, if so, how he generally dealt with feelings of being cheated, the conversation became animated and ultimately moved into the realm of disability, fathering children, and his life dilemma. That conversation, in turn, stimulated discussions about fairness and justice that moved other people to talk about their feelings of being cheated.

This father did not change radically through exploring
and discussing his feelings, but he continued to come to the
group and never filed a complaint. Ultimately, he came to
successfully adopt two more children. In talking with the
group facilitator years later, he shared (with humor) that
his adoptions were his way of "beating the system". As he put
it, "you can't keep a good man down". He also shared that he
was no longer feeling anger indiscriminately, but that he had
channeled it in such a fashion as to become moderately effective in influencing local legislators to back legislation that
facilitated the handicapped and their families! It was
obvious that this man had grown in such a manner as to have
a remarkably different internal sense of justice. The anger
he had felt effectively prompted change.

It is the rare professional who will be able to recognize
that parental anger is part of grieving and warrants acceptance and facilitation. Yet if the professional can tolerate
the displacement of anger and/or the parent talking negatively
about the child, such an interaction would be facilitative.
Parents who are able to talk with significant others about
their anger are less likely to become "abusive" parents.
Abuse, incidentally, can range from overprotection (denial of
the existence of anger) to extrapunitiveness within a socially
acceptable context (for instance, the parent who structures an
almost inhumane environment to work on language development
every waking hour of the child's life).

If allowed expression, if seen as acceptable, if indeed
incorporated as part of the normal process of grieving,
parents of deaf children will come to use the affective state
of anger to restructure their internal sense of justice and,
thereby, will move to yet another affective realm.

(e) Anxiety

Generalized feelings of anxiety are evidenced by parents
of impaired children who are grieving the loss of a dream.
This anxiety is related to how one balances responsibility
for the welfare of another human being with the right to have
an independent life of one's own. This balance requires a
most personal and internal adjustment. The event of having
a deaf child disrupts this internal adjustment.

Parents often report their shock and dismay at being their child's own medical manager. The child seems so vulnerable; the professionals often send messages that reek of emergency; there are conflicting messages. There is so much to be learned, and so much seems to hinge on learning it properly. All this new pressure and responsibility is heaped upon the already existing pressures and responsibilities of daily existence.

A parent once aptly described this state of grieving as feeling like one is juggling an overwhelming number of precious glass balls. The feelings of responsibility are overwhelming and the temptations to become a professional parent of a deaf child are very strong. This opposes the alternate temptation to run away and feel terrible guilt and pressure for not having acted in a fully constructive fashion. All of those pressures and pulls create a circumstance rife with anxiety. Of course, the attitudes of professionals and other parents of the hearing impaired can strongly influence the amount of pressure that a given parent feels and the amount of concrete responsibility one believes must actually be assumed. In truth, however, definitions of responsibility are an internal psychological process.

Parents who are experiencing anxiety as part of the grieving process are in need of significant others who will be accepting of such feelings. It is not helpful at all to give a parent an injunction requiring that he "calm down". This is a period when calming down is not only impossible, but maladaptive, for the anxiety itself facilitates a restructuring of one's attitudes concerning responsibility. It is, therefore, also a time when realistic expectations need to be clearly spelled out along with an understanding that parents have lives beyond their hearing impaired children, and further, that an unwillingness to do certain habilitative activities is acceptable and not indicative of destructive or non-caring parents. An overstressed, overwhelmed parent ends up doing nothing, while appearing intensly involved with doing everything. A parent who can build within his system a comfortable space to minister to himself and permission to skip or reject certain aspects of the habilitative process, will, in the long run, be a more effective child growth facilitator. Often a professional's overzealousness in saving the child will frustrate the parent's ability to comfortably come to resolve the anxiety phase of grieving.

(f)   Grief Counselling

The grieving process as described, is an affective process that permits the parent of a deaf child to separate from
the dreams and fantasies that the parent cherished for that
child.   The inability to successfully separate from such a
dream is devastating to both parent and child.   If the parent
does not generate new dreams that the child can fulfill, then
each day the child will be experienced as a disappointment
and failure in the eyes of the parent.   This parental disappointment will ultimately be communicated to the child,
leaving the child feeling as though he is indeed a disappointment and a source of pain to his parents.   If, however, the
parent is able to separate from the dream, there is the distinct possibility that the child will be accepted for who or
what he or she actually is.   Such acceptance is an important
prerequisite of attachment.   Such acceptance is an important
prerequisite of facilitating emotional development and
growth.   It is within this context of attachment and emotional
development that the concept of facilitating grief becomes an
important tool in the intervention and habilitation of very
young hearing impaired children.

It is the role of the significant other, a role that can
be fulfilled by a professional, that can facilitate or frustrate the normal grieving process.   Professionals who have
negative opinions or difficulty with the affective states of
denial, guilt, depression, anger, and anxiety are likely to
become inhibitors of the grief process and, thereby, detri-
ments to the ultimate habilitation of the child.   The professional who is able to convey an attitude of acceptance
towards such affective states will have a positive effect
upon the parents' role in attachment and in creating an atmosphere for the internalization of a sense of security on the
part of the child.   Without this, children cannot go on to
develop in the other areas (for example, language) that are
seen as tantamount to the successful habilitation of a deaf
child.

There is no point in a professional trying to become "a
grief diagnostician", since the affective states previously
described do not go in any order, nor are they mutually
exclusive.   That is to say, people feel what they're going to
feel when they're going to feel it, and ofttimes have two or
more feelings simultaneously.   Moreover, an attitude of
acceptance aimed at facilitating grief would be damaged by an
attempt to diagnose a person's grief state, since diagnosing

is by definition, a process of labelizing.

      The grieving process is far from a one-time occurrence.
Parents of deaf children repeat and rework the affective
states associated with grieving, even as the child matures.
Obviously, all parents seem to experience it at the point of
initial diagnosis. However, each time the child comes to a
major milestone that impacts the parent in a new way, grief
will, once again, be experienced. Common developmental points
when grieving reoccurs, are:

1)   when the child becomes "regular" school age (for that is
     a time when much comparison between children goes on);

2)   when the child becomes pubescent (and offers all the
     dilemmas that puberty generally offers, plus the complex-
     ities of a handicapping condition);

3)   when the child becomes high school graduation age and the
     disability negatively affects his ability to move on in
     a more independent manner of functioning;

4)   when the child comes to an age where the expectation is
     that he or she would indeed live totally independently
     (working on his own, perhaps married, etc.); and,

5)   when the parents come to retirement age and the nature of
     the disability is such that the child might interfere with
     their retirment and requires that arrangements be made
     beyond the lives of the parents.

It is positive to note that success with earlier grieving
facilitates later grieving. Also, each new process of grief
brings with it new insights and new strengths which were not
previously realized.

     (f) Coping

      Since grieving is an almost entirely affective or emo-
tional process, it is clear that there are other processes
that occur simultaneously, or in tangent with grieving. The
general rubric of "coping" covers most of the remaining
activities that require interaction between the parent, the
child, the child's environment, and the systems that serve
him. Although much has been written since 1960 about the
coping process, the most succinct and clear descriptions and

definitions of the process were offered by a rehabilitation
psychologist named Beatrice A. Wright (1960). In her book
which focused on the psychological processes of disability,
Wright highlighted four major coping processes. Each of these
impact the parent in such a manner as to precipitate a change
in one's value system. The four coping mechanisms are as
follows: containing the disability effects, devaluing
physique, enlarging one's scope of values, and converting
from comparative values to asset values.

When parents first begin to deal with the impact of having a deaf child, their tendency is to generalize the effects
of the disability. They are prone to see the entire life of
the child (and often of themselves) as ruined. It is not
uncommon for parents to say things like: "My child will never
marry, my child will never work, or my child will be dependent on me for the rest of my life." They conceptualize the
worst, and then deal with reality. Confrontation with reality
is facilitated through the process that prompts one to contain the effects of the disability. Such containment is done
attitudinally. That is, the parent does not permit the
concept of disability to contaminate those aspects of his
child that need not be (nor are not) affected by the deafness.
The professional can be extremely helpful during this facet of
coping by offering as clear and concise an assessment (or
diagnosis) as possible, particularly, an assessment that
emphasizes the competencies and assets that are not affected
by the disability. Parents who can be exposed to ordinary
deaf adults are also helped with this coping process.

The devaluing of physique, as a coping mechanism, attacks
one of the more painful blocks to successfully dealing with
handicapping conditions. Western culture seems to place high
value on appearance, ofttimes judging people according to
what is seen. Unfortunately, most handicapping conditions are
seen as ugly. Specifically, "deaf speech", hearing aids, the
use of sign language, and behaviours unique to deafness, are
ofttimes viewed negatively. The coping mechanism of devaluing physique deals with this issue. "Physique" is broadly
defined here as any detectable manifestation of the disability which might be judged negatively. One has seemingly
successfully coped with the issue of physique when one had
adopted a value system that focuses on those qualities and
competencies we associate with being human, and ignores or
devalues surface qualities.

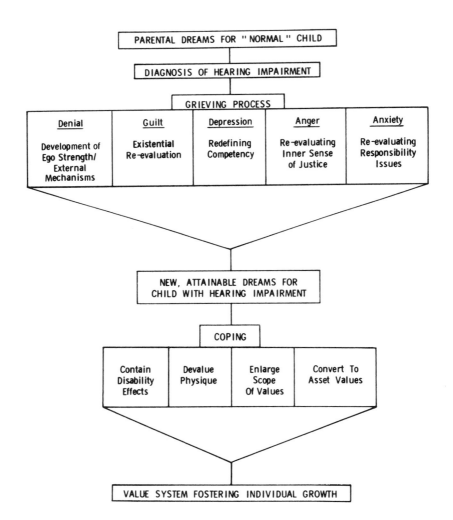

Enlarging the scope of values works on the premise that most people narrow their value system, experiences, interests, and associations as they age. This appears to be true for a great many people. Such narrowing poses a special problem when one has a deaf child whose disability precludes participation in the particular confined life style that the parents have chosen. If that is so, then to cope, thereby facilitating the child's growth, the parent must be able to enlarge his scope of values enough to genuinely accept whatever life style the child might persue. Such an exploration requires parents to examine their own values, often precipitating discomfort around what constitutes "the good life". If such coping does not occur, then both the parent and the child will feel as though the child's life style is, at best, second-rate and unacceptable.

The last coping mechanism involves the issues of comparison and competition. Western culture seems to put an enormous amount of emphasis upon winning, doing better than the next person, and comparing one person's performance to another. Such a comparative atmosphere can be uncomfortable for many non-impaired people. It becomes quite evident, however, that a comparative atmosphere is devastating to the impaired individual and his family. The parent must come to understand that how one does, compared with others, is far less relevant than the mastery of a skill or the demonstration of a competency. In the fields of hearing impairment, it is interesting to note that there are many measures (of a comparative nature) concerned with reading levels. Far less evident are measures (or even notations in reports) that speak to how the child uses his reading skills to enhance his everyday life.

The attitudes fostering these different views toward reading reflect substantively different value systems. The former emphasizes comparative values, the latter asset values. Ultimately, to cope with the child's deafness, the parent comes to value the child as he is, respecting each new achievement as an asset, without comparison to other children.

It is through such coping that the parent comes to primarily appreciate the child, and focus on the handicap secondarily.

Summary

     The growth and development of infants requires recipro-
cal interaction with caregivers to establish trust, and to
both initiate and maintain attachment. Parents are, most
commonly, the caregivers who can offer this nurturing and
stimulating relationship.

     The identification of deafness in an infant precipitates
grief in the child's parents. The process of grief can allow
the parent to constructively incorporate the emotional impact
of hearing impairment, and, thereby, cope with the demands
required for trust establishment and attachment. This, then,
allows the parent and child to engage in the many other tasks
concerned with growth in the context of deafness. Thus, the
successful habilitation of the deaf child is dependent upon
the parent's ability to grieve and cope. Professionals in
communicative disorders can have a powerful impact upon how
a parent traverses these important processes.

     It is the unconditional acceptance of denial, guilt,
depression, anger, and anxiety that constitutes the most
facilitative attitude that a professional can offer to a
parent: Such an atmosphere fosters parental coping which,
in turn, effects positive value changes which then strengthen
the competence of the parent, and facilitate child development.

     The parent who is actively gaining from the processes of
grieving and coping, shifts attitudes in ways best exemplified by the following parent's change around describing her
child: "I once could only see him as a deaf boy; now I see
him as a boy who is deaf".

DISCUSSION

DOCTOR IN THE AUDIENCE
     The most common cause of congenital deafness is genetics.
Many of these deaf infants have deaf parents. Would you
comment on that?

DOCTOR MOSES
       Often times parents who are deaf, who have a deaf infant,
deal with it better than parents who are not deaf, if,
indeed, they have worked through these issues for themselves.
The impaired individual grieves also and must cope in the
same fashion. If they come to accept their own values within
the limitations of the deafness, they are more likely to
accept deafness in their own children in more comfortable
fashion than those parents who are not deaf.

DOCTOR JOHN EADIE
       In many respects people "shop around" for a diagnosis
when they have a problem like deafness. Could you fit this
into your grieving process for me? Is it part of the
anxiety? Is it a sign that maybe things are getting towards
the end of the problem? How does this particularly affect
the deaf child and the parents?

DOCTOR MOSES
       It's an excellent question because this is, indeed, a
very common issue. I hear a bit of hope, "is the shopping
around indicative of the coming to an end" (I hope, I hope).
It's most interesting, we humans are terribly creative and,
therefore, just to confuse people like myself, we seldom
take a particular behaviour and have it be consistent to a
given grieving state. So that anything like "shopping" can
fit into any one of them. For instance, shopping around can
be denial of the existence of the deafness, and you're looking for a diagnosis that will confirm that indeed, it doesn't
exist. It can be undoing of guilt. "Now that I have this
child and I feel the guilt, I'm going to do everything I can
and shop the world over to undo the guilt." It can be
depression, a sense of impotence, and a sense of failure in
dealing with the impotence. ... I hope you're getting the
flavor of what I'm saying. We could go through all the
grieving stages and "shopping" can fit. Its effect upon the
child, of course, can be ghastly. I'm reminded of a family
that took a 12 year old, just pubescent, deaf daughter to a
psycho-surgeon in the Phillipines. A psycho-surgeon, if
you don't know what one of those is (I didn't), is a person
who does surgery by opening one's chest in a total septic
environment, without any anesthesia, and without any knife or
anything, just with their thumb. They find "yucky stuff" in
there that they throw away and that cures the people. Then

they close the patient without scars, and barely any blood.
Now that may be remarkable at first blush. Until, you decide
that it is total chicanery. It was written up, indeed, in a
book on quackery. They run their thumbs down and give the
illusion of opening the chest. They get some chicken liver
that they throw around a little bit, close up, and it works
very nicely for historical conversion reaction. However, it
does not work well for congenital, sensory-neural hearing
loss. The unfortunate thing, of course, was that these
parents took a very sensitive, just pubescent, adolescent
girl and had her go through this process, getting all the
messages that go with it. It's extremely difficult to find
the balance between accepting what a parent has to do, and
at the same time protecting the child. It takes, I think, a
particularly sensitive and empathic person to be able to
somehow send out that message that says, in essence, "look, I
know you as a parent have to do whatever you have to do, and
I respect that. But, while you're going through your struggle
to do what you have to do, let's also look simultaneously at
the struggle your child might be going through and let's see
if, somehow, we can find things that will work for both of
you." Perhaps taking the psycho-surgeon off the list might
be one of them.

MARY PAT MOELLER
    I wonder if you'd comment about the working mother. We
professional mothers are under some pressures from society.
I think when there's a deaf child, the problem must be even
more complex. I just wondered if you'd comment about that?

DOCTOR MOSES
    My wife is a working mother and, as some of you know, I
have a 2 year old impaired child - which was a bit of a sur-
prise after working in this field for over 10 years. There
is no place you are going to find a piece of research that
absolutely confirms what is the wrong thing to do or the
right thing to do. The types of complex things that one is
working with are as follows. Is it better for a child,
impaired or not, to have a mother out of the house, doing
what she needs to do, fulfilling herself, having a fairly
good quality period of time with the child, but one that is
very limited in terms of quantity. Or, is is better to have
more quantity, however, have a mother that feels thwarted,
perhaps resentful and limited? Well, which mother would you

like for yourself? I'd like a third option, if somebody
could offer it to me. The complexity becomes obvious. What's
often times being felt is the last area of grieving that I
was talking about, anxiety. Where each person has to - for
themselves, internally - restructure the limits of their
responsibility. To know how much you're going to cater to
yourself and how much you're going to cater to your child
and what you feel -- it's that redefinition (yourself within
yourself) of those issues of responsibility that must occur.

DOCTOR GEORGE MENCHER
     You referred to the fact that the child is also going
through a tough time. Is there any clue as to at what stage
the child becomes aware of the fact that it is, in fact,
different than the other people around it? Does it go through
the same kinds of grieving and adjustment patterns that the
parents do?

DOCTOR MOSES
     The last part I can answer quickly. Yes, the child goes
through exactly the same kinds of processes. Incidentally,
their displacement of anger is often times at the parent.
"How could you do this to me? Why didn't you save me? Why
did you have me if I was going to be this way?" That's a
real zinger. After you struggle for a number of years to get
a kid language, that's what comes out with the language!

     There is no specific point at which we can specifically
say, that, the "child" is aware of his differences. It
depends obviously, on how much the child is going out into
the environment, getting the feedback that other people
perceive a difference. One of the points when that seems to
happen fairly commonly is at entering school. So that, if
you haven't seen it in a child by around age 5 or 6, you're
likely to start to see it then. Often times you will get it
with very angry stories, or very angry jokes. It will come
out indirectly. Hostile jokes toward hearing people, making
fun of the hearing, etc. That can come as early as 5 or 6.
It does not come until the child is confronted with the
culture, and the culture begins to do terribly mean and
rejecting types of things that make them feel different.
Before that they're perfectly happy, the parents are not.

ANDRE LAFARGUE
    I was wondering if you could give us some idea how much
time you would allow for those stages. For instance, I'm
thinking of a case of a parent whose child has been diagnosed
as having a hearing problem and before action can be taken on
behalf of the child, how much time would you allow the parents
to go through that denial, or whatever stages ... .

DOCTOR MOSES
    I'm very pleased that you asked that question, because I
think that there's a thought in there that you implied from
what I said that I did not intend. I do not think that action
should be delayed 2 minutes. I think that you have a responsibility as a professional to do what you feel is correct,
and to continue doing it. I'm merely asking you to do it
sensitively, without rejection of what the parents feel and
how the parent deals with it. There is no "fixed" time
because there are a number of very complex variables included.
How significant is this loss to the parent? Has the parent
previously had a significant loss and successfully grieved it?
What is the support system around the parent to facilitate
grieving? Does it inhibit it, or does it facilitate it? etc.,
those things will have more to do with how long it takes than
anything else. But people do become arrested, and an arrest
is not so much identifiable with time as it is with the
quality of grieving. A person who's arrested is stagnant.
There's a dead quality to them. A person who is grieving is
active and affects the people interacting with them - either
moves them emotionally, or you want to get away from them
because they disturb and frighten you. If that's going on,
you've got a person who's actively grieving, they're not
stuck. If the person you're working with does not affect
you, and yet they're saying things you think would, you've
got a person whose arrested.

REFERENCES

Ainsworth, M.D.S., Bell, S.M. and Stayton, D.J. "Infant-
mother attachment and social development: Socialization
as a product of reciprocal responsiveness to signals,"
in Richards, M.P.M. (ed.) The Integration of a Child into
a Social World (New York: Cambridge University Press),
1974.

Arnold, L. Eugene (ed.) Helping Parents Help Their Children
(New York: Brunner/Mazel), 1978.

Bell, R.Q. "Contributions of human infants to caregiving and
social interaction," in Lewis, M. and Rosenblum, L. (eds.)
The Effect of the Infant on Its Caregiver (New York: John
Wiley & Sons), 1974.

Bowlby, J. Attachment and Loss (Volume I) (New York: Basic
Books), 1969.

Brazelton, T.B., Koslowski, B. and Main, M. "The origins of
reciprocity: The early mother-infant interaction," in
Lewis, M. and Rosenblum, L. (eds.) The Effect of the Infant
on Its Caregiver (New York: John Wiley & Sons), 1974.

Brody, S. and Axelrod, S. "Maternal stimulation and social
responsiveness of infants," in Lewis, M. and Rosenblum, L.
(eds.) The Effect of the Infant on Its Caregiver (New York:
John Wiley & Sons), 1974.

Buscaglia, Leo. The Disabled and Their Parents: A Counselling Challenge (Thorofare, New Jersey: Charles B. Slack),
1975.

Clarke-Stewart, A.K. "Interactions between mothers and their
young children: Characteristics and consequences,"
Monographs of the Society for Research in Child Development, 1973.

Eisenberg, R.B. "The development of hearing in man: An
assessment of current status," American Speech and Hearing
Association Journal, 12:119 - 123, 1970.

Erickson, E.H. Childhood and Society (Second Edition) (New
York: Norton), 1963.

Friedlander, B.Z., Sterritt, G.M. and Kirk, S.G. (eds.)
Exceptional Infant -- Assessment and Intervention (Volume
3) (New York: Brunner/Mazel), 1975.

Gordeuk, A. "Motherhood and a less than perfect child: A
literary review," Maternal Child Nursing Journal, 5:57 -
68, 1976.

Gordon, Sol. Living Fully: A Guide for Young People with a
Handicap, Their Parents, Their Teachers and Professionals
(New York: John Day Co), 1975.

Harris, A.E. "The development of the deaf individual and the
deaf community," in Liben, L.S. (ed) Deaf Children:
Developmental Perspectives (New York: Academic Press),
1978.

Heatherington, E.M. and Parke, R.D. Child Psychology (New
York: McGraw-Hill), 1975.

Kubler-Ross, Elisabeth. On Death and Dying (New York:
Macmillan Publishing Co.), 1969.

Levine, E.S. Youth in a Soundless World (New York: New York
University Press), 1956.

Levine, E.S. The Psychology of Deafness (New York: Columbia
University Press), 1960.

Lewis, M. and Freedle, R. "Mother-infant dyad: The cradle
of meaning," in Pliner, P., Krames, L. and Alloway, F.
(eds.) Communication and Affect: Language and Thought
(New York: Academic Press), 1973.

Lewis, M. and Rosenblum, L.A. The Effect of the Infant on Its
Caregiver (New York: John Wiley & Sons), 1974.

Lewis, M., Weinraub, M. and Ban, P. "Mothers and fathers,
girls and boys: Attachment behavior in the first two years
of life." Paper presented at the meeting of the Society
for Research in Child Development, Philadelphia, March,
1973.

Liben, L.S. "Experiential deficiencies: Developmental perspectives," in Liben, L.S. (ed.) Deaf Children: Developmental Perspectives (New York: Academic Press), 1978.

Meadow, K.P.   "The development of deaf children," in
    Hetherington, E.M. (ed.) Review of Child Development
    Research (Volume 5), 1975.

Mindel, E. and Vernon, M.   "They grow in silence -- The deaf
    child and its family," National Association of the Deaf,
    Silver Springs, Maryland, 1971.

Moses, K.   "Effects of Developmental Disability on Parenting,"
    in Rieff, M. (ed.) Patterns of Emotional Growth in the
    Developmentally Disabled Child (Morton Grove, Illinois:
    Julia S. Molloy Education Centre), 1977.

Paiget, J.   The Origins of Intelligence in Children (Cook, M.,
    Translator) (New York: International Universities Press),
    1952.

Robson, K.S. and Moss, H.A.   "Patterns and determinants of
    maternal attachment," Journal of Pediatrics 77:976 - 985,
    1970.

Schaffer, H.R. and Emerson, R.E.   "The development of social
    attachments in infancy," Monographs of the Society for
    Research in Child Development, 1964.

Schlesinger, H.S.   "A developmental model applied to problems
    of deafness," in Schlesinger, H.S. and Meadow, K.P. (eds.)
    Sound and Sign (Berkeley: University of California Press),
    1972.

Schlesinger, H.S.   "The effects of deafness on childhood
    development: An Eriksonian perspective," in Liben, L.S.
    (ed.) Deaf Children: Developmental Perspectives (New York:
    Academic Press), 1978.

Stewart, Jack C.   Counselling Parents of Exceptional Children
    (Columbus, Ohio: Charles E. Merrill Publishing Co.), 1978.

Webster, Elizabeth J.   Professional Approaches with Parents
    of Handicapped Children (Springfield, Illinois: Charles C.
    Thomas), 1976.

Wolff, P.H.   The Causes, Controls and Organization of Behav-
    ior in the Neonate (New York: International Universities
    Press), 1966.

Wright, Beatrice A. Physical Disability: A Psychological
    Approach (New York: Harper & Row), 1960.

Yussen, S.R. and Santrock, J.W. Child Development (Dubuque,
    Iowa: William C. Brown Co.), 1978.

THE MEXICAN APPROACH TO EARLY MANAGEMENT

Enelda Luttman
Orientacion Infantil Par Rehabilitation Audiologica, Mexico City, Mexico

How many children have we had under a year of age at OIRA in Mexico? Far too few, yet these few have been an eye opener and a delight. How essential it is to have more, to have the opportunity of starting work with the hearing impaired under one year of age. We have had a larger amount up to 18 months, which is still within the limits of the optimum period of growth in a child's development.

All and every one of these babies have, practically overnight, shown an undreamed of awakening. Not only were they insensitive to sound, but seemed to be delayed in all other sense modalities and skills that can be expected in the other infants of the same age. It is thrilling to see how quickly they respond to the reception of sound, thanks to the use of amplification.

What is more amazing is the effect the use of binaural amplification has on these infants. We attribute the day-to-day changes, the responses of the child, the growth of skills, the awakening to consciousness of the surrounding environment and to self, to the auditory input and stimulation received for the first time through the hearing aid. It convinces us what an important and vital sense hearing is. Advancement and progress starts with the use of amplification and the parents' active participation with, and correct stimulation of the baby. What else could account for the remarkable changes we see in our children? Everyone who observes these hearing impaired youngsters after several years of their specialized auditory therapy remarks that it seems as though we only receive children at our centre with a high IQ.

What a terrible handicap a hearing loss is. But we now know, thanks to the recent work of research psychologists, that constant stimulation from the mother during daily activities with the baby (e.g., singing, playing, dressing, bathing, feeding; and always talking, with constant verbalizing related to the activities and situations as they are taking place) not only helps the child catch up to the newborn who

279

hears, but stimulates all other aspects of the baby's
development. The advancement and progress observed is
breath-taking. How simplified and how logical every effort
and activity appears, once consciousness is drawn to the need
to supply stimulation and provide a normal auditory
environment.

The experts tell us how important the first 18 months of
life are to the human. They tell how the whole child's
potential can be enforced. What an unbelievable degree of
progress and learning the human child is capable of during
the first year of life. It is a level never to be proportion-
ately matched at any other period in ensuing growth.

From the actual birth day, a baby is active and alert
and development progresses in leaps and bounds.

Today we can tabulate what can be achieved. We know
what far reaching goals can be sought, what incredible
heights can be reached in later development and maturation,
if the first year of life offers adequate opportunities for
learning, stimulation, and encouragement to mental and
physical development.

At one time, the general belief was that the first year
of life was quite insignificant. That is, little or no learning took place before, say, two years. The baby is helpless
and dependent and, therefore, it is just wasted time to consider that any advancement of note can be developed or
achieved. And further, what in the world could you tell a
mother to do!

It is only within the last few years that the fundamental beliefs concerning an infant's development have changed.

The infant is born with survival skills. The ability to
suck appears generally before birth and is always present at
birth. With stimulation, this skill develops fully.

Researchers have demonstrated that most of the genetic
capacities of human beings develop or are activated only if
the correct stimulation is offered. There has to be a responsive environment or reflexes will disappear because of a
lack of stimulation.

It is absolutely essential that the parents of any infant know how important and vital the first year of life is, and that if the correct or appropriate stimulation for the development of cognitive abilities are not given, their child will become handicapped. The attitude of the parents toward the child is of great importance. The child's development can be hampered or encouraged by the parents' attitude.

Parents must be cognizant of the child's capabilities. Parents should be meticulously guided and should be given demonstrations of how to facilitate their own child's growth and development.

If this is so with all infants, how much more damaging and disastrous the lack of stimulation to a child born with a hearing impairment.

A child born hearing is able to detect the rhythms of speech and discriminate between music and speech sounds at birth. Responses to new sounds are by heartbeat deceleration. That response habituates easily. Shortly after birth, the child will respond only to new and different sounds, indicating a learning capacity. At two months of age, the baby can discriminate between "b" and "d", and shows preference to happy voices as opposed to angry ones.

Research psychologists have demonstrated that infants can be taught to choose between colors or sounds within the first few hours of life. Condon and Sander (1976) showed that babies modify their rhythm of thrashing to match the rhythm of voice.

A baby's communication starts early. It emits basic cries which the observant mother soon learns to interpret by the quality and tone of the cry. She relates a particular sound to the child's needs (e.g., stomach ache, frustration, anger, pain, hunger, joy.) Therefore, it seems that the only logical thing to do if the child is born with a hearing loss, is to supply the infant with binaural amplification, thus providing auditory input as soon as the loss is detected. As a result, the child loses as little time as possible in covering the normal sequence of development of listening, language, and speech skills. Specialists indicate there is an optimum period for learning or enforcing skills and, if the child is not stimulated and those skills used at the appropriate time, it is a much more complicated and difficult

task to learn later, and the child will probably never be as
well developed.

By 7 - 9 months, all normal infants move from sensory-
motor intelligence to intelligence influenced by language.
It is for this reason that it is hard before that age to
depict the IQ potential. The tests utilized with children
that young are based mostly on learning names for things.

At 10 - 12 months, the baby's understanding of language
is based on pitch, intonation and stress. A parent of a hearing impaired baby should be aware of using much vocal expression and intonation, stressing these qualities and utilizing
a voice with inflexion.

An infant has great capacity for learning and memory.
Old behaviour is used by the infant to develop new. New
behaviours depend upon the maturation of the central nervous
system and the physiological state of the child.

In our experience in Mexico, most, if not all, of the
hearing impaired babies of one year or less we have had the
fortune to know and help guide, have had a severe or profound
loss and parents in the higher educational and socio-economic
level. Invariably it has been the parents themselves who
have persisted and not been satisfied with the doctor's
suggestions to wait. Unfortunately, we are heartbroken to
have a much larger list of parents who did not hear of OIRA
or the Auditory Approach when deafness was first suspected
and later confirmed. They and their children lost precious
time investigating what to do and where to go. They, and I,
personally, cannot forgive the specialists for misinforming
or not caring enough to guide the parents correctly. Sometimes it is lack of knowledge. In this day and age, this
should not be. Doctors and other specialists easily forget,
unless constantly reminded, how essential correct help and
guidance is for parents. Habilitation should commence
immediately that habilitation is possible.

In most cases, the parents are young and emotionally
very unhappy and disturbed. Their high aspirations for their
offspring, their dreams and hopes for a better life, if
possible even higher goals than their own, seem shattered.
What deafness is, what it means, how much of a handicap it
can be, is still not clear. Few have had the experience of
knowing a deaf person. We have had various families whose
first child was hearing impaired, and then have had subsequent

offspring born with hearing defects.   Those younger children,
therefore, had the advantage of commencing habilitation
earlier.   However, the blow of realising that deafness is an
hereditary impediment is often a shock that some parents find
hard to face.   Though they are conscious of, or suspect a
hearing impairment, accepting it as a fact is such a night-
mare that the onset of habilitation becomes postponed.

The Initial Interview

        The first interview with a parent is very important.   It
is advisable that the individual who conducts the introductory
interview be experienced, self assured and well informed
about the techniques of the auditory oral approach, child
development, and infant care.   The person should be genuinely
dedicated to, and deeply interested in, the habilitation of
the hearing impaired.   It can be of help to have been a mother
oneself, but most certainly, the interviewer should be fully
aware and knowledgeable about infant care and development and
the importance of the parents' role.

        If possible, there should be a comfortable private room
from which outside interference can be excluded.   The room
should not be somber.   It should have happy colours, flowers
in a vase, good pictures, curtains which let in the light but
allow for privacy, and it should have a carpeted floor for
warmth and comfort.   Toys of various types should be kept on
a low shelf easily accessible to the child.   A box of tissues
should be provided in easy reach of the parents.

        A few direct questions often help the parents come to
the point.   It is hard to have the courage to state, without
breaking down and appearing a fool, "I suspect, or know, that
my child is deaf."   It is important that the interviewer
should be relaxed, appear to have plenty of time to listen to
and talk with the parents, and be able to encourage them to
tell as much as they can.   It is important to determine what
they know about when deafness was first suspected, by whom,
how, and what they did about it.   How did they feel, and what
have they done up to now are important questions.   What does
deafness signify to them?   If they have already been through
an audiometric evaluation and confirmation of loss, they are
obviously more informed.   Usually if the baby is very young

and assessment is missing, it is important to explain what a
hearing impairment is and why something should be done about
it right away. Very often it has to be clarified that, though
a child seems to hear certain ambient sounds when loud enough
and near, this still would not guarantee enough hearing for
the reception of voice and speech sounds and, ultimately, for
speech development.

It is crucial to stress how important the time element
is and to explain why every day lost has a very strong impact
on the baby's facility for learning and developing good
auditory verbal communication. One needs to stress that a
child will not learn to speak if he does not hear, therefore,
it is essential that he should have amplification so that he
can hear and learn to listen. Parents need to know immediately how important the first year of life is, and why. They
need to know that responsibility for the habilitation is
basically theirs, but shared and guided by specialized therapists on a one-to-one basis. It is a team approach, but the
fulfillment of everyday stimulation and development is in
their hands. It should be carried out, throughout the day,
in the natural home environment and amongst the family members,
with later stimulation through attendance in regular kindergarten and regular school. It is important to show confidence
in the prognosis if the basic requirements are carried out.
The parents must have full consciousness of what is being done
and why it is important. The specialized teacher will guide
and suggest according to the needs of the child at the present time, helping the mother modify activities according to
the progress of development and personal requirements.

At the very beginning, too much information can be confusing and can make a mother depressed. This is particularly
true if one stresses too many future activities. The important thing is to show confidence in the mother and her capability to carry out what is expected of her and what is, in
fact, her rightful responsibility. Also, it is important to
show confidence in the child's future and treat him as
"unique".

It is helpful to enquire about the siblings, how they
were brought up and what are the customs and ways of life and
type of home for this particular family. In Mexico we have
such a varied difference amongst the social classes that the
socio-economic and educational status is important to know.

It is necessary to learn how much knowledge the mother has in child care; how she looked after her other babies; how old they are; what developmental level they have reached; and, how close to the "norm" they are. Invariably one finds that a great deal of guidance can be given which will also prove helpful to the siblings of the hearing impaired child.

Initial Management Sessions

The first sessions should concentrate on establishing good rapport with the parents and learning as much as possible about the family, their way of life, their outlook, and their expectations. Comments made during the course of the conversation may clarify their misconceptions or queries. The main objective of the interviewer/therapist is to give to the family definite guidelines, a positive attitude, and an optimistic prognosis based on their fulfillment of basic requirements.

The importance of taking advantage of the great learning capacity of the first year of life, which will never again be equalled, cannot be stressed too strongly. The mother needs to be told that she must always be cognizant of:

1) the current level of the child's development;

2) which steps have already been reached;

3) which areas must be stimulated to bring the child up to par; and,

4) how to help the child in those areas where there might be delay.

It should be explained that when a hearing handicapped child receives amplification for the first time, he is at the level of a newborn - just starting to learn to listen. So, we know where to start and what activities the mother should devise to stimulate listening skills. It should be indicated to the mother that she will learn through demonstration and active participation with her child. The object of the individual therapy session is to teach her and to suggest pertinent activities by re-enforcing the known and introducing the new (roughly at a quota of 90% learned to 10% new). The mother's information will progress with the child's progress. She will always know where she is heading and why, what the

next steps up the developmental ladder are and that it is
detrimental to try and skip any step. The therapist must
often help the parent become comfortable with the child.

The parent should understand that deafness is only one
aspect, that the needs and requirements of the whole child
have to be met.

It is important that the parent understand that the constant use of a proper functioning hearing aid throughout the
child's waking hours is essential. For a child to learn
aurally, he has to be hearing repeatedly. This mechanical
device will aid and supplement residual hearing. Alone,
without the correct stimulation, the child will not learn to
listen and process language. The parent must understand
that her child has to follow the same steps a normal child
has had to cover. We know babies hear at birth, but they
have to learn to listen, to identify sounds, and to relate to
sounds which are meaningful to them. They will learn them
and memorize their characteristics by hearing them often. A
hearing handicapped child will have to hear so much more
often to retain that memory.

The mother must consciously learn to talk to her child
in short, relevant sentences, in a normal voice. The therapist, being too conscious of the technical aspects of language production, tends to forget that parents of deaf children must be trained to use language with normal voice
qualities. The therapist must use normal spoken language in
the class session and only use isolated speech sounds for
specific corrective exercises, which should not be applied
until basic spoken language has developed.

If the situation in the session is artificial and highly
technical, the mother will tense up and feel incapable. The
guidance given by the therapist should be based on the
mother's reports of home situations and concrete activities
that are relevant and applicable at that particular stage and
level of development. If this is done, the mother soon sees
the beneficial results of her activities.

A therapist should learn much about the particular
child's family, their activities, way of life and home, and
then adjust her guidelines and program development to that
environment and cultural and economic situation. It is a
good idea to invite the siblings of the child to class so

that they, too, can understand how to participate and how to take a positive role in the habilitation of their hearing impaired siblings.

Obviously there are basic activities required for the development of auditory verbal communication. Fundamentally, they are:

1) the earliest possible use of appropriate amplification (usually binaural);

2) one-to-one teaching;

3) the development of auditory self-monitoring of speech, spoken language, and communication learned through hearing natural sounding spoken language;

4) attendance in regular schools from the beginning;

5) expecting the child to function independently in the most normal learning and living environment possible;

6) periodic evaluation of language development and speech production, articulation skills, language structure and general child development.

The therapist who works with young babies should learn all about baby care and child development. Ideally, she should herself have had experience and active participation before she is qualified to demonstrate and guide. Work in the habilitation of the hearing impaired child should, in fact, be general parent guidance, parent training for specialized needs and parent orientation on how to observe and evaluate the progress of their child. Simultaneously, the professional will undertake responsibility for providing moral support and help in reprogramming according to the specific needs of each individual, and then applying the specialized exercises which are needed for corrective purposes. I hope the future will offer the commencement of habilitation for all hearing impaired children before they are one year of age.

The Mexican Model

Mexico, as you know, is a country in development and rich in contrasts and ways of life. There are a great variety of mores. Amongst the rural people, there still is a rigid acceptance of old traditional behaviour, but as schools are expanding, this is being changed. Illiteracy has greatly diminished, but still many parents have had very little school education. Their knowledge about child development and child rearing is handed down in a slipshod manner and usually falls back into the habits and behaviour patterns of their own childhood and their parents' treatment of them. Unfortunately, and particularly amongst lower socio-economic educational levels, a child exists and grows and develops as chance permits. Parent interaction is usually only evident if a child displays bothersome activity to the adult; such as, making too much noise when father is tired, or disturbing mother in her daily activities. Discipline is carried out as a relief from pent-up disturbances or annoyances often caused by other than the child's activities. Invariably, it is not consistent, causing great confusion to the child. Unfortunately that is a problem in many other parts of the world too.

The ABC's are taught in school. Work skills are developed with aims towards self-economic support. Human interaction, marriage relationships, child rearing, normal child development, including the need to stimulate, guide and develop the correct environment for the growing child and the knoweldge of constructive disciplinary methods, are completely ignored.

It was with great delight that I received from Nicholas J. Anastasiow of the Institute for Child Study, Indiana University, a monograph entitled "Preventing Tomorrow's Handicapped Child Today", in which project FEED is presented. The document is a middle grade (7 - 8) curriculum experience which focuses on assisting young people to learn, before they become parents, about child growth and the development of infants and preschoolers.

In Mexico, even though there is free education, it is only the very low income families who send their children to the government schools. Most middle class families find it necessary to incorporate their children in private schools.

This is encouraged by the government as a means of leaving
room for those who cannot pay in the government schools. The
demand is so great that there are morning, afternoon and
evening shifts offered in the free schools.

Classrooms have no less than 60 children. In all fields
of education, normal and special, there are not enough facilities to go around. The tax payer in Mexico does not take
for granted that the Government will provide free the innum-
erable services that are required. The minimum wage earner
does not pay taxes. Supposedly those who do, cover the needs
of the non-tax payer. There still are insufficient services
to go around. This situation has developed parents who know
that the responsibility for covering the needs of their offspring is entirely theirs. Once they have grasped what is
required and have been convinced of the benefits derived,
and that they can receive the guidance and orientation
necessary, they will try through all means possible to comply.
The parents who have attended OIRA have, in varied degrees,
learned that the responsibility for the successful habilitation of their hearing handicapped child is theirs. We have
encouraged the parents and expect them to face up to that
responsibility and solve the problems. We have encouraged
them to provide the necessary requirements, to look for good
regular school placement, and to orient the regular classroom teachers who, together with actively interested parents,
work on the scholastic curriculum. The parents train the
teachers to be responsible for informing the other students
about what a deaf child is, why one is incorporated in their
classroom, and how to be conscious of the role they can play
in easing the adjustment of the deaf youngster by helping him
face up to school requirements.

The parents know they can apply to OIRA if they need
help in solving problem situations. Usually they ask guidance
and receive suggestions and know they are always free to
discuss and plan as a team, but that the final decision and
execution is in their hands. It is not easy, it is hard work.
At times, school placement is unsatisfactory, teachers are
not co-operative, and studies seem to be getting out of hand.
Nevertheless, I salute the majority of parents I have been
privileged to meet and know, for their unselfish dedication
and their ability to solve problems inspite of seemingly
insurmountable odds. They take it in their stride as part of
being a parent and do not consider themselves exceptional or

unique because of their dedication and responsibility. Some
are luckier than others and have an easier time. They all
know, however, that they have a responsibility towards their
children until those children are on firm ground and develop
into mature, responsible, capable, self-assured human beings.

From the very first day a family enters OIRA, the
parents' role is very clearly defined and work and collaboration and full responsibility for the child is expected. In
turn, they receive understanding, guidance, full orientation
and the security of knowing that they have this support
behind them, if they ever feel they are floundering. The
parents accept this as a matter of course.

REFERENCES

Anastasiow, N.J. Preventing Tomorrow's Handicapped Child
Today. (A middle School Child Development Curriculum).
Institute for Child Study, Indiana University, June, 1977.

Condon, W.S., & Sander, L.W. "Synchrony demonstrated between
movements of the neonate and adult speech." Child Development, 45:446 - 462, 1974.

Griffiths, C. Conquering Childhood Deafness (New York:
Exposition Press), 1967.

Ling, D. Speech and the Hearing-Impaired Child: Theory and
Practice (Washington, D.C.: A. G. Bell Association), 1976.

Northcott, W.H., (ed.). Curriculum Guide: Hearing-Impaired
Children, Birth to Three Years, and Their Parents, revised
edition (Washington, D.C.: A. G. Bell Association), 1977.

Pollack, D. "Acoupedics: A unisensory approach to auditory
training." Volta Review, 66:400 - 409, 1964.

DISCUSSION

DOCTOR MENCHER
Ms. Luttman, I have both a comment and a question.

Throughout the entire address the primary emphasis has been
on the mother. I appreciate the fact that the mother is, of
course, the primary care provider in the young baby, but as
a father, I would like to see the father involved as much as
the mother. I wonder if you would care to comment.

MS. LUTTMAN
    I started out by talking about the parents, and fathers
are involved. As a matter of fact, my daughter who read
through my paper, said, "Why are you always saying mother?"
I said, well I keep thinking about the baby and unfortunately,
the father is out very much. The father often doesn't have
as much interest in small babies. If the father doesn't
voluntarily come - we, personally - even if he is an employee
and says, "I can't, my employer won't let me quit work to
come to each session" (we have about two 50 minute sessions a
week) - we encourage him. We have found a very marked difference between the children whose mother and father have
assisted, not to mention the siblings too, and those whose
entire family does not get involved. The father does play a
very important role. The mothers get together and have meetings, but the fathers themselves say, O.K., our wives have a
great opportunity. They have all the guidance, we don't.
So these fathers get together and form a fathers' club and
they get together in the evenings. It is very vital that
fathers participate.

DOCTOR MENCHER
    Both Nan Phillips in her comments, Doreen Pollack in her
comments, and now you in your comments, have alluded to the
fact, if I can use what may appear to be a negative term (I
don't mean it to be), that the clinician in effect "marries"
into the family in terms of helping the family through the
situation and through the dynamics of adjustment. Would you
care to comment? What is the effect of that on the interaction within the family? Does the family become dependent
upon the clinician for this guidance and, thus, lose its
ability to be able to guide itself? One has the feeling of
this counsellor becoming (again, this sounds more negative
than I mean it to be), manipulative of the family. What does
that do to the dynamics of the family and its ability to
survive by itself in this situation?

MS. LUTTMAN

It depends on what you call guidance. I mean teacher guidance to parents for participation. I think one of the things to watch out for is that when there is a therapist working with a child, they want to show and prove to themselves and others what they can do to develop this child. It is important that this not become excessive. If you have an habilitation centre like Doreen's and others like it, in which they are using hearing as the first process for developing language, usually the children come twice a week for 50 minute periods. Obviously, no matter how good the therapist or the teacher can be, if you haven't really trained the parent to be able to carry on in an everyday situation at home, it won't work. We always indicate to the parent that it is their responsibility and we're there to guide. The therapist is there to guide and tell them. They usually solve their own problems. In Mexico we don't have a large sect of specialized personnel. We don't have the money to have the people to be able to visit the private schools. Parents have to solve all their problems themselves. They come to ask advice and guidance and discuss things at the centre, but they're the ones who have to chose the schools. If this school is not adequate, they're the ones who have to speak to the teachers in the regular schools. They're the ones that have to make all the decisions, but they always feel they have this support behind so that they can discuss. I think it's very important that things should not be held back from them. They should understand. They should know how much hearing their child has, or does not have. They should know everything they can. Clinicians should not underestimate the capacity of a parent, and I am coming from Mexico where we have had parents, some of whom have been illiterate, who have no schooling, and words alone don't suffice. That's why I talk so much about active participation. If you have a parent who has arrived and who is very emotionally upset, it doesn't matter how many degrees she might have, when it's her own child she is dealing with, she isn't processing what she is being told. It goes in one ear and disappears. Not until you are actually participating - until somebody actually shows you - what it is you have to do; shows you how to play with your child; how to sit on the ground and play ball, and how you can be talking about what you are doing, does it make sense. Just talking, whatever degree of education or whatever socio-economic level they might come from, doesn't help emotional, disturbed parents, as they all are when they first come.

EARLY MANAGEMENT OF HEARING LOSS IN A PARENT EDUCATION CENTRE

Edgar J. Lowell
John Tracy Clinic, Los Angeles, California

The title "Early Management of Hearing Loss" means different things to different people, based I would suspect, on their professional training and the setting in which they are employed.

From the point of view of a Parent Educator, early management of hearing loss is seen as one important component of a total parent education program. We are concerned with instructing the parents in the role they can play in their child's education, with offering them counselling help as they deal with their feelings about having a child who is different, and, of course, with providing the child with an educational program which will facilitate the development of speech and language.

The goals of John Tracy Clinic are to find, encourage, guide and train the parents of young deaf children, first to reach and help the child to understand language and to speak, and second, to help the parents themselves. Thus, we have a clear committment to early identification and management of hearing loss. Note, however, that the primary goal has to do with parents. We believe that this makes a number of differences in our early management plans.

This paper will attempt to concentrate on those special emphases in our early management of hearing loss program that result from our location in a Parent Education Center.

Importance of Parental Understanding

Our plan for early management of hearing loss places a major emphasis on parental understanding. Just as we feel that early education of the hearing impaired child to be maximally effective must involve the parents, so we feel that the early management of hearing loss to be maximally effective, must involve the parents.

We want the parents to understand as much as possible about the diagnostic procedures that are used with their

293

child. If the initial visit to the clinic is the first time
the parents have learned that their child is deaf, it is
generally not an appropriate time to be concerned about what
the parents have learned. We do want them to see all of the
test procedures, and ultimately to understand how those procedures relate to their child. The emphasis on parental
understanding is, obviously, a continuing one that is built
into all of our contracts with the parents.

Involving parents presents at least four major challenges for our management team. First, we deal with parents
who may, understandably, be emotionally involved in either
the initial diagnosis or its confirmation by our testing.
As we know from studies of all parents of handicapped
children, there is a period of grief. Parents work through
grief in many different ways. It does take time and during
that time it may be difficult to contribute very much to the
parents' understanding.

Second, we are dealing with some fairly complex concepts
in our evaluations and educational planning. It is easy to
fall into technical jargon which may be completely incompre-
hensible to the parents. I am reminded of this every time I
go to a doctor and then return home and have my wife ask me
questions about what the doctor said. I realize that,
although I nodded my head at what I am sure were the appropriate times, I actually did not come away with a very clear
picture of what the doctor told me. I am generally not
familiar with the medical terms used, and can rarely remember
them very long after my visit to the doctor's office. When
you couple emotional confusion and technical complexity, the
challenge becomes formidable.

The audiologist, the psychologist and the teachers who
form our management team have a continuing and direct responsibility for parental understanding. The content is broken
into essentially cognitive and affective components. The
audiologist and teacher deal with the development of communication skills, and the psychologist helps the parents deal
with their feelings.

The information is imparted in both scheduled individual
conferences with the parents, and in formal classes which are
held weekly in the evenings, so that fathers can attend as
well as mothers.

The third challenge concerns motivation. We are dealing with parents who have different motivations for becoming involved in their child's education. As students, they are not working for grades or degrees or, in some cases, even because they want to know about the education of young deaf children. Some are eager to learn and apply what they learn toward helping their child. For others, avoiding becoming involved may be the way of dealing with a painful situation.

Our fourth challenge is that we are dealing with parents with widely different abilities to absorb the information being offered. Some are college graduates with advanced degrees, and others have minimal education. This diversity presents our staff with an enormous challenge. We must continually ask ourselves, "Are the parents just nodding their heads at what they hope is the right time, or are they really understanding what is being said?"

We must also put all of our material to the test, "is this the next most important thing for this parent to know?" That is not always easy. It is surprising how many times something that might be included in a college course because it was theoretically interesting or background, has to be excluded because it does not meet this test.

Lack of Diagnostic Urgency

Coupled with our feelings about the importance of parental understanding is a lack of diagnostic urgency. The clinic is primarily an educational center and, just as we view education as a continuing process, we view the evaluation of a hearing loss as a continuing process. We normally do not feel any sense of pressure to complete an audiological examination immediately, as we must do when a family comes to the clinic from out of town and is not planning to stay in the city for any length of time.

Most families remain with the clinic for a considerable period of time, so that there are ample opportunities to see the child for repeated visits. Our service program is organized so that any family with a child under 6 years of age can make an appointment to come to the clinic for a hearing evaluation. If the child has a nonmedically correctable or sensory-neural hearing problem, the family is invited to participate in all of our educational services.

One of those services is the Demonstration Home, where
the mother and child come on an appointment basis to a home-
like setting within the clinic building. They meet with a
teacher of the deaf who shows the mother how she can begin to
incorporate language training into everyday household activities. Another service is our Friday Family School, where new
families are invited to attend a weekly group meeting. The
children are in the nursery school with our trained teachers,
while the parents attend classes in the development of
communication skills and group discussions led by our psychologist. These visits provide convenient opportunities for
the audiologist, psychologist and teacher to see the child
as often as necessary. It is also possible to re-schedule
the family for a full audiological and psychological
(developmental assessment) re-evaluation visit when more
time is required.

Comments about the lack of diagnostic urgency should not
be interpreted to suggest that we are leisurely about our
evaluations. Of course, it would be nice to have a complete
and reliable pure tone audiogram (both sound field and from
separate ears under phones), bone conduction results, speech
testing (depending upon the child's age), and impedance testing (including tympanograms and acoustic reflexes) during the
first evaluation. In many cases, however, where there is a
multiple health problem or an infant, it is not possible to
obtain all this information in a single visit.

Free Services

The whole issue of providing free hearing management in
a society that is used to paying deserves more than passing
consideration. There are some very positive aspects to free
care. Staff need never be concerned about the cost of service being provided or the parents' ability to pay. There
need be no hesitation in recommending additional services, as
there might be if the parents' ability to pay was a consideration. At the same time, we must be sensitive and recognize
that some people have feelings about accepting free service
because it seems like charity. The increasing number of
insurance and other third-party payors is reducing the likli-
hood of this situation arising, but there are still some
families who are uneasy with free service.

There is a related problem. That is, how to manage the
caseload in a free service situation where the number of
families we can serve is limited. We view the clinic's
diagnostic service as primarily an intake service for the
clinic's educational program, so that top priority is given
to serving young children who may be in need of our educational services, or to follow up those children already in
our care. To the extent possible, we offer service to other
families. The waiting period may be longer, however, if for
example, the child is enrolled in another educational program
and the parents merely want a re-evaluation.

Feedback from Educators and Parents

The entire management program is subject to a great deal
of feedback from both educators and parents because of our
parent education setting. Exchange of questions and information is encouraged, and both teachers and parents feel free
to question the audiologist about any perceived change in the
child's response to sound. The fact that the diagnostic
team, the teachers and the parents are working together in
the same setting and interacting regularly, makes this type
of exchange quite easy and natural. Given the difficulty of
testing very young children, this type of feedback to the
diagnostic team is an important part of our management plan.

Hearing Aid Loaner Bank

Another way in which our parent centered program may
differ is in our hearing aid loaner bank. The clinic does
not dispense hearing aids, but we do maintain an extensive
number of loaner aids for children to use until permanent
hearing aids are obtained or, as they are needed in emergency
situations. Because of our tax laws, it is sometimes advantageous for people to give hearing aids to the clinic. As a
consequence, we have collected a great many aids. Those in
need of repair are put in operating condition. We are able
to loan several different types of aids to families, for
extended periods, or even give them to families when that
is appropriate.

When a hearing impaired child's education can begin
during the early critical years, chances for full integration
into society are greatly improved. The child with a hearing

impairment is at a profound disadvantage unless effective
amplification and language stimulation are provided during
the very early years. A program developed to offer early
management of hearing loss operates from the belief that
parents are the child's most natural first teachers and can
provide early listening and language experiences. An interdisciplinary professional staff, including an audiologist,
psychologist, teachers of the hearing impaired, serves both
the child and family. The ultimate objective of the program
is to have each parent think of each child as a normal person
who happens to have a hearing impairment, not a hearing
handicap.

DISCUSSION

DR. ROBERT RUBEN
     Dr. Lowell has raised a number of interesting issues.
I'd like to ask a rather small question. How do you picture
the advocacy role of who's ever doing the intervention,
audiologist, psychologist, physician, secretary, etc., etc.
Who is the child's advocate, and what is - if we cannot use
the term "moral responsibility" - what is the legal responsibility to the child. From what you described, one has the
feeling that we'll make excuses for the people who have the
legal responsibility, the parents. It used to be called
"moral responsibility", but now we put teeth into it, so it's
legal responsibility. I'd like you to expand on that if you
could.

DOCTOR LOWELL
     Well, from our point of view, any step other than placing
the responsibility where it belongs - with the parents, the
people who are most concerned - is abdicating responsibility.
Parents are expected to be educated enough to participate in
an IEP conference. But they often don't know what the words
that you are using, mean, and when they called about multi-
cultural, unbiased evaluation procedures, it became a joke.
So, I think we have a very serious job to do, and, I think
we are not geared up to do it. We are kidding ourselves if
we think that we're bringing parents into the IEP conference
and, hence, into the legal advocacy arena, when we are not
providing them with the proper background. We are generally

not organized to provide that kind of education, but it's so
obviously needed. So, in answer to your question, I think
it's got to be the parent, and the "advocates" that go into
the IEP conference* and sit right up to the table ought to
be sitting back against the wall and become consultants to
the parents, when the parents want them.

DR. KEVIN MURPHY
     Dr. Lowell, I find myself in a quandry about all the
papers I have listened to up to now. They all seem to have
middle class, literate, highly verbal patients. Now I know,
and you know too, that we both have patients that are not
like that. I wonder if you could say how the program which
you initiated for socially disadvantaged parents has been
structured so that communication really occurs between the -
let's call them the officials - and the parents? How have
you programmed this? Is there a pattern of communication
from which one can tell whether they're disadvantaged
because they have a deaf child, or disadvantaged through
other things, that the parents really are in a position to
comprehend and to absorb whatever measures you put to them?

DOCTOR LOWELL
     Well, our attempt, as you know, was to alter our goals.
Again, I think this may not have been fair to the parents,
but certainly we have had to readjust them. I think there
are two ways that we have tried to evaluate this. One, as
you know, is in our demonstration home program where we
actually have the parents perform the same kinds of activities
(i.e., demonstrate the kinds of skills that we are trying to
teach). We think that is one of the ways of looking at
communication. The other is direct feedback. I think that
for many years we were working under the mistaken notion
that because we said something to parents, they understood it.
I think we still do work with that assumption. I think that
most of the speakers, myself included, assume - we assume -
that you know what I'm saying after I've said it. But what
we've been trying very hard to do, and it's been terribly
embarrassing and time consuming, is to ask the parents what
we've said. Assumptions don't always apply. I don't think
there's anything that will shrink your ego more.

---

*   Individual Educational Programs. See Nober, "The Effects
    of New U.S. Legislation on Services to Very Young Hearing
    Impaired Children and their Parents," this volume.

ACOUPEDICS: AN APPROACH TO EARLY MANAGEMENT

Doreen Pollack
Porter Memorial Hospital, Denver, Colorado

Acoupedics is a comprehensive program of management for young children with hearing losses, which was initiated 30 years ago in response to the technologic improvement in hearing aids. It was so named by the late Dr. Henk C. Huizing of Holland to describe a new philosophy of teaching those children whose hearing losses were detected at an early age.

For several centuries, educators have tried to alleviate the handicap of deafness through manual and visual methods of communication with results which have been well documented in terms of low educational and vocational achievements (U.S. Govt. Report, 1964; Office of Demo-Studies).

The deaf infant of today, however, does not have to 'grow in silence' (Mindel and Vernon, 1971). With the power and fidelity of modern hearing aids, even a profoundly deaf child can hear and learn to interpret conversational speech, can identify a whisper, and can use a telephone.

From its inception, there are two main goals for an Acoupedic program: the first is to integrate audition into the total personality development of the prelingually deaf infant, so that sound is an important and meaningful part of everything experienced and learned. Fortunately, total deafness is very rare.

The second goal is to prepare the deaf individual for full participation in our society as an independent person. That is, the child is not being prepared for special education and communication through interpreters (Pollack, 1970).

This is not a denial of the problems associated with deafness; rather, it represents a philosophy that a handicap can be overcome and need not circumscribe a person's whole life. The infant is not a 'deaf' person, but a person who has a hearing loss.

There are four major components in an Acoupedic program:

1. The earliest possible intervention, with ongoing manage-
    ment by a medico-educational team, preferably within the
    same organization. This team includes the child's physi-
    cian and otologist; an audiologist; an occupational
    therapist; a speech and language specialist; a family
    counsellor and a psychologist.

2. Optimal utilization of residual hearing. Unless contra-
    indicated, two well fitted hearing aids are worn during
    all the child's waking hours.

3. A program of intensive auditory education based upon the
    sequential and interrelated development of normal
    auditory, speech and language skills.

4. A complete change in the learning environment. This
    includes families as partners in therapy; individualized,
    1-to-1 teaching, and mainstreaming.

    The first Acoupedic program was started in 1948 at
Columbia Presbyterian Hospital in New York City, and the
second at the University of Denver. Since 1965, it has been
part of the Speech and Hearing Services of Porter Memorial
Hospital in Denver, Colorado (Pollack, 1974).

    There is no selection process for the children involved.
They have been routinely referred by physicians or other
agencies, such as Public Health. Their average hearing losses
are the same, if not greater than those reported by national
programs for the deaf in the National Demographic Surveys
(see Figures 1, 2 and 3).

    We do, however, have a higher incidence of multiple
handicaps, in proportion, in the acoupedic group:

	Denver	National
Additional handicapping conditions:	41	21,424
Total students	54	49,427
Number with additional handicaps	28	29,427

Handicaps include brain damage, cerebral palsy, epilepsy,
heart disorder, visual problems, perceptual-motor disorders,
retardation, symbolic learning disorders, emotional problems
and so on.

FIGURE 1:   DEGREE OF HEARING LOSS OF CHILDREN IN THE
            ACOUPEDIC PROGRAM

	Acoupedic Program Per Cent	National Per Cent
Total known information	100.0	100.0
Normal (under 27 dB)	0.0	2.4
Mild (from 27 to 40 dB)	3.8	4.0
Moderate (from 41 to 55 dB)	5.7	8.2
Moderately Severe (56 to 70 dB)	17.0	13.3
Severe (from 71 to 90 dB)	24.5	26.3
Profound (91 dB and above)	49.1	45.8

It is difficult to discuss management of children labeled 'deaf' and 'hard of hearing' in simple terms: they are a very diverse group. Even in the absence of severe problems, the occupational therapist has found that hearing impaired children frequently have immature reflexes, poor eye control, poor sensori-motor integration and display problems in the vestibular area up to 3 years of age.

FIGURE 2:   AGE OF ONSET OF HEARING LOSS OF CHILDREN ENROLLED
            IN ACOUPEDIC PROGRAM

	Acoupedic Program Per Cent	National Per Cent
Onset at birth	81.4	76.7
Under one year	9.3	6.7
One year	9.3	6.6
Over one year	0.0	20.0

FIGURE 3: ETIOLOGY OF HEARING LOSSES OF CHILDREN ENROLLED
IN ACOUPEDIC PROGRAM

	Acoupedic Program Per Cent	National Per Cent
Causes At Birth		
Maternal Rubella	43.3	33.7
Heredity	26.7	16.9
Complications of Pregnancy	0.0	5.7
Prematurity	3.3	8.3
RH Incompatibility	6.7	4.7
Trauma at Birth	0.0	4.3
Other	6.7	4.7
Causes After Birth		
Meningitis	3.3	10.7
Mumps	3.3	0.8
Measles	3.3	3.0
Otitis Media	3.3	2.7
High Fever	3.3	4.7
Infections	3.3	3.3
Other	3.3	4.8

Information not reported (24 students)

Age Span Within The Program:

In spite of a neonatal screening program within the area,
the majority of infants are not enrolled until they are
between their first and second birthdays. They remain in the
Acoupedic program for as long as they need supportive help,
some into their teen years. This has provided 15 years of
consistent collection of data, so that a number of observations can be made about early management.

1. Neonatal Screening and Follow-up

There has been excellent co-operation on the part of
physicians and parents. (For example, 465 babies were
brought back for follow-up in 1979). Less than 1% of all
babies are born with a profound hearing loss. The majority
are in the high risk category, but a significant number of
babies have middle ear effusion, and some developed permanent
sensory-neural loss after their first birthday in spite of
excellent medical care. There seeems to be an early progressive factor in congenital deafness which could explain the fact
that children are rarely enrolled in habilitative programs
until the second year of life.

We have found that the normal hearing infant orients to
the human voice at very low levels - 5 to 15 dB - around 6
months of age, so that atypical responses are easily charted.

A group of parents who reported "etiology unknown" gave
birth to a second hearing impaired child several years after
the first. Three of the rubella children were also in that
category.

2. Audiologic Assessment

Audiologic testing at Porter's has been carried out in a
sound suite by certified audiologists using such test strategies as behavioural, visual reinforcement audiometry, (V.R.A.)
play conditioning and Auditory Brainstem Evoked Response
Audiometry (ABR), depending upon the maturity of the child.

With due respect to the expertise of clinical audiologists, several findings were pre-eminent:

A. *The initial audiogram, obtained before an*
    infant has received a program of amplified
    auditory stimulation, can be misleading
    and should never be used as the determining
    factor for the selection of communication
    systems or educational management.

Infants with severe to profound losses frequently
inhibit responses to sound when it is meaningless to them,
and, such losses may also appear to be more severe because
of a conductive overlay caused by persistent respiratory
and middle ear problems. There are also problems with ABR
interpretation. One example will suffice (see Figure 4).

FIGURE 4: CASE D.M. AN EXAMPLE OF MISLEADING INFORMATION
            FROM INITIAL AUDIOGRAMS

		250	500	1000	2000	4000	Speech Threshold
First Audio	Rt Ear	N.R.	125	N.R.	N.R.	N.R.	No Response
	Lt Ear	N.R.	125	N.R.	N.R.	N.R.	No Response
Audio After Training	Rt Ear	75	90	105	N.R.	N.R.	Aided Speech Awareness 55 dB
	Lt Ear	65	80	105	110	105	Aided Speech Reception 40 dB

This child was seen for Auditory Brainstem Evoked Response Audiometry at 7 months of age. No response was seen in
the left ear, and a minimal response at 100 dB was reported
for the right ear, according to the materials received from a
center with a national reputation. Five months later, after

wearing amplification, he responded at 55 dB in the left ear. One year later he was speaking in 3- and 4-word sentences and had a pleasant voice. However, there was still minimal response in the right ear!

B. *Hearing aids may be used as soon as possible, but a final selection should not be made until a program of diagnostic therapy has been carried out because of the changes in response which may occur.*

Contrary to certain current reports, our studies of children wearing high powered hearing aids over a period of 10 years or more, do not show statistically significant damage (Ott, Balkany and Pollack, 1980; Libby, 1980). However, a Maximum Power Output (M.P.O.) of 130 dB SPL appears to be an optimal output for very severe hearing losses. The majority of children show greatly improved speech discrimination with a true binaural fitting. See Figure 5 for examples.

FIGURE 5: EXAMPLES OF IMPROVED SPEECH DISCRIMINATION SCORES WITH TRUE BINAURAL AMPLIFICATION

		Pure Tone Average	Aided Discrimination
Case R.A.	Rt. Ear	103 dB	52% at 70 dB HL
	Lt. Ear	110 dB	48% at 70 dB HL
	Binaural		68% at 70 dB HL
Case M.B.	Rt. Ear	85 dB	60% at 60 dB
	Lt. Ear	92 dB	56% at 60 dB
	Binaural		80% at 60 dB

3. The Development of Auditory
    Verbal Communication

    The auditory pathway is the natural and most effective
way to learn speech and language, in addition to providing
all the other auditory information from our environment, such
as, music, doorbell, bird song and so on. Hearing is the one
sense which, whether we are awake or asleep, provides us with
information in the dark, or about what's going on behind our
backs, or around corners. However, it is not sufficient to
hang hearing aids upon an infant and talk to him. Listening
has to be learned.

    Furthermore, there appears to be a critical period for
learning to listen after which it becomes increasingly difficult for the brain to process sound and develop an auditory
feedback and feedforward system. Traditionally, educators
have not placed emphasis upon developing an auditory function
but, rather, have diverted the child's attention to watching
a speaker's hands and face. If an auditory function is not
successfully developed, auditory stimuli are meaningless and
are ignored. For that reason, many older deaf children will
discard their hearing aids.

    Neurologists have long known that weaker signals are
inhibited by the reticular system in the brain so that we can
pay selective attention (Negus, 1963). That voluntary attention, according to Vygotsky (1956), is also a social act
depending upon the interaction between adult and child. However, Luria (1973) states that this information takes place
only in the most simple conditions; namely, when there are no
distracting objects in the external field of vision. That is,
a spoken instruction cannot overcome factors of involuntary
attention competing with it; and not until 4½ to 5 years of
age is the ability to obey a spoken instruction strong enough
to invoke a dominant connection.

    Although the infant with a hearing loss must eventually
integrate and use all the cues available, the emphasis in
Acoupedics is placed initially upon listening and responding
to sound, to the extent that the speaker's mouth is covered
where necessary. The child is encouraged to imitate and
process sound and, above all, is taught that he/she lives
in a world full of sound where people use sound for
communication.

Long before a normal hearing baby learns language, there are thousands of hours spent listening. Auditory skills are developed sequentially. The deaf infant who is wearing hearing aids must follow the same sequence:

The Interrelated Development of Auditory, Speech and Language Skills

Audition	Speech	Language
Understanding	Spontaneous Speech	Receptive and Expressive Language
	Articulation Development	
Processing Patterns	Jargon	Development of Syntax
Sequencing	First Words	Symbolic Language; Concrete and Abstract
Auditory Memory Span	Blowing and Whispering	Functional Words, Often associated with gestures
Auditory Feedback	Echolalia	
Discrimination	Babbling and Lalling	
Localization	Vocal Play	Sounds have meaning
Distance Hearing	Cooing and Smiling	
Attention or listening		
Awareness	Crying	Sound is used for Communication

(Self Monitoring — bracket alongside Sequencing through Auditory Feedback)

After becoming attentive to a variety of sounds, the infant should be trained to turn in the direction of sound. Luria (1973) has said that the manifestation of the orienting reactions are among the essential conditions for the formation of a conditional reflex, which will be slow to develop if the conditioning takes place in the absence of an orienting reflex.

It takes a considerable amount of listening time, depending upon the degree of residual hearing, before an infant will
begin to discriminate and recognize different sounds. This is
true even though the mechanism for this task comes into operation very early (Eisenberg, 1976). At the same time, the
infant is trying to localize the source of sounds from different directions and from increasing distances, and is, thus,
becoming a part of the world of sounds. When sound becomes
meaningful, the child is ready to learn spoken language
(Levine, 1956). During this period, which occurs during the
first 6 months of life or the first months after being fitted
with a hearing aid, an infant is listening not only to
environmental sounds, but also to his own sounds and is
establishing auditory feedback and an auditory memory.

During the next 6 months, the child is actively involved
in vocal play, laughing, 'singing', babbling and echoing, so
that soon the vocalization sounds like the child's mother
tongue. That is, a French baby begins to sound French, and
an English baby English. The infant is beginning to monitor
his own sounds through his auditory feedback system, so that
what comes out of his mouth resembles the sounds which are
going into his ear.

As the child begins to imitate and process patterns of
sound, a functional vocabulary emerges. It is usually part of
a routine experience, such as "bye bye". Once there is the
realization that experiences and objects can be labeled, the
child is ready to learn symbolic language.

One of the most important auditory skills to be developed
and one which is never mentioned in deaf education, is auditory memory span. That skill enables us to understand how
words are grouped together so that the syntax of the language
can be learned. This, too, follows certain developmental
sequences, such as: the one word phrase, followed by the two-
word phrase, during which time we acquire the concepts of
verbing, negation and possession (Brown, 1973).

It has been customary in deaf education to bypass most
of the early stages just described, particularly those
involving vocal play and the development of auditory feedback
and feedforward. Customarily, training began at the level of
symbolic language with primary emphasis placed upon visual
perception and visual memory. That approach was, of course,
necessary before the advent of the modern hearing aid.

Following normal developmental sequences, as is done in Acoupedics, requires individualized 1-to-1 stimulation and correct timing so that an infant's immediate feelings, needs and experiences are verbalized without interruption or delay. For example, if an infant and its mother and building blocks together, mother cay say: "Up!" or "... fall down". With a visual or manual approach, the infant has to look up and away from the activity and stop building blocks in order to communicate.

An Acoupedic program does not group children with hearing losses together. If we are educating children to listen and imitate, their models must be normal speaking models. Therefore, Acoupedic children are also encouraged to attend preschools with normal hearing children. Further, as has already been mentioned, children with hearing losses frequently have additional problems which can best be remediated on an individual basis so grouping can be counterproductive.

4.   The Role of the Family

The fourth component of Acoupedics is an emphasis upon the responsibility of the family. When parents set the goal for their child of full participation in the hearing world as an independent person, they are, in fact, charting a long-term program of commitment for themselves. A clinician or teacher can develop the skills which underlie auditory-verbal communication, but they have to be integrated into every aspect of the infant's life. For example, hearing aids must be constantly maintained, and an environment has to be created in which the child is expected to listen, is shown how to respond, and is encouraged to speak.

This is accomplished in different ways: family members are coached or guided through childhood activities; parent meetings and home visits are conducted; family counselling and financial support are provided as necessary. Parents are encouraged to help other parents. In Denver, the parents have formed an organization known as the LISTEN Foundation, which has offered workshops and has also purchased a house where families can stay when their children need intensive help.

The majority of parents are willing partners when a positive approach is used. Unfortunately, they complain that professional people tend to be negative, and to emphasize what the child will <u>not</u> be able to do because of his hearing

loss. Parents also complain that very few physicians or
audiologists describe the different options available to them.
It is very important to the success of a program that parents
have visited other programs and have made a choice.

THE RESULTS

Several findings are apparent as we inspect the record of
children who stayed with an Acoupedic approach:

1. Ninety-five per cent developed auditory verbal communica-
    tion and more than 50% were successfully mainstreamed
    before P.L. 94-142 mandated education in the least
    restrictive environment. For example, there were 49
    children of school age attending Porter's on a weekly
    basis in 1978 - 1979. Of that group, 11 were in normal
    hearing preschools, 27 were in normal hearing elementary
    and Jr. High Schools, and 13 were in special classes.
    Most of the latter group of children were multiply handi-
    capped. The children in regular schools did not require
    interpreters, but some received itinerant help.

Severity of the hearing loss and a child's communication
and educational progress cannot be equated. For example,
S.H. (with an average loss in both ears of 103 dB) who was
enrolled in an Acoupedic program when she was 17 months of
age, became a law student and a finalist for the Rhodes
Scholarship. Intactness of the central nervous system and
the quality of parental involvement are far more important
factors than the audiogram in predicting a successful outcome.
However, the configuration of the audiogram has to be taken
into consideration.

The age of 3 is not a magical number for the development
of language. Although the earliest possible start is preferable, and particularly for the profoundly deaf, many prelingually deaf children who entered the Acoupedic program at
3 years of age are now successfully integrated into normal
hearing schools and colleges. Figure 6 illustrates Case C.M.
as an example. It should be noted that this child is also
legally blind and her general knowledge about the world was
restricted by her visual handicap. She is representative of
the large group of intact children whose hearing losses are
severe (or better). With today's hearing aids and an auditory
approach, there should be no need for teachers to resort to
manual communication.

FIGURE 6:   AUDIOMETRIC AND PEABODY INDIVIDUAL ACHIEVEMENT
            TEST RESULTS OF CASE C.M.

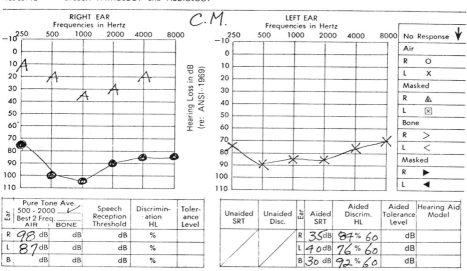

PORTER MEMORIAL HOSPITAL

739-001-73   SPEECH PATHOLOGY and AUDIOLOGY

	1976	1977	1978	1979
Math	7 – 9	4 – 9	9 – 6	12 – 9
R. Recognition	4 – 7	4 – 8	5 – 8	8 – 9
R. Comprehension	3 – 2	3 – 1	4 – 4	5 – 5
Spelling	3 – 6	4 – 4	6 – 0	7 – 7
G. Information	0 – 3	3 – 4	6 – 0	5 – 6
Total	3 – 6	6 – 3	6 – 0	7 – 7

Peabody Picture Vocabulary Test

1977	1979
7 – 3	12 – 10

313

FIGURE 7: AUDIOMETRIC AND INDIVIDUAL ACHIEVEMENT TEST RESULTS OF CASE D.S., NOW INTEGRATED IN A NORMAL SCHOOL

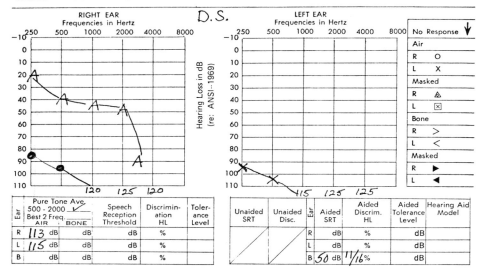

Peabody Picture Vocabulary Test: C.A. = 6-6; Mental Age = 3-10

Carrow Test for Auditory Comprehension of Language:
                          78 out of 101 items correct

Detroit Test of Oral Commissions: 7 out of 8 correct

Houston Test of Language Development: Language age = 5-5

Boehm's Basic Concepts Form A1:   22 out of 25 correct

FIGURE 8: AUDIOMETRIC AND INDIVIDUAL ACHIEVEMENT TEST RESULTS
OF CASE J.L., NOW INTEGRATED IN A NORMAL SCHOOL

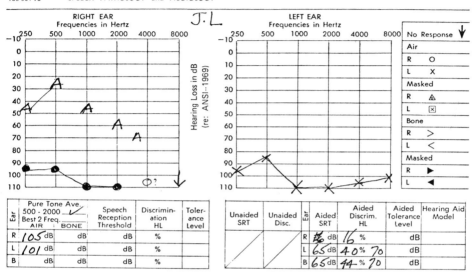

PORTER MEMORIAL HOSPITAL

739-001-73   SPEECH PATHOLOGY and AUDIOLOGY

Peabody Individual Achievement Test

Math	3 – 7
R. Recognition	4 – 8
R. Comprehension	6 – 2
Spelling	5 – 6
G. Information	3 – 9
Total Test	4 – 6

Peabody Picture Vocabulary Test

C.A.	10 yrs. 6 mths.
M.A.	9 yrs. 1 mth.

The next two cases (Figures 7 and 8) have profound losses,
and were fortunate to have excellent parental involvement.
Both children attend schools for the normal hearing.

No single program can meet, to the same extent, the needs
of a group as diversified as the hearing impaired. It is
essential to have a number of different educational options,
but the early years are well spent developing auditory verbal
communication if the objective is full particiation in our
society.

DISCUSSION

DOCTOR J. JACOBSON
May I ask you the criteria you use for defining profound
deafness?

DOREEN POLLACK
The same as the national demographic survey to which we
subscribe. That is, an average loss of the speech frequencies
in the better ear of 91 dB.

DOCTOR R. RUBEN
Miss Pollack, an interesting presentation. Two things,
however, are missing. The first is an objective presentation
and analysis of the failures. The second thing is an analysis
of selectivity. I've been around too long to get upset about
an audiogram that's been missed. Any of us working in this
field knows that a child will develop and will learn to attend
to sound. What I find disturbing about the presentation is
that it is anecdotal and does not have an analysis of
successes and failures. I am compelled to speak, for I think
that not to mention that would leave one with the feeling,
"Aha, all children would do this well." That is patently not
the case. One also must challenge the logic of the statement,
"All children should have the opportunity to learn how to
speak". But there is another side to that coin. What is the
price which is paid by that substantative large number of
children who, for either physiological, anatomical, social or
psychological reasons, cannot obtain speech and then have no
language and no communication. On which side of the coin do
you do the least damage, and on which side of the coin do you
do the most help?

DOREEN POLLACK
    We have voluminous files on each child, with standardized
tests of the usual kinds - speech, language development and
intelligence testing, etc., etc., etc., - all this data is
there. Some of our children do not do well. Some of them
have very grave symbolic learning problems. However, these
children are not necessarily failures, you know, because they
have these other problems. In spite of all their problems,
we have managed to break through. If you have auditory
information, you have information for which there is no
substitute; information which helps open up the doors to
much learning. But no, I did not say all children could do
this either. I said this was never put forth as a panacea
for all deaf children. But every young child deserves this
opportunity because, for too long, we have made excuses for
our inability to teach these children and, I think, this is
really not so any more. But there are many multiply handicapped children who cannot learn and we need all the talent
and the knowledge in the world to deal with them.

DOCTOR R. RUBEN
    I'd like to make one other comment. An analysis of what
happens in the classroom in a School for the Deaf, by someone
like an efficiency expert, was very interesting. Approximately 22 minutes during the day there was useful teaching
going on. Twenty-two minutes of a 5 hour day. That might
explain a lot. For those of you who aren't following my
argument, let me clarify. What I'm saying is, that in a
highly personalized, a highly motivated program, instead of
getting 22 minutes a day, the child may get an hour and a
half.

DOREEN POLLACK
    Well, I appreciate your comments because the children who
can do well are always very rewarding and delightful. But
there just ought to be more of them if they have the opportunity. The children bring to us many problems, including,
as Dr. Lowell says, the problems of the break-up of the old-
time family patterns. We're dealing with that too. The
majority of our mothers today are working and/or single
parents and this has changed the situation too. So we have
many, many things to deal with. But this does not mean that
we should start out setting limits upon the child.

REFERENCES

Brown, R.   A First Language (Cambridge: Harvard University
    Press), 1973.

Eisenberg, R.   Auditory Competence in Early Life (Baltimore:
    University Park Press), 1976.

Levine, E.   Youth in a Soundless World (New York: New York
    University Press), 1956.

Libby, E. R.   Binaural Hearing and Amplification (Chicago:
    Zenetron), 1980.

Luria, A.R.   The Working Brain (New York: Basic Books), 1973.

Mindel, E. and McCay, V.   They Grow in Silence (Maryland:
    National Association of the Deaf), 1971.

Negus, V.E.   "Purposive Inattention to Olfactory Stimulation"
    Acta Otolaryngology, Supplement 105, 1958.

Office of Demographic Studies: REPORTS, including:
    Communication Patterns and Educational Achievements of
    Hearing Impaired Students, Series T2.   Washington.
    Gallaudet College. 1974 - 1978.

Ott, B., Balkany, T. and Pollack, D.   "Long Term Effects of
    High Power Hearing Aids" Paper presented at the Neuro
    Otology Conference, Palm Beach, California, 1980.

Pollack, D.   Educational Audiology for the Limited Hearing
    Infant (Springfield: Charles C. Thomas), 1970.

Pollack, D.   "The Denver Acoupedic Program" The Peabody
    Journal of Education 51:180 - 185, 1974.

United States Advisory Committee on the Education of the Deaf:
    The Babbidge Report. 1964.

Vigotsky, L.S. "Selected Psychological Investigations" Izd.
    Akad. Pedagog. Nauk RSFSR, Moscow, 1956.

EARLY SPEECH DEVELOPMENT

Daniel Ling
McGill University, Montreal, Quebec

Introduction

The ability to communicate through speech is of enormous value. It provides a range of opportunities and options in personal, educational and social life, as well as in employment, that cannot exist through any other form of interchange. Accordingly, it is of the utmost importance to ensure that, if at all possible, hearing-impaired children develop effective spoken language skills from early infancy.

In the 1970's there have been substantial, if not widespread, advances in the early identification of hearing impairment. Admission to early management programs is, thus, becoming feasible for an increasing number of children. Given such realities, can we look forward with confidence to a decade in which many more hearing-impaired children will learn to speak intelligibly and grow towards a full, independent adult life through the early use of spoken language? The answer to this question is resoundingly negative. Few more are likely to do so, though many more could. The rationale for this view is presented in the following sections, in which studies favoring early oral programs are reviewed, obstacles to the widespread provision of such programs discussed, and the achievements of profoundly hearing-impaired children who have had effective early oral treatment reported.

No one method or collection of methods can possibly be appropriate for all children. Thus, group comparisons receive mention, but their weaknesses and their potential to mask individual differences are recognized.

Obstacles to Appropriate Programming

There appear to be four major obstacles to generally improved standards of speech development in hearing-impaired children who are presented for treatment in early infancy. These are: (1) lack of program availability;

319

(2)   uncritical acceptance of prevailing philosophies;
(3)   unmet research needs in the areas of evaluation and
intervention; and,   (4)   an inadequate number of appropriately
trained professionals.

(1)   Program Availability

     There is abundant evidence that early parent/infant
programs can help advance the linguistic and academic performance of normally hearing children (Bronfenbrenner, 1975).
The value of early parent/infant programs aimed at developing
spoken language skills in hearing impaired children is not,
however, generally recognized.   Accordingly, few such programs exist.   Workers in those that are in operation have
not, in general, reported their results or attempted to
undertake or publish adequate evaluation and follow-up studies.
Thus, there are relatively few data that can be used to
justify the funding of these and further oral programs.

     Public and professional confidence in early oral programs
has also been eroded by biased, inaccurate and adverse reporting.   For example, the purpose of a study by Vernon and Koh
(1970) was to compare the attainments of deaf children of
deaf parents with those of deaf children of normally hearing
parents.   An unrepresentative sample of 32 matched pairs of
subjects aged 11 to 20 years was involved.   Only 10 of the
deaf children of normally hearing parents had had extensive
early oral education.   Five had had none.   Because the deaf
children of deaf parents were about a year ahead academically,
the outcome was interpreted -- and continues to be interpreted -- as evidence that early oral education is ineffective.
Even the finding in favor of the deaf children of deaf parents
was subsequently shown to be in error by Balow and Brill
(1975) who did an extensive study of the achievements in
reading and arithmetic of 590 children drawn from the same
population.   They found that deaf children who had attended
an early oral program scored significantly higher than those
who had not.   Apparently, the effects of early oral training
were so strong that they persisted even after several years
of education in a non-oral school.   This study has not been
widely cited.

(2) Prevailing Philosophies

In the past decade, thousands of children in North
America have been educated through a simultaneous (total
communication) approach. The trend has reached into early
parent-infant programs. So far, no results have been published to support the notion that the early introduction of
sign language (except for hearing-impaired children of deaf
parents, cf. Stuckless and Birch, 1966) has any advantage
over early oral education. The possibility that any linguistic advantage may persist and lead to academic superiority
in later school life is seriously challenged in a recent
study by Messerly and Aram (1980). Among many, Moores, Weiss
and Goodman (1978) have claimed that certain such advantages
exist, but they have provided no evidence to support their
position. Indeed, in their extensive studies of several programs described in a series of technical reports, there was
only one significant finding; namely, that orally taught
children have significantly better speech articulation skills
than those exposed to total communication (Fuchs et al, 1979).

Unless one can show that speech, academic achievements
and adjustment are, over a long-term period, fostered to a
greater extent by simultaneous teaching (total communication)
than by oral training, there can be no justification for the
trend to discard an oral approach in both early and later
education. Jensema and Trybus (1978), reporting on numerous
programs in the U.S., showed that the use of signs among
school aged children tended to replace rather than enhance
speech development. Indeed, among the 657 children studied,
those who signed most used speech least. Further, subjects'
academic achievements were shown to be negatively correlated
with sign language use but positively correlated with speech
in every one of the 20 conditions studied (Table 19, p. 17,
of Jensema and Trybus, 1978). In the calculations of these
correlations, the influence of program type, hearing loss,
preschool attendance, use of hearing aids and parental income
were partialed out. Thus, the evidence does not support the
notion that total communication yields results that are
superior to those obtained with speech. In fact, they show
the opposite.

It could, of course, be argued that in a large study
such as that undertaken by Jensema and Trybus (1978) the
results obtained in exemplary oral or total communication
programs would be obscured. However, results obtained by

Hanners (1977), who contrasted exemplary programs of each
type, showed that the academic achievements and the level
and variety of language skills of oral children were vastly
superior to those of children trained through total
communication.

Hanners' (1977) study, together with work reported by
Ling and Milne (1980), suggests that speech is best developed
from early infancy. Indeed, the extensive survey of speech
in numerous programs undertaken by Jensema, Karchmer and
Trybus (1978) indicates that when training is begun at a
later stage, children rarely become fluent talkers. Among
the 978 children they studied, no trend towards improvement
was observed with age or duration of treatment in special
education programs. In common with several other studies and
in accordance with the predictions of Carson and Goetziner
(1975) the authors found that speech intelligibility was
positively and significantly related to the use of speech in
teaching and everyday communication. They also reported
strong negative correlations between speech intelligibility
and the use of signs, finger spelling, gestures and/or
communication through writing. In view of the apparent need
to develop spoken language through the exclusive use of oral
procedures from early infancy, if speech is to become a
highly efficient system of communication, it is reassuring
to have the confirmation provided by McLean and Becker (1979)
that effective oral education is compatible with good psycho-
social adjustment. Even further, it is reassuring to note
that it does not cause the mental health problems that
Schlesinger and Meadows (1972) found common among children in
alternative types of programs.

To suggest that speech development is best fostered by
early and exclusive interaction through spoken language is
not to claim that all children either can, or should be
expected to develop high level speech communication skills
through the use of residual hearing. It would be ridiculous
not to support the use of Cued Speech (a visual-oral system)
with those children who have little or no useful audition or
fail to develop verbal skills adequately through an early
auditory-oral approach. As demonstrated by Nicholls (1979),
such children can achieve exceptionally high levels of speech
reception and spoken language through this system. It would
be equally absurd not to support the use of sign language
with those children whose parents wish it; with those who
cannot learn to communicate by speech; with those whose

spoken language cannot, given exemplary teaching, be developed
sufficiently to realize their potential both academically and
personally; and with those who, having acquired high levels
of oral skills, wish to become "bilingual" in speech and sign
and, thus, be able to communicate with their non-oral peers.

Current evidence, then, indicates that effective speech
development is incompatible with the early and continued use
of sign language. In this regard, it is significant that
after more than a decade of total communication in our schools,
not a single study has been published reporting that children
within this system have learned to produce speech that, on
objective measurement, is intelligible. Further, it seems
unlikely that, even if such data were published, it could be
shown that such children were representative or that they
could not have achieved even better spoken language if signs
had not been used.

(3)   Unmet Research Needs

The principal factors that underlie the successful and
early acquisition of spoken language skills have been isolated
but are certainly not adequately understood. It is now clear
that one cannot, on the basis of currently accepted measures,
predict at the time of diagnosis which children will fail and
which will succeed in the task of learning spoken language
skills. Such prediction, initially proposed by Northern and
Downs (1974) has not proved to be feasible (Downs, 1976).
Although initial diagnostic information is essential to the
teacher/clinician who works with hearing impaired children and
their parents, it is not sufficient either for the selection
of the most appropriate type of program or the choice of
habilitative procedures to be used. For most children, these
have to be determined in the course of ongoing, evaluative
treatment in an oral program (Ling and Ling, 1978). As shown
in Figure 1, numerous factors, both intrinsic and extrinsic
to the child, determine whether and/or how well abilities
relating to speech communication can be established. Some of
these factors have been arbitrarily assigned intrinsic or
extrinsic status. In fact, successful treatment involves
considerably more interaction of variables than can be shown
in simple diagrammatic form.

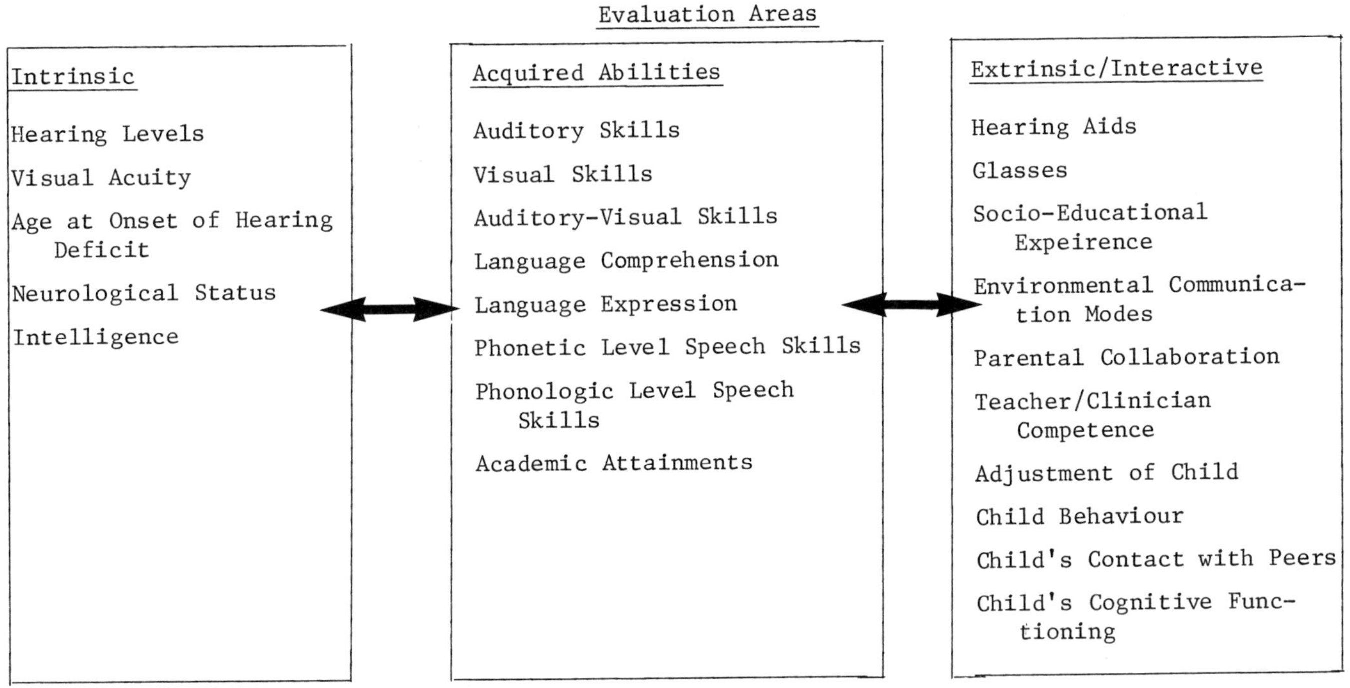

Evaluation Areas

Intrinsic

Hearing Levels
Visual Acuity
Age at Onset of Hearing Deficit
Neurological Status
Intelligence

Acquired Abilities

Auditory Skills
Visual Skills
Auditory-Visual Skills
Language Comprehension
Language Expression
Phonetic Level Speech Skills
Phonologic Level Speech Skills
Academic Attainments

Extrinsic/Interactive

Hearing Aids
Glasses
Socio-Educational Expeirence
Environmental Communication Modes
Parental Collaboration
Teacher/Clinician Competence
Adjustment of Child
Child Behaviour
Child's Contact with Peers
Child's Cognitive Functioning

FIGURE 1: The major intrinsic and extrinsic/interactive factors that determine what modality-related skills and levels of achievement can be acquired by hearing impaired children placed in early oral education programs.

The acquired abilities shown in the center box of
Figure 1 are the essential features of oral education: the
dependent variables which should be frequently measured to
determine each child's levels of skill, rate of progress and
immediate learning needs. To ensure adequate assessment of
every infant, research towards the development of better
measures of these variables should be given high priority.
But one cannot wait. Unless we use the rather coarse instruments that we currently have, there is a danger that children
will be left to languish wastefully in ineffective programs --
ineffective perhaps only because the extrinsic variables that
adversely affect a child's progress may remain unidentified
and, hence, unmodified. This topic has been pursued in considerable depth by Ling (1980a) to whom the reader is
referred for further discussion.

Pragmatic assessment in the course of training requires
that one should focus upon the measurement of a child's
acquired abilities. However, better measures of each of the
factors intrinsic and extrinsic to the child as listed in
Figure 1 are also required. Thus, for example, research is
needed on hearing aids and better fitting procedures; the
effects of socio-educational background; the influence of
communication modes (type, quality and quantity) on oral
progress; improved procedures for providing parents with the
three basic components of management for their hearing
impaired children -- counselling, education and directive
guidance -- and the measurement of their effects; the competencies required of the teacher clinician who is to work
effectively in early oral education and specifications of
the procedures that he should use to nurture optimal
acquisition of abilities by the infant. The list is not
exhaustive.

Further research is also required to specify how rates
of progress of children in early oral programs can be
increased and what rates of progress must be considered as
too slow to justify continuation of attempts to establish
spoken language communication in early infancy. A necessary
adjunct to such research would be the definition of factors
that would allow children who fail in early oral programs to
succeed in Cued Speech or in sign language programs. These
factors have not yet been adequately studied. As a result,
children may be transferred from early auditory-oral or
visual-oral provision in which they are not doing well, to
programs using alternative approaches in which, unless there
is systematic evaluation and treatment, they may also fail.

Many hearing impaired children can, of course, acquire
spoken language at a normal rate and at a normal developmental
stage if efficient habilitative treatment is begun well before
one year of age. However, children who are brought for treatment later in life and most who have hearing levels averaging more than 90 dB (ISO) usually lag behind normally hearing
children in their development of speech communication skills,
and are best helped through structured speech and language
intervention. For several such children, generalization of
spoken language skills from specific training to general use
may be a serious difficulty. This problem, regarded by Guess,
Baer and Sailor (1978) as "one of the most current and pressing of all aspects of teaching communication skills", is
particularly evident in children of school age (Ling, 1980b).
Our initial approach to research on generalization was to
examine transfer of training within and between each of the
six levels of processing depicted in Figure 2 (Ling, 1980a).
Studies currently being carried out are concerned with relating phonetic and phonologic skills, while controlling the
major underlying variables listed at the bottom of this
Figure. It is not within the scope of this paper to review
the considerable amount of work on generalization that has
been done with normally hearing children. No substantial
investigation of the topic has been undertaken with those who
are hearing impaired. Such investigation is urgently required.

(4)   Appropriately Trained Professionals

There is a widespread lack of professionals specifically
trained to develop speech communication skills in hearing
impaired children from early infancy. Three groups have
peripheral interest in the work: teachers of the hearing
impaired, speech/language pathologists and audiologists. For
none of these groups does traditional training provide the
essential expertise, although in general, teachers of the
deaf appear to possess more of the necessary skills than most
members of the other two professions. Speech pathologists, by
and large, have neither the pedagogical nor the audiological
skills that are required and few audiologists know much about
speech, language and education. There are some exceptions.
Thus, the field abounds in "experts", most who see but one or
two sides of a multifaceted discipline, a small number who
have themselves successfully nurtured the development of
spoken language skills in hearing impaired children.

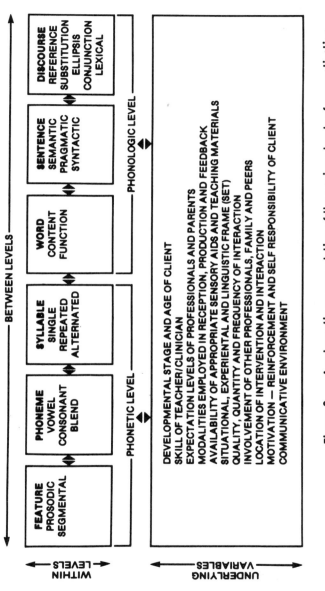

Figure 2. A schematic representation of the various levels of generalization that are involved in the acquisition of spoken language.

327

A commonly proposed solution when there is a lack of
true expertise is to try a 'team' approach. This is a poor
alternative to the preparation of competent professionals
(see Ling, Ling and Pflaster, 1977). Opinions expressed by
a number of people whose professional training is but peripheral to the task are not likely to have much validity.
Multiple sources of advice can be very confusing to parents
who are grieving after the diagnosis of their child's deafness and an excellent excuse for administrators who wish to
avoid taking action (Ling and Ling, 1978). Fortunately,
there are a few university programs which prepare specialist
teacher/clinicians for this work and a sufficient number of
exemplary early oral education settings in which their few
students may learn and practice their skills. Many more
university programs to prepare specialist teacher/clinicians
must be created for work through speech communication with
hearing impaired infants and their parents before any significant increase in the quantity or improvement in the quality
of early educational settings can be expected. The time
required to design such programs, the vested interests of
various professionals dabbling in the field and the present
state of the economy should all, unfortunately, conspire to
ensure that the 1980's will not be the decade in which the
majority of young hearing impaired children will receive
appropriate early opportunities for speech development.

Speech Production by Profoundly Hearing Impaired
Children: Results of an Effective Early Auditory-
Oral Program

The speech of profoundly hearing impaired children
(those with average hearing levels of more than 90 dB (ISO)
in the better ear) is usually less than 30% intelligible.
It also contains numerous typical errors (Ling, 1976;
Nickerson, 1975). These findings suggest either that deafness is an insuperable barrier to clear speech, or that
current programs are not adequately geared towards speech
training. The writer's view is that the latter is the case.
The purpose of this section is to report studies that provide
supporting evidence for this view.

The subjects in this study were 7 children, 3 boys and
4 girls, with hearing impairment of more than 90 dB (ISO) in
their better ears. They were drawn from a population of 9
such children who had attended the McGill Project for Deaf
Children from early infancy over a period of three years or

more from 18 months of age, or less. None had handicaps
addition to deafness. Following their early parent/infant
training program, they were placed in regular schools. When
this study began, they were between 6 and 12 years of age and
all but 1 (Subject 3) was functioning at or above the grade
level appropriate for his age. Subject 3 was one grade below
age level in reading skills.

Each subject was engaged in a conversation which was
recorded. The recordings were then analyzed and five sentences from 5 to 9 words each were dubbed onto another tape
for the purpose of rating intelligibility. Every tenth or
nearest to tenth sentence of this length was extracted to
ensure, (1) that the speech was representative of the child's
production; and, (2) that listeners received no contextual
cues. A control group of children with no history of deafness or communication problems, matched in age and sex, was
then drawn from regular school classes. Conversations with
each of them was recorded, analyzed and dubbed in the same
way.

A group of 17 incoming graduate students in Communication Disorders was given the task of listening to the recordings and writing down what each child said. The number of
words correctly identified in each sample was then tallied
and expressed as a percentage score for each child. A comparison of speech intelligibility of the two groups was
carried out. Results are shown in Table I. Pairs (hearing-
impaired versus normally hearing) are shown opposite to each
other. Thus, Subject 1 was paired in age and sex with Subject 8, or Subject 2 with Subject 9, and so on. The mean
scores for each group are shown in the bottom row.

Statistical tests indicated that the hearing impaired
subjects were no less intelligible than their normally hearing peers. Such results indicate that profound hearing
impairment is not an insuperable barrier to clear speech and
suggest that the widespread failure to attain highly intelligible speech reflects inadequate training strategies rather
than children's inability to learn. Not all 7 children had
normal sounding speech. Four showed a few of the faults
typically associated with "deaf speech". However, the program
which was initially provided for these children was in its
experimental stages and helped to shape the framework of the
system of training later proposed by Ling (1976).

The final stage of this study was completed 3 years later. During this period, all 7 of the subjects described above received occasional speech training according to their needs, as specified by phonetic and phonologic evaluations and procedures defined by Ling (1976). Spontaneous speech samples were recorded and later played back to 18 listeners unfamiliar with the speech of hearing impaired children. All subjects were 100% intelligible.

TABLE I

Percent Intelligibility Scores for all Fourteen Subjects

Hearing-Impaired		Normally Hearing	
Subject	Score	Subject	Score
1	91	8	95
2	98	9	95
3	74	10	93
4	78	11	92
5	91	12	90
6	95	13	75
7	56	14	71
Mean	81.9	Mean	87.1

Conclusion

In conclusion, I have outlined the four major obstacles to effective early oral programming and speech development for hearing impaired children. I have also shown that normal levels of speech communication can be achieved, even by profoundly hearing impaired children. That these children could acquire such natural speech communication skills, demonstrates that others can do similarly providing that the obstacles discussed above can be overcome to the extent that present day knowledge permits.

Acknowledgments

The writer is grateful to Muriel Milne, who collected the initial data on the intelligibility of the children, and to Dr. Agnes Phillips, who supervised much of their early diagnostic training. The results reported would not have been achieved were it not for the parents' collaboration over many years. Finally, my thanks are due to the children who have so willingly participated in every aspect of this work.

REFERENCES

Balow, I.H. and Brill, R.G. "An evaluation of reading and academic achievement levels of 16 graduating classes of the California School for the Deaf, Riverside," Volta Review, 77:255 - 266, 1975.

Bronfenbrenner, U. "Is early intervention effective?" in B. Z. Friedlander, G.M. Sterritt and G.E. Kirk (eds.) Exceptional Infant (Volume 3) (New York: Brunner/Mazel), 1975.

Carson, P.A. and Goetzinger, C.P. "A study of learning in deaf children," Journal of Auditory Research, 15:73 - 80, 1975.

Downs, M.P. in J. Alpiner (ed.) "Report of the ARA Committee on Research," Journal of the Academy of Rehabilitative Audiology, 9:34 - 35, 1976.

Fuchs, D., et al. "To the Editor," American Annals of the Deaf, 124:799 - 802, 1979.

Guess, D., Baer, D. and Sailor, W. "A remedial approach to teaching speech deficient children," Human Communication, 3:55 - 69, 1978.

Hanners, B.A. A Study of Language Skills in 34 Hearing-Impaired Children for Whom Remediation Began Before Age Three. Unpublished Ph.D. dissertation, Vanderbilt University, 1977.

Jensema, C.J., Karchmer, M.A. and Trybus, R.J. The Rated Speech Intelligibility of Hearing-Impaired Children: Basic Relationships And A Detailed Analysis (Washington, D.C.:

Office of Demographic Studies, Gallaudet College, Series R, Number 6), 1978.

Jensema, C.J. and Trybus, R.J. Communication Patterns And Educational Achievement of Hearing Impaired Students (Washington, D.C.: Office of Demographic Studies, Gallaudet College, Series T, Number 2), 1978.

Ling, D. "Integration of diagnostic information: implications for speech training in school-aged children," in Subtelny, J. (ed.) Speech Assessment and Speech Improvement for the Hearing-Impaired (Washington, D.C.: A.G. Bell Association), 1980a (in press).

Ling, D. "The integration of speech and language teaching," Paper to be presented at the International Congress on Education of the Deaf, Hamburg, August 1980(b).

Ling, D. Speech and the Hearing-Impaired Child: Theory and Practice (Washington, D.C.: A.G. Bell Association), 1976.

Ling, D., and Ling, A.H. Aural Habilitation: The Foundations of Verbal Learning in Hearing-Impaired Children (Washington, D.C.: A.G. Bell Association), 1978.

Ling, D., Ling, A.H. and Pflaster, G. "Individualized educational programing for hearing-impaired children," Volta Review 79:204 - 230, 1977.

Ling, D. and Milne, M.M. "The Development of Speech in Hearing Impaired Children," in F. Bess (ed.) Amplification in Education (Washington, D.C.: A.G. Bell Association), 1980 (in press).

McLean, G. and Becker, S. "Studies of the psychosocial adjustment of the hearing impaired," Canadian Journal of Psychiatry 24:744 - 748, 1979.

Messerly, C.L. and Aram, D.M. "Academic achievement of hearing-impaired children of hearing parents and of hearing impaired parents: another look," Volta Review 82:25 - 32, 1980.

Moores, D.G., Weiss, K.L. and Goodwin, M.W. "Early education programs for hearing-impaired children," American Annals of the Deaf 123:925 - 936, 1978.

Nicholls, G.H. Cued Speech and the Reception of Spoken Language (Washington, D.C.: Gallaudet Office of Cued Speech), 1979.

Nickerson, R.S. "Characteristics of the speech of deaf persons," Volta Review 77:342 - 362, 1975.

Northern, J.L. and Downs, M.P. Hearing in Children (Baltimore, MD: Williams and Wilkins Company), 1974.

Schlesinger, H.S. and Meadows, K.P. Sound and Sign: Childhood Deafness and Mental Health (Berkeley: University of California Press), 1972.

Stuckless, E.R. and Birch, J.W. "The influence of early manual communication on the linguistic development of deaf children," American Annals of the Deaf 111:462 - 462, 1966.

Vernon, M. and Koh, S.D. "Early manual communication and deaf children's achievement," American Annals of the Deaf 115: 529 - 536, 1970.

BILINGUALISM: AN ENVIRONMENT FOR THE DEAF INFANT

Sanford E. Gerber
Carol A. Prutting
University of California, Santa Barbara, California

We begin our discussion with the expression of some philosophical decisions with respect to the title of this paper and the subject matter of this conference. First, we take a stand that to deny any person -- child or adult, hearing or deaf -- any mechanism to communicate, is intolerable. After philosophical positions, we turn our attention to educational positions, and then to language and bilingualism in the context of the deaf community.

Philosophical Positions

Although the philosophy we present in this paper is a contemporary issue, the debates on this subject span centuries. There seems to be a climate of readiness or acceptance which may be attributed to the fact that the deaf community has become more visible with regard to educational issues and needs in general. Particularly, we have been influenced by the thinking and writing of theorists Gregory Bateson and Norbert Wiener. It was Wiener (1954) who considered that "communication and control belong to the essence of man's inner life ...". Ruesch and Bateson (1951) had similarly claimed that "communication includes all those processes by which people influence one another". It is not the fact that we communicate with similar animals, but the complexity and arbitrariness of the code we choose for this purpose, which is significant. With Wiener, we consider that "language" is another name for communication itself. We view our narrow habit within a larger context, one which Wiener considered to be justice. He said that there are three requirements for justice:

> "The liberty of each human being to develop in his freedom the full measure of the human possibilities embodied in him; the equality by which what is just for A and B remains just when the positions of A and B are interchanged; and a good will between man and man that knows no limits short of those of humanity itself."

The other philosophical position is the one for which we
are indebted to Bateson. Bateson observed that distortions
arise whenever the products of one system are superimposed
upon those of another. Consequently, he correctly observed
that "the logician's dream that men should communicate only
by unambiguous digital signals has not come true and is not
likely to." If a discrete digital code -- whether or not an
ideal language -- is not to be achieved, then how can we tell
if a given symbol system is a language? And, furthermore,
employing a notion mentioned above, if it is not a language,
then it does not communicate. That may be a little too
simple, however, because it implies that that which communi-
cates is perforce a language; although, that is probably true
for us human animals. But if we do not speak, then how can
we tell that communication has occurred?

If we adopt, and we do, the philosophical positions
taken above, then how do we know which form (manner, style)
of human expression counts as communication? Bateson considered "communication" and "behaviour" as synonyms. That
these are "an aggregate of data perceptible and meaningful
to other members of the same species." Certainly, we communicate in Bateson's sense to other members of our species without the use of the larynx. Consequently, it is our position
that, while speech, that is the auditory-vocal mode, is the
greatly preferred mode of communication in contemporary human
society, it is certainly not the only mode, nor is it in all
respects superior to others. Gleason (1979) noted that
language is a function of the brain, not the tongue or the
larynx. One of the basic premises upon which language
universals rest is the notion that no language is any more
complex than another. Languages are related by their underlying similarities to one another, rather than their surface
differences.

The question, then, which has been addressed by several
contemporary linguists (notably Bellugi and Klima) has been
to assess the linguistic (i.e., communicative) value of
systems which are visual/gestural. Information theory deals
with truth by exclusion. That is to say, this theory teaches
us that we are limited in the choices we make and frequently
come to necessary conclusions by observing what some phenomenon or set of phenomena is not. Bateson reminded us that
"the notion that language is made of words is all nonsense".
So, language is not words, and, hence, communication is not
composed of words. That is not to say that we cannot employ

words to communicate, but only that it is not essential.
Words, communication, or language are not necessarily English
or French, or either, or both. As before, then, what is
language communication? One of us (Prutting, 1979) observed
that the communicative system involves two people interacting,
switching back and forth in speaker and listener roles. Further, that the components of the communicative system -- the
presuppositions, the linguistic rules, and communicative
rules -- represent the shared knowledge acquired by the members of the communicative dyad in order to communicate.
Communication, according to Prutting, is a vehicle by which
we initiate, maintain, and terminate our relationships with
others. It should be noted that communication and its meaning is found in its use. Philosophers such as Pierce, James,
and Wittgenstein spent their lives theorizing about linguistic expression and all concluded that the essence of language
is in its utilitarian focus. In fact, communication acts are
based (if not totally contained) within Bateson's notion that
language is first and foremost a system of gestures. This is
not to exclude the oral gestures, nor is it required to
include only oral gestures. A language is defined by the
culture which uses it. It is a social system used to carry
on the everyday affairs of a language community.

Educational Positions

     The foregoing has been a summary of some of the main
contentions in the philosophy of language. In this section,
we present an educational philosophy. Foremost is the notion
that every child has a right to a full, complete, and early
education. Recall the earlier quotation from Wiener about
"the liberty of each human being to develop in his freedom
to the full measure of the human possibilities embodied in
him". Note that Wiener referred to the human possibilities
embodied in the person, not the human possibilities embodied
in a classroom teacher or the board of a local school district.
Furthermore, Wiener observed that languages (not language) are
epiphenomena, and are not themselves the phenomena of education or communication.

     In our part of the world, namely the southern part of
California, we have a large Spanish-speaking population.
Here in Canada, there is a large population of native speakers
of French. No one suggests that the learning abilities of
Spanish-speaking or French-speaking children are improved by

instruction in a foreign language. To be sure, both of
these groups are surrounded by an English-speaking milieu,
and they have some obligation to them. The purpose of education is self-contained. Dewey observed many years ago that
the only purpose of education is more education. If children
have a right to education and more education, they have a
right to be educated in their native language, reflecting
their own culture and values whether Spanish, French, or
Signs.

In particular, the research of Bellugi and Fischer
(1972) and of Cicourel and Boese (1972) has shown without
question that the language of Signs is the native language
of the deaf. However, just as we expect our Spanish-speaking
population of California and our French-speaking population
of Canada to be bilingual, we have every right to expect that
of the deaf as well. As socially competent adults, they
should be able to code-switch as needed. It is reasonable
for us, when it is possible, to ask the deaf to acquire
English as a second language. As it is reasonable for us to
expect the Chicano child to become a Chicano adult and the
Quebeçois child to become a Quebeçois adult, the deaf child
becomes a deaf adult, and like those other populations,
becomes a member of that community. The fact is, as Schlesinger (1978) has reminded us, "most deaf adults do ... acquire
mastery of language". Since, as we mentioned before, Bellugi
and Klima (1978) have shown clearly that the American Sign
Language has all the properties of natural language, it
therefore, meets the same criteria of a language such as
English, Spanish, or French. In addition, it is the language
preferred by and used by the deaf community. In fact, it is
the fourth most widely used language in the United States.

Of course, those who speak Spanish or French as a first
language in the English-speaking world frequently find it
important, even necessary, to speak English. For this reason
it is sensible for the deaf child to acquire English either
as a second language or, preferably, simultaneously with the
development of the native language of Signs. The use of
Signs and English is bilingual and bicultural to the same
extent and in the same manner as the use of English and
Spanish or French is to any other person. The work of
Schlesinger and her colleagues is illustrative. She has
observed that bimodal language acquisition shares much with
the acquisition of spoken language. Furthermore, she has
observed that each of the children in her studies acquired

the language of its mother, whether it was Signs or English.
In other words, the deaf children she has studied "have
demonstrated the capacity to learn one language in two modalities or even two languages in two modalities." What we are
saying is that the deaf child should be viewed not in terms
of auditory limitations, but in terms of the rights and
privileges of social fulfillment as a minority group.

ASL as a Language

McCall (1965) and Bellugi and Klima (1978) have observed
that the American Sign Language (ASL) has developed into a
language with all the systematicity and hierarchical organization which characterize other human languages. ASL is
characterized by stable, conventional hand movements, postures
and facial expressions which convey concepts shared by the
deaf culture. Sign language is a language which is independent of spoken language. Sign language makes systematic use
of the following parameters: orientation, configuration,
movement, and location or place of articulation. In addition,
ASL has all of the components of a language -- namely,
semantics, syntax and pragmatics. As in all languages, the
rules at each level, as reflected by the surface structure,
may be unique to that particular language. For instance,
pluralization in ASL is marked by reduplication of the Sign,
rather than with a morphological ending. Paralinguistic
features such as intonation for spoken language are conveyed
in ASL by facial expressions, while posture is utilized for
such semantic notions as affirmation, negation, and question
forms. Pragmatic rules for interaction such as turn exchanges
between partners, are signaled by a pause as the hands return
to an at rest position near the lower portion of the signing
space. The syntactic rules of ASL have been noted to be
ordered freely, nevertheless, ambiguity among native Signers
does not take place any more often than it does with spoken
English. At all levels, there are systematic rules for
interaction with ASL. They just do not happen to be the same
rules found in oral communication. The important point is
that ASL meets the criteria of a natural language and is
used by the deaf culture. Arguments in favor or against the
use of Sign language in the education of deaf children should
not include the linguistic status of the language, as value
judgments are no longer credible.

The Bilingual Deaf

    Experience with congenitally deaf adults has lead vir-
tually all observers to note that such people are bilingual
and bicultural. The point is communication, not English or
French or Spanish or ASL. Hardy and Hardy, in their collected essays (1977), observed that "... every reasonably normal
youngster develops a language learning system ...". This
system permits the learning of any language or languages.
For example, Penfield and Roberts (1959) supplied considerable evidence indicating that bilingualism or even trilingual-
ism is acquired with considerable ease if done at the earliest
time of life. Nevertheless, we all know that many people are
able to acquire a second language in adulthood. For example,
Schlesinger observed that hearing mothers of deaf children
have little difficulty acquiring American Sign Language. The
fact that the severely hearing impaired youngster develops a
language learning system permits the acquisition of visual/
motor language just as a hearing child acquires language in
the oral/aural mode.

    Bateson attributes to Lamarck a comment, presumably made
in 1809, that one cannot attribute psychological capacities
to a creature for which it has no organs. It is unreasonable,
at best, to demand an oral/aural mode of communicative competence of a creature which has no functioning auditory
organs. Of course, the vast majority of the profoundly
hearing impaired do have some residual hearing and it is
encumbent upon us to make maximum and optimum use of it.
But that optimum use requires the visual/motor mode. In fact,
the California courts, in what we believe is the first case
of its kind in the United States, have ruled that a deaf
child has a legal right to a bilingual education and the
local school district must provide it (Mclellan vs. Santa
Barbara County Schools, 1980). Furthermore, the state of
Texas includes ASL in its bilingual education programs.

    For quite a long time, the claim has been made that the
use of visual/motor communication interferes with the development of oral/aural communication. But this claim is without
substance. As a matter of fact, there has never been any
research to substantiate the claim, and all the research on
the issue has led to the opposite conclusion. How can this
be? Sperling (1978) hypothesized that "the more language
people know, the easier it is for them to learn still more
language". This leads to conjecture that acquisition of a

visual/motor language should be expected to enhance later
development of oral/aural language. The evidence supports
this contention. Moores (1978), writing in the same volume
as Sperling, noted that American deaf children who acquire a
Sign language from birth, develop skills in English usage
superior to those of deaf children who do not have the Sign
language skills. Sperling reviewed experimental data showing that young children who sign develop articulatory skills
at least as good as those who do not. This observation is
reminiscent of Quigley's (1969) experimental finding that
children who learn to fingerspell at a very early age develop
phonological skills superior to those of deaf children who do
not. We concur with Moores (1978), that it is an essential
goal of the education of the hearing impaired to promote
children who may become proficient in speech and speech
reading. The fact remains, however, that proficiency in
speech and speech reading depends, to a large extent, upon
proficiency in communication and, of course, on having something to say and having someone to say it to. Furthermore,
Moores correctly observed that a rigid adherence to an oral/
aural method, "even with the best of auditory training, is
self defeating for many deaf children". It is clear that
communicative competence has its origins in visual/motor
behaviour and is a prerequisite to auditory-vocal behaviour
(Bates, 1979).

We advocate, therefore, a means of early management
which is genuinely total. We are well aware that there has
been considerable lip service paid to the notion of total
communication. By total communication, however, we mean a
pedagogic method which is total and not partial. No moral
person who deals with profoundly hearing-impaired infants
would deny all acoustic and auditory means initially. Equal
morality demands that we never deny visual-motor means of
communication as well. The point is that the child must
learn to communicate. Having learned to communicate effectively, such a child could and should be expected to develop
into a bilingual adult, one who functions successfully in his
deaf community and also interacts with a larger hearing
community. The implications of all this for early management
should be self-evident. The only acceptable management procedure is one which is genuinely total; one which is visual/
motor and which is oral/aural. Nothing else can or should be
tolerated. A total program is an acceptance of deafness.

REFERENCES

Bates, et al. The Emergence of Symbols (New York: Academic Press), 1979.

Bateson, G. Steps to an Ecology of Mind (New York: Ballantine Books), 1972.

Bellugi, U. and Fischer, S. "A comparison of sign language and spoken language" Cognition, 1:173 - 200, 1972.

Bellugi, U. and Klima, E.S. "Structural Properties of American Sign Language," in L.S. Liben (ed.). Deaf Children: Developmental Perspectives (New York: Academic Press), 1978.

Cicourel, A. and Boese, R. "Sign Language and the Teaching of Deaf Children," in C.Cazden, V.John, and D.Hymes (eds.), Functions of Language in the Classroom (New York: Teachers College Press), 1972.

Gleason, J.B. "Gestural linguistics," Science, 205:1253 - 1254, 1979.

Hardy, W.G. and Hardy, M.P. Essays on Communication and Communicative Disorders (New York: Grune and Stratton, Inc.), 1977.

Liben, L.S., (ed.). Deaf Children: Developmental Perspectives (New York: Academic Press), 1978.

McCall, E. A Generative Grammar of Signs. Unpublished masters thesis. University of Iowa, 1965.

Moores, D.G. Educating the Deaf: Psychology, Principle, and Practices (Boston: Houghton Mifflin Co.), 1978.

Moores, D.G. "Current Research and Theory with the Deaf: Educational Implications," in L.S. Liben (ed.). Deaf Children: Developmental Perspectives (New York: Academic Press), 1978.

Penfield, W. and Roberts, L. Speech and Brain Mechanisms (Princeton: Princeton University Press), 1959.

Prutting, C.A. "Promoting Pragmatic Behavior." Mini-seminar presented for the annual convention of the American Speech-Language-Hearing Assn., Atlanta, 1979.

Prutting, C.A. and Skarakis, E.A. Communication Development. in S.E. Gerber (ed.). Audiometry in Infancy (New York: Grune & Stratton, Inc.), 1977.

Quigley, S. The Influence of Fingerspelling on the Development of Language, Communication, and Educational Achievement of Deaf Children (Urbana: University of Illinois), 1969.

Ruesch, J. and Bateson, G. Communication, the Social Matrix of Psychiatry (New York: W.W. Norton), 1951.

Schlesinger, H.S. "The Acquisition of Signed and Spoken Language," in L.S. Liben (ed.). Deaf Children: Developmental Perspectives (New York: Academic Press), 1978.

Simons-Martin, A. and Calvert, D.R., (eds.). Parent-Infant Intervention, Communication Disorders (New York: Grune & Stratton, Inc.), 1979.

Sperling, G. "Future Prospects in Language and Communication for the Congenitally Deaf," in L.S. Liben (ed.). Deaf Children: Developmental Perspectives (New York: Academic Press), 1978.

Wiener, N. The Human Use of Human Beings (Garden City, New York: Doubleday and Co., Inc.), 1954.

DISCUSSION

DOCTOR MacLEAN

    I had to take copious notes because the speakers were presenting a great deal of information in a very short time. One can hardly disagree with anything that they have had to say, except perhaps that the deaf community very often resents having hearing people as advocates. May I suggest to the organizers of this program that they might want a

deaf person to attend when they hold further conferences
that address some of these issues. The Quigley study in the
mid '60's was occasioned by the lag that graduates from
schools for the deaf showed in their ability to read and
write English. Do the speakers have any comments on the use
of signed English and reading? If English is the second
language, and we all advocate that the child learn to read
in his first language, how do we do this with ASL?

DOCTOR GERBER
     The answer, of course, is that you don't. Consider two
things - one is that the proposal we are making is a bilingual proposal, not a monolingual one. Secondly, that this
conference deals with infancy. I don't know any infants -
even hearing infants - who know how to read, so I don't see
that as a primary issue. If we are dealing with bilingualism, we will expect the child to learn to read and write in
the language of the melieu (e.g., English, French, Spanish).
In any case, we don't expect him to do it before the age of
2 years.

DOCTOR MacLEAN
     What about some kind of signed English as a formal first
language. Since hearing mothers of deaf children tend to be
able to learn signed English rather easily, is it better?

DOCTOR GERBER
     I suppose, however, as Doctor Rubin suggested this
morning, there is a horrifying lack of data. I would suppose
that signed English would be a very nice way to get from ASL
to English, but it is not another language, it is English.

     I would like to make a comment about the issue of who
Signs. It is unfortunate, as Schlesinger observed, that
although hearing mothers of deaf infants can learn to Sign,
they usually don't. In contrast, hearing children of deaf
parents learn to Sign very early, with no difficulty at all.
They are fully bilingual.

DOCTOR IN THE AUDIENCE
     We have talked about the end product being speech/lang-
uage, reading comprehension, etc., etc. In the beginning,
that's almost like the hole in the donut. You have to get

to it through the donut itself. The donut is really the process called socialization, or how does a family communicate.
How do you express such things as love, hate, anger, fear,
etc., etc. I wonder if the last two authors, and perhaps
the previous two authors, may want to comment. How does this
family communicate with one another during the first 18
months?

DOCTOR GERBER
    You mean here and now, or in the next 2 days?! I think
that's one thing we will want to share among all of us. I
think all of us have had different experiences with deaf
children and their families. What have I observed? It is
certainly my experience, and it may be a chicken and egg
process, that when I see the deaf babies in our parent program, they've already taught their parents to Sign.

DOCTOR LING
    I think Drs. Gerber and Prutting have very successfully
polarized the issue in the field. I think they've done it on
the basis of the type of advocacy that is, in fact, not very
helpful, because it is not advocacy that is supported by
anything more than theorizing. It's the sort of polemic that
we've heard from the deaf for a long time; the sort of pro-
paganda that we've heard from the deaf for a long time.
That is, the complaint that the literature to support the
notion that speech develops well in the presence of Sign is
not quoted or is claimed to be non-existent. This is simply
not the case. What is the case is that, not any time has
there been a study that has demonstrated that objectively
rated intelligible speech can be developed by children who
have simultaneously been exposed to speech and Sign. It
would have been impossible to demonstrate, as in the case of
Schlesinger and Meadows, that these children could not have
learned to speak equally well, and learn language equally
well, without the use of sign. I think that this is a rather
important point because, obviously, Sandy Gerber and I and
Carol Prutting and I read the same sort of literature and get
a great deal that's different out of it.

    As far as deaf advocacy is concerned, I think that
there's some terrible assumptions that are being made, particularly, that the deaf really ought to be in a deaf community. I think that this is sort of global type thinking that's

very weak and wrong. One might as well say that all mentally
deficient people should be in a mentally deficient community;
physically handicapped people in a physically handicapped
community, and so on. To say that, in fact, one should
really regard the deaf as having a guideline possibility for
where deaf education and early treatment should go is crazy.
Because I breath, I am not an expert in pulmonary medicine.
If I were mentally deficient, I would not be able to specify
what should be done for mentally handicapped children.   I
think you've done an excellent job in presenting what is, in
fact, a non-scientific, highly emotional, highly polemic
discussion which has, in fact, polarized the way in which I
think would be to really discuss things in the portion of
this conference that lies ahead.

DOCTOR GERBER
     I think it quite correct to say that the deaf should not
decide what's best for them, and, of course, that the
mentally deficient should not be segregated among the mentally deficient. While that is correct, I think it's the
wrong sociological position. If I were black, I would say,
"Honky, get off my back!"

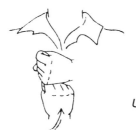

"ADVOCATE"

Carol A. Prutting
Sanford E. Gerber
University of California, Santa Barbara, California

In light of the acceptance of deafness as indicated by
Gerber and Prutting in this volume, we can state with certainty that American Sign Language (ASL) meets the criteria
of a natural language and is used by the majority of the deaf
in the United States and parts of Canada. Further, as a
generalization based primarily on the results of scientific
research of the last two decades, we can also say that ASL
does not restrict or educationally interfere with the acquisition of cognition or competence in spoken English.

Science, Findings and Responsibility

Bronowski (1977) stated that science can be practiced
only "... if we value the truth. The activity of science is
committed to truth as an end in itself." The findings, therefore, can be neither good nor bad. The scientific community
endeavors to set experience in some kind of order. Science is
predicated on the assumption that scholars know what the world
is like (Kuhn, 1970).

We now know more than ever before about the social, cognitive, psychological and linguistic world of deafness.
There are responsibilities across disciplines which come with
this knowledge. Continued advances rest on the interface
among professionals in deaf education, speech/language pathology, linguistics, audiology and psychology, to name a few.

Fuller (1975) has stated:

"We are in an age that assumes the narrowing trends
of specialization to be logical, natural, and desirable. Advancing science has now discovered that all
known cases of biological extinction have been caused
by overspecialization, whose concentration of only
selected genes sacrifices general adaptability."

Fuller goes on to say that:

"In the meantime, humanity has been deprived of
comprehensive understanding. It has also
resulted in the individual's leaving responsibility for thinking and social action to others."

We live in a credentialed, over-specialized society.
The lack of articulation between hearing and deaf individuals
and within and across those fields interested in the welfare
of the deaf is all too evident. The challenge is to break
down the divisions among areas and to view our common goal:
being "Advocates" for the deaf. An advocate is one who argues
for, defends, maintains and recommends a cause or proposal.
A document published by the United States Department of
Health, Education and Welfare (1965) indicated, "Deaf people
generally look upon themselves, not in the negative terms of
their auditory limitations, but in the positive terms of their
rights and privileges for social fulfillment as a minority
group." That is how the deaf view themselves; more importantly, what are our attitudes toward the deaf? The most
pressing work to do across all disciplines is in the area
of the rights and privileges of the deaf.

Identification of the Problem

The foundation upon which this paper is developed is
two-fold. First, that when an individual has a speech, language, and hearing problem, it is one's social identity which
is affected. Goffman (1963), in his book Stigma, discusses
the various aspects of social acceptance and compensations
made by individuals when a diminished social identity exists.
The core of the deaf person's difficulties manifest themselves in social problems as well as auditory ones.

The second assumption is that successful education is a
process of socialization, not a preparation for it. Dewey
discussed this aspect of education in 1897:

"Education being a social process, the school is
simply that form of community life in which all
those agencies are concentrated that will be most
effective in bringing the child to share in the
inherited resources of the race, and to use his

own powers for social ends. Education, therefore, is a process of living and not a preparation for future living."

Socialization revolves around communication. An individual's language is a reflection of a particular social group
or culture. Acceptance of one's language is an acceptance
of that person and the culture from which the language
evolved. It has been common to find ethnic minorities fight-
ing for their identity and acceptance as a group through the
centuries. Almost always, the focus was on the use of their
own language. This has also been true of the deaf culture.
For example, young deaf children have been found to generate
their own esoteric sign systems to code and share their
experiences with others. The reliance on non-verbal communication, as well as verbal behaviour, has been reported even
in settings where only spoken English was being developed
(Curtiss, Prutting and Lowell, 1979). In Canada, in the
Province of Quebec and the City of Montreal, the merging of
three cultures created French Canadian Sign Language (FCSL),
a combination of ASL and two spoken languages, English and
French. The language was created clandestinely by students
at the Institute des Sourds and Muetes so that they could
communicate more effectively than they could with the spoken
language they were being exposed to at the same time
(Mayberry, 1978).

In the novel written by Greenberg (1972), In This Sign,
there is a description of how the deaf come to associate the
use of Signs with the smell of urine, since the only place
they were allowed to Sign was in the lavatory. All of these
examples depict the fortitude and compelling drive which the
deaf have had in order to maintain their identity through the
use of language. If spoken English alone had met their needs
for socialization, there would have been no need to create,
generate, and maintain their Sign language, even under the
most adverse conditions.

The Deaf Culture

In order to be an advocate for the deaf, it is necessary
to understand this unique culture and the problems which face
it. The deaf, as any minority group within a country, live

in two cultures, the deaf and the hearing. They are different worlds and, in passing from one to the other, one must
become acclimated. The Norwegian psychiatrist, Basiler (1973)
stated:

> "When I accept another person's language, I have
> accepted the person ... When I reject a language,
> I have rejected the person because the language
> is part of ourselves ..."

The deaf know subtle aspects of deafness that we do not
always understand. Wright (1969) in his book, Deafness,
wrote:

> "The deaf do not, because they cannot, deal in
> the nuances - particularly the verbal nuances -
> of personal relationships. Their dealings are
> direct - may appear outrageously direct; their
> handshakes are ungloved. They have a naivete,
> and also a plain honesty of intent, that makes
> the polite wrappings up of ordinary people seem,
> by contrast, hypocritical."

Wright goes on to discuss some of the most difficult
communicative problems which the deaf face:

> "Not being able to overhear, rather than not being
> able to hear, is the real turn of the screw. Being
> overheard is a related problem, for I have no judg-
> ment of how far the voice can carry, or of what
> noises may mask it. In crowds, or where people
> are about, the instinct is to lower the voice -
> particularly when what I have to say is not meant
> for the general ear. Conversely, my impulse is to
> raise it in empty places or where no one is around.
> So, I have an involuntary and maddening tendency to
> whisper at parties but shout in churches."

In the recent play, Children of a Lesser God, a deaf
actress commented that a hearing actor's use of signs suggested he was using ASL with a hearing accent. These are unique
comments which could have been made only by the deaf.

Few hearing people know ASL. When using spoken English
with the deaf, they tend to talk slower, be more careful, and
to exaggerate lip movements and facial expressions. By the

same token, few deaf people can produce and comprehend spoken English well. Each half of the dyad, the deaf and the hearing, must absorb a part of the impact of the communication breakdown. It has been reported that hearing parents do not learn Signs while their deaf children are growing up. All of these facts add up to a frustrating situation for both the deaf and the hearing.

Toward Advocacy

Across disciplines there is a need to represent and acknowledge the deaf culture. Acceptance is intimately tied to their language, ASL. While linguists have already begun to describe the semantic and syntactic rules of Sign language, information is needed concerning the pragmatic aspects of ASL. That is, details are required concerning the use of the language, its rules for managing discourse interactions such as turn-taking topic maintenance, and the physical proximity as communicative partners. Viewing the pragmatic aspects of ASL will bring us closer to understanding the social behaviours and values within this culture.

Pediatricians now view themselves as advocates for the child. We should view ourselves as advocates for the deaf. Professionals such as teachers of the deaf, speech/language pathologists, audiologists, otologists, and psychologists need to come to philosophical grips with ASL. Whether you test a deaf person's hearing, counsel parents about educational placement, teach academic material or assess and remediate speech and language, it will be necessary to learn about and thereby acknowledge, the deaf culture.

Academics involved in the leadership of various programs in which students are being trained to work with the deaf need to ensure that ASL is included in the curriculum. In a recent general survey of both the fields of educators of the deaf and speech/language pathology and audiology, we found that only 10 universities out of 100 programs offered ASL as a course. Only one offered a course related to the social-cultural aspects of deafness.

Bilingual programs such as Teaching English as a Second Language (TEASL) in the future, will offer us a wealth of information. This discipline has already dealt with the core issues of bilingual education with other minority groups in the United States. The recent appraisal of successful

programs indicates that a functional, utilitarian emergence
of both languages during infancy is most desirable. We can
utilize the ground work already laid down by this field for
our own purposes.

    In order to be advocates for the deaf, we will need to
turn our efforts to a joint interdisciplinary venture and
deal with all the issues which bilingualism raises. Many of
us entered our chosen career field to work with the deaf,
only to find that at the time, we were involved in very
different issues than we are now. Today we are in the business of social change and the promotion of human welfare
involving a minority group with all the rights and privileges
of any group. To be an advocate for the deaf now is to be
political.

    We, therefore, recommend that all professionals who deal
with the deaf assume the advocate's positive attitude,
namely, to accept the deaf infant. We are not talking about
ears, but children, and our attitudes toward them.

REFERENCES

Bronowski, J. A Sense of the Future (Cambridge: MIT Press),
    1977.

Curtiss, S., Prutting, C., Lowell, E. "Pragmatic and seman-
    tic development in young children with impaired hearing,"
    Journal of Speech and Hearing Research, 22:534 - 552, 1979.

Fuller, R. Synergetics (New York: Macmillan), 1975.

Goffman, E. Stigma (Englewood Cliffs, New Jersey: Prentice-
    Hall, Inc.), 1963.

Greenberg, J. In This Sign (New York: Avon Publishers),
    1972.

Anonymous. Interpreting for Deaf People (Washington, D.C.:
    U.S. Department of Health, Education and Welfare), 1965.

Kuhn, T. The Structure of Scientific Revolutions (Chicago:
    The University of Chicago Press), 1970.

Mayberry, R. "French Canadian Sign Language: A study of
   Inter-Sign Language Comprehension," in P. Siple (ed.).
   Understanding Language through Sign Language (New York:
   Academic Press), 1978.

Wright, D. Deafness (New York: Stein and Day), 1969.

MANAGEMENT AND FOLLOW-UP OF EARLY DETECTED HEARING IMPAIRED CHILDREN

Lilly Tell
Moshe Feinmesser
Chaya Levi
Hadassah University Hospital, Jerusalem, Israel

Early detection of hearing impaired children is extremely important for establishing an appropriate habilitation program.

The parents, the clinician and the social worker are the persons involved in pursuing the program. However, first they have to cope with the problem of deafness itself and its influence on their own personality.

The parents of the deaf child are the key persons during the child's infancy and early childhood. They are the ones who are most in need of assistance when faced with the diagnosis of deafness - usually before the child reaches one year of age. They are in a state of shock and confusion which can be alleviated only by constant help received from professional personnel (Table I).

TABLE I: PARENTS' EMOTIONAL STATUS

Despair, disappointment, disbelief

Lack of understanding of the problem

Appeal to various consultants

Gradual understanding parallel with child's progress

Cooperation in the habilitation program

Interaction between the parents, the clinician and the social worker enables the family to see the child primarily as a child and secondly as a child with a problem; namely,

hearing impairment. These perceptions help to reach a
balance between the normal physical and psychological
development of the child, and the need to use every opportunity for contact with the outer world through residual
hearing, vision and innate intellectual endowment.

1. First Stage

     The clinician starts the actual work with the child and
parents in the Speech and Hearing Center while taking several
factors into consideration (Table II).

TABLE II: SPEECH AND HEARING CENTER, DETERMINING FACTORS IN
           PLANNING THE HABILITATION PROGRAM

The child's age

The child's degree of deafness

The child's psycho-motor development

The family's intellectual level

The family's socio-economic status

     Usually early management of the hearing impairment is
influenced by the kind of reactions exhibited during the
first hearing tests, general health status and the child's
behaviour during the process up to the final diagnosis.
Sometimes management is dictated by these factors and may
follow a natural sequence of procedures if deafness occurs to
an otherwise normal child. If the child has other problems,
the help of the neuropediatrician, the geneticist and the
child's psychologist is enrolled.

     In the initial stage, parents visit the Audiology/Speech
and Hearing Center once or twice weekly for a mean period of
6 months. Every child is given the same opportunity in the
standard habilitation program. At this stage, early

amplification is started by fitting the children with individual hearing aids, teaching them to adjust to those devices,
and training them to an auditory awareness of sounds and
visual contact with the people in their surroundings.
Emphasis is placed on developing vocalization, babbling and
incipient communication. The clinician tries to estimate
each child's general development and emotional disposition.

The routine work in the Speech and Hearing Center conducted by the clinician with the support of the social worker
helps the parents to familiarize themselves with their
child's deficiency, but at the same time, encourages them to
see the child's positive traits which will enable him to
compete in the world of the hearing in spite of deafness
(Table III).

TABLE III: SPEECH AND HEARING CENTER, HABILITATION PROGRAM

Fitting of hearing aids

Developing the child's: auditory awareness, eye contact,
                          attention span, imitation ability,
                          vocalization, babbling, communication

Evaluation of the child's readiness for referral to Micha
Center

---

2.   Second Stage

The second stage in the management is the Micha Society
for Deaf Children

In our country, the Micha Centers are the most important
habilitation institutions before pre-formal education is
started at the age of 3 years. The program of Micha is
geared towards the development of communication, either oral
or total, and endeavours to help the child to speak and
understand speech. The program is two-pronged for the child
and the parents. The Centers utilize electronic amplification equipment to help the child to make maximal use of

residual hearing. Transportation is provided to and from
the Centers, and a large number of volunteer teachers' aids
are employed to offer additional help to underprivileged
parents or new immigrants. The personnel of Micha are in
continuous contact with the clinicians in the Speech and
Hearing Center. By the time a child is 2½ - 3 years of age,
the clinicians have obtained an accurate audiogram and re-
evaluated the kind of hearing aids the child has been using.
This information is transferred immediately to Micha.

The years spent by the child in Micha will be the basis
for the whole educational program. The goal of the preformal
training is to help develop the ability to acquire the
necessary language to cope with hearing children in a suitable educational framework. The child begins to function
according to those innate special gifts which will enable
him, a little later on, to demonstrate his full potential.

At the same time, the parents mature with the child's
problem. They become more determined to work in close co-
operation with the professional personnel to achieve the
goal to habilitate their deaf child. The child's progress is
due not only to the teacher, but also to the parents who
sometimes have to change their habits at home, renounce their
mother tongue and find a way of life devoted to their deaf
child without damaging their attitude towards their other
children (Table IV).

TABLE IV: MICHA CENTER

CHILDREN	PARENTS
Individual and group auditory training	Individual and group guidance and counselling
Developing speech and language	Lectures by professionals Audio-visual aids
Detecting special gifts	Home-training, if necessary
Teaching group interaction in communication and play	Active participation in the training program
Evaluating suitable school frameworks	Participation in evaluation
Social workers' and Volunteers' services	

3. Third Stage

In the third stage which represents pre-formal teaching,
the hearing impaired children are integrated in a kindergarten for normal hearing children. The professional supervision continues to be under the auspices of Micha Center.
Especially trained kindergarten teachers assist the regular
kindergarten teachers. There are 4 integrated kindergartens
in Jerusalem. In 2 of them, emphasis is placed on Jewish
customs and practices, as required by a group of religious
parents. There are 7 - 8 hearing impaired children to 20
normal hearing children in each kindergarten. All the indoor
and outdoor activities are geared to enrich the vocabulary
of the hearing impaired child, expressive language, and
adjustment to normal hearing peers who provide a natural
stimulating environment. Each hard-of-hearing child has two
individual training periods during the day in addition to the
common group activities with hearing children. In the
individual sessions, the special kindergarten teachers try
to prepare the hard-of-hearing children for the story-telling
hour or for any specific subject matter to be discussed in
the classroom with all the children. They also take care of
the auditory training and speech correction they need.

The rate of progress in language acquisition and the
ability to use speech determines who will succeed orally and
who will require total communication. The specially trained
kindergarten teachers are proficient in both methods and try
to adapt them according to the children's needs.

During the years in kindergarten, each child begins to
show an innate trend for the kind of education for which he
will best be suited. This natural trend - oral or total
communication - determines also the parents' attitude and
their own aspirations for their children. Some of the parents
easily accept the fact that their sons and daughters will
continue their education among deaf peers, while others
decide to fight for oral-auditory integration, even if their
own children do not exhibit the necessary gifts or
intelligence (Table V).

At the end of the kindergarten period - around 6 years
of age - several parameters are taken into consideration by
a team of professionals in order to decide the most suitable
educational program for each child. These include:

1) The ability to function through hearing

2)   The quality of speech production;

3)   The language level as measured by formal language tests;

4)   Results of formal Intelligence Tests;

5)   Behavioural and social maturity.

   The eventual educational framework for the deaf child
will vary with the factors outlined. Included in the
current possibilities are individual integration in regular
schools, group integration in regular schools, individual
integration in special schools, School for the Deaf, retarded
classes in School for the Deaf, and institutions.

TABLE V: PARENTS' ATTITUDE TOWARDS EDUCATION

Relentless efforts for oral communication	Satisfied with any kind of communication
Higher standards of achievements	Basic skills for daily needs

READY FOR   -   changes in family customs   -   NOT READY

              Not Deterred By: Deterred By:
                    a.   socio-economic drawbacks
                    b.   number of siblings
                    c.   number of deaf siblings

| Choice of education and career through integration | - End Goal - | Material Security not minding segregation |

4. Fourth Stage

    Deaf children found suitable for individual integration
in schools for hearing children of normal intelligence participate in all school activities including subject matters,
sports and social events. This participation is dependent
upon 3 - 5 weekly sessions of special instruction provided by
the educational authorities outside the school's schedule.
In these sessions, special teachers for the integrated deaf
children assist in mastering new school material, correcting
speech defects and taking care of other needs. This is done
under the guidance of a supervisor responsible for the education of the deaf. An experiment is carried out to integrate
3 - 6 deaf children in a regular class of 30 - 35 hearing
children. In this kind of integration, children participate
only in certain activities - mainly skills or sports - and
are given special help in subject matters by specially
trained teachers.

    Deaf children with serviceable residual hearing, but
with dull-normal intelligence, are still benefiting from
integration. However, they are enrolled in special schools
(e.g., schools for mentally retarded or emotionally disturbed
hearing children).

    Deaf children with additional problems (such as cerebral
palsy), but of normal intelligence, are integrated in special
schools, also for hearing children.

    The School for the Deaf is the most suitable educational
facility for those children who function best in small groups
(7 - 8 children in a class). These profoundly deaf children
often suffer from additional problems. During the 8 years
spent in the School for the Deaf, the Principal and the
teachers try to accommodate every child according to special
needs.

    The curriculum in the School for the Deaf and the text
books are similar to those in regular schools, but the educators use many additional special materials in order to adapt
them to the level of the children. Subjects are taught for
the main purpose of enriching language and correcting speech.
Daily news, current events, political actualities, personal
and family happenings, are discussed in classrooms. Most of
the children are guided towards crafts and manual professions
at the end of the elementary school. A new experiment is

taking place right now; namely, the foundation of a high
school for deaf graduates in which formal education will
continue.

Results of our Program

   We shall describe the results of the management of 69
children diagnosed as hearing impaired by the clinicians in
our Speech and Hearing Center and by different educational
services in Jerusalem. The 69 children were detected out of
40,000 newborns in Jerusalem during the period September 1,
1967, to September 1, 1974. The oldest child is now approximately 12½ years, while the youngest is 6 years old.

   Forty-six children were detected during the first year of
life, 8 in the second year, 6 in the third year, and 9 with a
moderate degree of deafness, when they were older than 3 years
of age. The detection was performed using the methods which
were reported in previous papers (Feinmesser and Tell, 1976a;
Feinmesser, Tell and Levi, 1977a; Tell, Levi and Feinmesser,
1976b). The hearing impaired children were divided into four
categories according to their degree of deafness (Goudman,
1965; Silverman and Davis, 1970).

   Accurate audiograms (see Table VI) were obtained from 60
children; the remaining 9 were assessed as hearing impaired by
results recorded in a free field testing situation by impedance audiometry and by Electric Response Audiometry tracings
(Tell, Levi and Feinmesser, 1978; Sohmer, Feinmesser, Tell,
Levi and David, 1972; Leiberman, Sohmer and Szabo, 1973;
Sohmer and Feinmesser, 1974).

TABLE VI: DEGREE OF DEAFNESS IN 69 CHILDREN ASSESSED BY:

	Reliable Audiogram	Free Field Response ERA Tracings
Profound	22	7
Severe	20	1
Moderate Severe	6	1
Moderate	12	–
Total	60	9

Follow-up and Comment

Out of the 69 children, 2 died before the age of 1 year and another 2 left the country at the same time. Sixty-five out of 69 children could be followed up systematically from the time of detection until the present time (Figure 1).

As pointed out in this paper, early detected children were given the same habilitation opportunities, but progress in acquiring language was not the same for all of them, no doubt, due to the effects of the factors seen in Table II.

Three children had to be institutionalized before the age of 1 year, because they suffered from multiple handicaps in addition to deafness. Fourteen of the children were enrolled in the School for the Deaf, two of whom were in a class for retarded deaf children. Of the remaining 12, 9 were of borderline intellectual ability, their language level being poor and their parents' co-operation insufficient.

It is noteworthy that 3 profoundly deaf children and 1 severely hearing impaired child who were referred to the School for the Deaf could have been integrated had their parents chosen to do so and co-operated towards this aim. However, there were deaf siblings in the family and the parents preferred segretagion to integration because they could not cope again with the efforts previously required (Downs, 1972).

Twelve profoundly and 17 severely deaf children were found suitable for continuing their education in regular schools. Two of them were in special schools for mentally retarded and/or emotionally disturbed hearing children. One other child had become deaf in the third year of its life because of illness and the habilitation program was initiated immediately. Normal intelligence, very encouraging parents, and well established speech and language before the child became deaf, helped in its integration. In all, normal or above normal intelligence, complete dedication of the parents and good progress in language acquisition made possible the successful integration of the 29 children. Two additional advantages contributed to the ability of this group to compete in regular schools:

1)   an innate gift for language acquisition; and,

2)   continuous, gradual educational progress from the

FIGURE 1: EDUCATIONAL FRAMEWORKS FOR 65 DEAF CHILDREN

EDUCATIONAL FRAMEWORKS FOR 65 DEAF CHILDREN

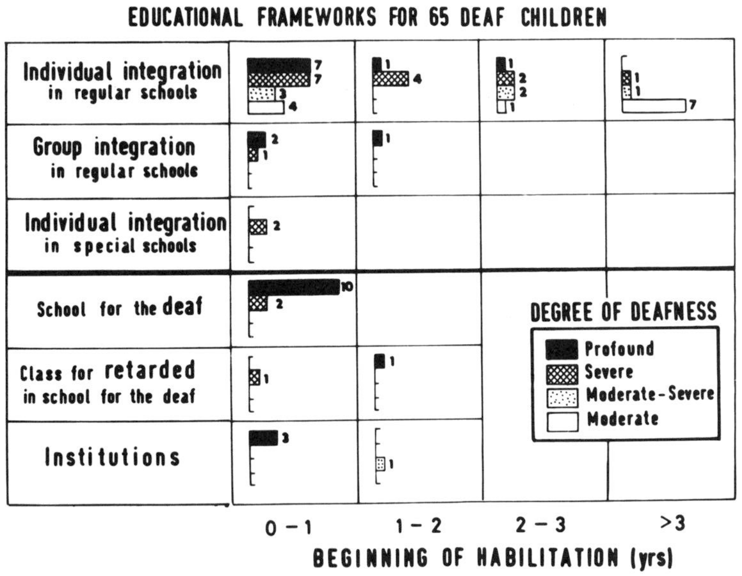

starting of the program until enrollment in a suitable
school framework.

Eighteen children needed only auditory amplification and
educational help in schools. The hearing impairment of this
group was of a moderately-severe or moderate degree. They
succeeded in studying in regular schools, also due to normal
intelligence and their parents' endeavors.

One child with a moderate-severe degree of deafness had
to be institutionalized because of severe mental retardation.

According to the reports of the teachers in the regular
schools, the integration of the hearing impaired children is
satisfactory, both in school subjects and in school social
activities. Efforts are made to facilitate contact between
them and their hearing peers during the after school hours
by establishing common clubs with different programs.

Conclusions

The success of the habilitation program with the aim of
integration is secured if the following three conditions are
fulfilled:

a) Parents' complete dedication to this goal;

b) Normal or above normal intelligence of the child;

c) An innate gift for language acquisition.

Children with severe hearing loss may be successfully
habilitated and integrated even if they are detected in the
second or third year of life. Profoundly and severely deaf
children can ultimately succeed, only if there is no interruption between the time of detection and complete integration
in the course of their struggle to acquire language.

Profoundly or severely deaf children of below normal
intelligence and those who do not have the benefit of very
cooperative parents have to be referred to the School for
the Deaf, even though the habilitation program was started
immediately after early detection.

DISCUSSION

PERSON FROM AUDIENCE
     I have two points I'd just like to highlight in terms of
what you've brought up. I'm a little bit concerned about the
possibility for either bias or judgment to come in. Numerous
times during the presentation you mentioned the issue of
normal intelligence as a pre-requisite for selecting children.
I'm really quite interested in how that is determined and why
that is focused on in the fashion that it is. Especially
when we know that that's often times confusing with the non-
impaired child. Secondly, you mentioned issues of an innate
gift or innate type of function either for capacity for
language or otherwise. Again, that is something that seems
very open to bias and judgment to use to separate different
children. I'd appreciate your comments on those areas.

LILLY TELL
     When we at the Speech and Hearing Centre have worked
with the child, we see his rate of progress. If he has
intelligence, he will progress according to a certain program.
In addition, they are given formal intelligence tests by
objective authorities, psychologists at the Municipal Department of Education. We tried to integrate every child, but we
did not succeed until we realized that only those children
who were of normal intelligence succeeded in competing with
35 to 40 children in a classroom. This is a fact.

     Now for the question of those innate gifts for language.
Do we all have, all of us here in this room, the same innate
gift for language? We do not. The same is true for deaf
children. If I am starting to work with the child and the
child's progress is at a special rate because there is
something intangible, something that I cannot measure, I say
he has a special talent. Like I see, and Picasso sees, and
so on. So, there is a special gift for this.

PERSON FROM AUDIENCE
     You mentioned that most of your presentation was about
children from Jerusalem. I was curious as to what happens
to the other children from around Israel, from other areas;
what happens to them? Do they stay with their families and
are they treated within the families, or do they have to come
for their pre-kindergarten program to your center?

LILLY TELL
    No. I'm proud to say that similar programs are all over
my country. I brought the one here from Jerusalem because I
have very strick follow-up data starting September 1 and to
this date, and I know exactly what happens to all of my 69
children. But similar programs are in the North of the
Country, around Tel Aviv, and in the South of the Country.
The detection and the means of diagnosis are not exactly the
same. They are best in our capital which is my Jerusalem.

REFERENCES

Feinmesser, M., Tell, L. "Evaluation of methods for detect-
    ing. hearing impairment in infancy and early childhood"
    in Mencher, G.T. (ed.) Early Identification of Hearing Loss
    (Basel: Karger), 1976.

Feinmesser, M. and Tell, L. "Neonatal screening for detec-
    tion of deafness" Archives of Otolaryngology 102:297 - 299,
    1976.

Feinmesser, M., Tell, L. and Levi, C. "Screening for hearing
    impairment in early childhood" ORL 39:227 - 232, 1977.

Tell, L., Levi, C. and Feinmesser, M. "Screening of infants
    for deafness in baby clinics" in Bess, F.H. (ed.) Childhood
    Deafness (New York: Grune & Stratton), 1977.

Goodman, A. "Reference zero levels for pure-tone audiometers"
    ASHA 7:262, 1965.

Silverman, S.R. and Davis, H. "Hard of hearing children" in
    Davis, H. and Silverman, S.R. (eds.) Hearing and Deafness
    (New York: Holt, Rinehart & Winston), 1970.

Tell, L., Levi, H. and Feinmesser, M. "The Hadassah Program
    for Early Diagnosis of Hearing Loss" in Gerber, S.E. and
    Mencher, G.T. (eds.) Early Diagnosis of Hearing Loss
    (New York: Grune & Stratton), 1978.

Sohmer, H., Feinmesser, M., Tell, L., Levi, A. and David, S.
    "Routine use of cochlear audiometry in infants with uncer-
    tain diagnosis" Annals of Otology 81:72 - 75, 1972.

Lieberman, A., Sohmer, H. and Szabo, G. "Cochlear audiometry
    (electrocochleography) during the neonate period" Develop-
    mental Medicine and Child Neurology 15:8 - 13, 1973.

Sohmer, H. and Feinmesser, M. "Electrocochleography in
    clinical-audiological diagnosis" Archives O-R-L 206:91 -
    102, 1974.

Downs, M. "Basis for choosing the appropriate habilitation
    program" paper presented at the ASHA convention in San
    Francisco, California, November, 1972.

THE BLIND-DEAF MULTIPLY DISABLED INFANT

Kevin P. Murphy
Royal Berkshire Hospital, Reading, Berkshire, England

David J. Byrne
Borocourt Hospital, Reading, Berkshire, England

I. Introduction

This paper is designed to illustrate that multiply disabled children are difficult, but not impossible to help. Diagnosis of function will be shown to be distinct from diagnosis of sensory sensitivity or acuity. The relationship between causation and therapeutic management will be emphasized and strategies of therapy will be presented. Many of these strategies will be supported by newly developed equipment and will be related to a proposal for a more closely integrated pattern of diagnostic therapy involving the parents as the logical and natural therapists, with the professionals as counsellors, assessors and educators.

The population of audio-visually disabled children, of which we have had most recent professional experience, has presented problems for therapy derived from the following:

1) Incomplete indices of auditory function;

2) Incomplete indices of visual function;

3) Neuromotor inco-ordinations relating to cerebral palsy, specific crippling disorders, or failure of early training;

4) Emotional disturbance;

5) Severe mental subnormality;

6) Heart lesions;

7) Metabolic disorders, often derived from or resulting in serious feeding difficulties;

8) Causation   (i)   Genetic
                 (ii)   Intrauterine trauma
                (iii)   Meningitis, encephalitis, non-specific
                         febrile episodes.

The commonest result of such mixed symptomatology has
been a tendency on the part of paediatricians and developmental psychologists to confuse acuity or "sensitivity", to
use the North American expression, with function. The child
may be given behavioural tests of vision or hearing which
seem to reflect depressed performance and, hence, there may
be false assumptions about acuity. Such pessimistic scoring,
with all the attendant consequences of faulty labelling,
cannot but modify prognostic statements and discourage all
but the most independent parent from engaging in the early
therapy so vital to progress. At the other extreme, there
can also be a danger of over-optimistic counselling based on
thresholds derived from evoked response audiometry and visual
evoked potentials, or similar tests of end-organ and brain
stem function. It is essential to stress, therefore, that in
the case of multiply disabled children, modification of
function must be the basis for therapy, while modification
of acuity provides the caveats upon which prescriptions of
prostheses are based and towards which therapy must ultimately
be directed.

Hence, the three D's of Disability (Detection, Diagnosis
and "Dealing with") assume a different time scale in relation
to function. In the case of multiply disabled children,
detection is rarely a problem except for those circumstances
where mild sensory deficits supervene upon severe intellectual
or neuromotor disabilities. If auditory training has any
meaning as a term and any validity as a procedure, it can
only be so because we recognize that there is a real difference between acuity and function, and so between impairment
of sensory sensitivity on the one hand and the handicap which
we aim to prevent or minimize by therapy on the other.
Diagnosis and dealing with (or, to use the English term,
"management") are overlapping procedures, particularly in
relation to multiple disability.

Multiply disabled children usually present an even
greater shock to their parents than do those hearing impaired
children without additional problems. Parent counselling,
diagnosis and therapy are continuous and co-terminous and
therapy is seen both as diagnosis and as "preventive medicine".

We aim to prevent the cyclic degeneration which typifies the multiply disabled child unless therapy is prompt and efficacious as soon as detection occurs.

We would be unprepared, therefore, to accept the notion that diagnosis can be completed before a multiply disabled infant reaches the age of 3 years. Function must depend on harmonious integration of sensory and neuromotor behaviour with associated cognitive development. Since cognitive development is so vulnerable to early training, therapy has to be aimed at a number of targets. An abbreviated and incomplete list of targets for early therapy would include:

1) Completion of diagnosis of function;

2) Bases for parent counselling;

3) Foundations for early intervention with patient and family;

4) Prevention of cyclic underfunction;

5) Prevention of stereotypic behaviour;

6) Maintenance of emotional and psychological integrity.

If we begin by assuming that the child has been fitted with some near adequate prosthetic devices relevant to his various disabilities, therapy may be designed to promote cognitive and emotional growth and, as a result, increased efficiency of sensory and intersensory learning. In the course of these early therapies, the relevance and accuracy of the original prosthetic fittings will be examined and their use maintained, changed or withdrawn accordingly. Main strategies will use near senses to replace the distance senses as monitors. Small portable vibro packs and bone conductors will be used to inform the infant about the presence of others, of the location of objects within reach. Simple walkways will be constructed which can be placed between the door and the highchair so that, in the case of blind children, they can be alerted to the approach of others. Vibro devices which can help to identify distant and near objects, or to encourage crawling, standing, stepping with support, stepping self-supported by furniture and eventually purposive walking or climbing, will be utilized. Curiosity, pride in achievement, strategies of exploration, continued voicing and responding

to sound are all vital to progress. Therapy should be
designed to encourage their use and, by so doing, to improve
the quality of that usage.

     Much of this paper will be designed to show that the
multiply disabled child presents a series of complex problems
which are not simply the arithmetical sum of the consequences
of blindness, deafness, locomotor malfunction or intellectual
deficit. We are faced with an exponential equation, many of
whose variables, though theoretically predictable, cannot be
calculated in the time scale during which early therapy must
occur. Indeed, the basic problem which we cannot avoid is
that the child and his family are here before us. How and
where are we to begin? How are we to avoid the trap of doing
anything in order to do something? Let us look at our
targets once more.

(1) Diagnosis of Function

     The development of neuromotor function is not seen as an
end in itself for children with audio-visual disabilities.
In the normal infant, the whole body is pressed into the
service of the visual processes. Vision leads to reaching,
crawling, climbing, walking, the achievement of self-initiated
goals, conceptual structures like object permanence or object
function. Notions of cause and effect help the child to
identify that he is separate from others and with power over
his environment. Until one meets infants with impairments of
sensory or locomotor function, it is easy to forget the inter-
dependence of these two functions. For instance, random hand
and arm movement is unlikely to develop to purposive reaching
and grasping without visual information and motivation. In
turn, visuo-motor behaviour reinforces cognition and leads to
improved visual learning and, hence, to the deployment of
visual attention.

     The child with under-developed visuo-motor function may
be mis-diagnosed as "apathetic" or "intellectually retarded",
when in fact immaturity of function, though acceptable in the
younger normal child is, without therapy, likely to lead to
cyclic degeneration. Even mild modifications of audio-visual,
audio-motor or audio-visual-motor function can be undiagnosed
sources of deprivation and stress, loss of confidence and
irritability, to such an extent that parents become distressed
or alienated and bonding is threatened.

Speech teaching with deaf children is onerous enough. In the case of visual deficits, the child does not only miss the 'how' of speech, but also the 'why'. Without vision, the notion of signalling needs and wants, the need for communication, and object reference points, are lost. The normal child is helped to communicate by his recognition of his needs and wants. The child with visual impairments may not be aware of objects or situations which he could need or want. Hence, the notions of needing, of wanting, of specific demanding, do not become apparent. The child is unable to discern parents or siblings as potential sources of satisfaction for such needs and wants as he does identify. As a result, the motivation to vocal or gestural signalling is not present. Much speech development is based on visual acuity, both for speech reading and for motivation. In its absence, specific steps have to be taken to help in signal motivation, signal reception and signal response. Without these, signal emission is unlikely to develop.

Absence of vision is not only a source of deprived visual and social learning, but also of emotional learning. Vision can provide pleasure, reassurance, and the basis for bonding and security on the one hand; or, on the other, to list but a few, aggression, fear and withdrawal. Learning to cope with frustration is an important lesson in life, as are interest, curiosity, construction, manipulation, building and dismantling, all of which help cognitive development. Modified vision may preclude or delay the development of such skills and, hence, produce cognitive delays or, more importantly, delay the development of the cognitive foundation upon which subsequent learning would normally be based. Thus, a downward spiral in the development of motor skill may occur. Fine motor development, for instance, is unlikely to emerge in finger-thumb prehension without reach and grasp. Similarly the sounds associated with such activity, and normally an integral part of such learning, are not heard, decoded and stored for comparison and recall. Skill development does not exist in its own right. It is fed by, and in its turn feeds, visual and auditory experience.

In other words, sensory experience must mature alongside, and integrate harmoniously with, developing neuromotor function. Where such integration is threatened by modified sensory, sensory-motor or neuromotor function, the consequences are cyclic; malfunction leads to maldevelopment, which in turn leads to restricted cognitive and emotional

development. These factors lead to modified attention, modified curiosity and, hence, to further modification of function. Our first target, then, is to identify and develop
function; function for its own sake and as a basis for further diagnosis.

(2) Parent Counselling

     We find that parents of multiply disabled children tend
to be pulled asunder by the multiplicity of specialists who
see their role to be of primary importance. Later in this
chapter we identify the ideal environment in which diagnostic
therapy can be developed and in which the dignity and integrity of the family can be maintained and their pre-eminence
as therapists can be assured. We will summarize at this
stage by saying that the child belongs to the parents. They
delegate therapeutic responsibility to us and this delegation
must never abrogate their rights or responsibilities.

(3) Foundations for Early Intervention

     All too often the diagnosis has emphasized deficits; we
talk of hearing loss, impaired vision, locomotor underfunction. Therapy begins by listing capacities and skills.
Parents are shown or encouraged to demonstrate assets, skills,
and residual capacities. First steps are designed to illustrate what the child can do. What are the assets upon which
a programme can be built? Parents are encouraged to compile
registers of even the most minute developing skills and are
trained to identify them as bases for accurate fitting of
prosthetic devices, for realistic prognoses, and for extended
therapy. They are taught to give encouragement of voicing
by audio-tactile inputs. There should be encouragement of
locomotor function (especially sitting upright in the baby
chair, which will become the child's laboratory and classroom),
and encouragement of searching for objects, (especially food
and drink, by sense of smell, residual vision and vibro-tactile
inputs). They are taught about development of locomotor
skills by means of vibro crawlers, crawl and walk-ways, and
development of fine motor skills by squeeze blocks and bars
which produce audio-tactile stimuli. Creation of consistency
by the careful monitoring of domestic stimuli is essential,
and by selection of stimulus modes relevant to the specific
aims of therapy. For instance, as deaf educators, we are

accustomed to the idea of what we have described in other
papers as "kitchen-sink therapy". Here the domestic events
of a normal household are given therapeutic significance and
purpose. The same applies to multiply disabled children.
Feeding, dressing, bathing, handling, cuddling, can all be
utilized but need careful organization to avoid confusion
and bewilderment. The role of the parent-therapist requires
careful guidance, careful monitoring and considerable support.

(4)   Prevention of Underfunction

     As we have illustrated, malfunction leads to underfunc-
tion, which leads to pessimistic prognoses. Fortunately,
once parents are given clear goals and the means to achieve
them, this problem does not become as severe as it would
otherwise have been. At the same time, realistic goals and
sympathetic management can easily be lost when therapeutic
enthusiasm is allowed to run riot. Hence, the careful
delineation of targets requires close collaboration between
parents and domiciliary teacher, and in turn, between teacher
and therapeutic team. Case conferences must be carefully
planned, clearly documented, and all concerned must see such
steps in progress as have occurred. In particular, the
minutiae of progress which may appear minimal to the clinical
observer must be identified for what they are. That is, not
simply as indices of attainment, but rather as the outcome of,
and the rewards for, hours of hard work on the part of parent
and domiciliary teacher.

     The attached schedule may be seen as a summary of those
items which we ask parents to record and which our therapists
use in working with their patients and pupils.

                    Developmental Schedule
                         (Summary)

Gross Motor: Primitive body movement
                  Crawling position
                  Crawling movement
                  Sitting
                  Balance in sitting
                  Standing with support
                  Balance in standing
                  Forward movement (standing)
                  Walking independently

Fine Motor: Grasping object placed in hand (primitive
                           palm reflex)
                       Grasp in picking up for exploration
                       Grasp in letting go
                       Reach and palm grasp (search or visuomotor)
                       Shaking. Beating. Push-pull.
                       Pincer (finger-thumb opposition)
                       Self-occupation by pincer manipulation

Self-Help: Application of gross and fine motor skills
                           to feeding, drinking, caressing, etc.;
                           (e.g., two-handed palmer grasp of feed-
                           ing cup leading to unilateral palm with
                           some pincer).
                       Finger feeding
                       Beginning of spoon feeding aided and mini-
                           mally aided with specific built-up
                           spoon handles
                       Water play as preliminary to bathing and
                           washing
                       Bowel training

Socialization: Contact with others, responding to voice or
                           vision or handling
                       Beginnings of voicing
                       Physical exploration

Communication: Demand-Response arc (primitive)
                       Beginning of sophisticated signalling
                       Gross tactile signs
                       Responding to tactile cues (e.g., Tap under
                           arm for 'stand', tap behind knees for
                           'sit'; rub on head for priase; finger to
                           side of mouth for 'food'; shaping child's
                           hand into cup form to sign 'drink').

(5)   Prevention of Stereotypic Behaviour

     Stereotypes are not only distressing to the observer,
they are also processes of auto-distraction. When the child
is actively involved in a therapeutic programme, it may be
less likely to develop. But the emergence of some stereotypics, (light play, finger-flicking, head banging, tooth
grinding, rocking, to cite just a few) has to be expected,
especially in bored or understimulated infants. Steps must

be taken to provide activities which will avoid them, or
attempt to reduce them if they do develop.

(6) Maintenance of Emotional and
     Psychological Integrity

     So much of what we have described appears to ignore the
role and function of the child himself. If we are not careful, we will begin to regard him as a lay figure, a flawed
receptacle into which we pour our therapeutic offerings.
Parents are encouraged to recognize the signals the child
emits, where relevant, to answer them accurately and speedily,
and to restrain themselves from over-indulgence when their
own emotional satisfaction becomes their primary goal. Pity
is shown to be a negative virtue. Consistency, reinforcement,
encouragement, insight are needed for the child and family's
sakes. It is too easy for the whole house to become subordinate to the child. The child has needs, true; but so do the
family. The needs, wants and rights of parents and siblings
have to be considered. Once the family can see this, the
integrity of the child as one member of the family can be
developed. Love and care should never lead to smothering or
to the substitution of facile expressions of emotion for the
encouragement of independence and self-help. The temptation
to maintain the child in a form of infantile dependence can
be overwhelming. The encouragement of independence, management of tantrums and of all the ploys which keep the child
securely in control of the whole household require considerable support and counselling. The family needs to be reminded
that such skills are characteristic of even the severely disabled child, and to be alert for their own and for the child's
sake, to the danger of facile compliance.

     The family is encouraged to identify assets, to per-
ceive and record progress, to recognize their vulnerability
to manipulation and, in particular, to take time out. This
last measure needs to be developed from the beginnings of
therapy. Selected baby-sitters, brief periods in therapeutic
centers in which family role may be temporarily reduced,
involvement of neighbourhood services for baby-minding, or
where feasible, in actual therapy, will not only lighten the
load for the family, but also, hopefully, reduce the omni-
present pressure to be continuously involved, or to become
so exhausted and disillusioned that all hope is lost and the
therapeutic regime collapses.

At the end of the day, if we are realistic, we see our
role as designed to remove the family and child from our continued care. We recognize that the child belongs to the
family and we are a support service. It is essential to keep
this point in mind, particularly in the United Kingdom where
the National Health Service has such a potentially intrusive
role. Independence based on confidence, competence and
courage will lead to patterns of co-operation which are far
more effective than those situations in which family dependence is implicit in the therapeutic regime.

II. Strategies of Co-Operation

We describe the learning patterns of some multiply disabled, educationally sub-normal children as "chaotic". This
term is selected because it illustrates the fact that the
child has not only failed to develop any pattern or structure
to explain his experiences to himself, but has also failed to
develop consistent relationships with society by means of
which he can exchange information. That is, he has little or
no ability to receive or pass on information, with dire consequences for the parents and himself. As Lillywhite has
stated, the parent needs "feedback" from the child. Failure
to respond to parental overtures in a consistent or predictable manner is not only likely to cause distress and anxiety,
but also a deprivation of emotional reinforcement as a result
of which the emotional links between parent and child are put
under considerable strain, often distorted, and sometimes
severed. It is difficult for a family to develop a normal
emotional pattern of family life and relationships if one
member does not fit a pattern or, more particularly, if one
member begins to develop a pattern of social behaviour which
is likely to be disruptive and unpredictable. In addition,
it may demand a degree of compliance from the whole family
which creates a disruption of their own previous life style,
a deprivation of emotional communication, anxiety, guilt,
fluctuations of patterns of management, and a modification
of their own image of themselves. The normal closely knit
family not only fosters its own internal emotional integrity,
but gives an appearance of contentment, satisfaction, justifi-
able pride and stability. Serenity in such families takes
for granted that the child will respond, will express
pleasure, affection or needs, and by doing so, will build
emotional bonds with the rest of the family.

When families are deprived of the mutual support that
comes from shared affection and predictability of behaviour,
there is a tendency to replace the normal emotional system
with various compensatory processes. Some parents build
false hopes. Others refuse to see hope. Some compensate by
"babying", others by claiming degrees of skill and amounts of
progress in their disabled child which are clearly exagger-
ated. Frustration often leads to variability in tolerance or
to increased irritability. For instance, continuous loss of
sleep will lead to acute fatigue. Possibly, parents may have
to work out some kind of shift system, taking turns to cope
with disturbed nights. However, because the husband is often
the wage earner, the mother is left to carry the major burden.
So, a vicious cycle of fatigue, irritability, guilt, and
failure to plan, (all disruptive of domestic life and harmony)
emerges, and the capacity for a constructively planned
approach to the care and education of the child is seriously
impaired.

By the time the child is brought to assessment, the
parents will have experienced most, if not all, of the conditions mentioned above. Hypersensitive, defiant, seeking
almost any source of pride in their child, they may well have
run the gauntlet of well intentioned but potentially wounding
questions in a variety of waiting rooms. Visits to general
practitioners, paediatricians, specialists of one kind or
another dealing with sensory acuity, locomotor capacity,
orthopaedic integrity, neuromotor function, heart condition,
psychological state, etc., not only produces the hazards
inherent in telling your story time after time to a variety
of people, but also the necessity of sitting, often for hours
at a time, with other people and their bored, fretful, often
hyperactive children. The enforced social contact with other
disabled children at a time when the parents are finding
difficulty in coming to terms with their own child's problems,
may sometimes serve as an anodyne. It is more likely, however,
that it will add to the stress, that it will reinforce self-
classification within a parental sub-class, and continue the
assault upon natural pride which the parent takes for granted
until it is threatened. No matter how gently a genetic history is taken, the majority of parents have to steel themselves against an intrusion into family cupboards which are
usually kept locked - often even from themselves. Where
there is a genetic link, parents may have to discover this for
the first time from their own distressed parents or grandparents. The side of the family from which the genetic link

with the disability has been identified may be made to feel
guilty or inadequate and, consequently, marital relationships
may be brought under stress. The situation does not necessarily improve when no genetic linkage can be found. Parents
seek for causes, study the tealeaves almost, in a search for
explanations. Finding none, they are bewildered, frustrated
and naturally fearful of future pregnancies.

Ideally, therefore, the assessment centre will see itself
as a place in which parents can feel at ease; where they can
reverse the roles and ask questions instead of answering them;
where they can put the pieces together again of a child who,
up to that point, seems to have existed - or at least to have
been investigated - as though made up of a distinct and dis-
tinctive parts. Ideally, they will be able to ask how Dr.
A's report fits with Dr. B's, and how the whole picture is
emerging. They should have access to a single authoritative
interpreter who can utilize their information and experiences,
in addition to the clinical records before him, as a basis
for an outline plan for diagnostic therapy. Ideally, there
will be time for parents to talk, to display the child's
skills, for the child to relax, and for privacy in which to
reflect on and to develop the working relationships conducive
to the earliest possible familial relief and support. Eventually there will be time for parents who so chose, to meet
other parents with similar problems and to share their own
hard-won patterns of expertise. As confidence develops,
parents may assume some aspect of therapy with another child
in which their own emotional state is less intrusive. Hence,
increased confidence is encouraged in parent and child alike
through successful progress.

It should be clear that bringing a child to assessment
has its own therapeutic quality for the parents. Foundations
of successful intervention depend on the care with which the
earliest contacts are planned. Relief that something is
likely to happen will rapidly dissipate unless something is
seen to be happening. Feedback of information must be planned
with scrupulous care. Parents are arriving as outsiders to a
system which has its own in-group structure. Often such
systems are unaware of their exclusivity until they find
themselves resenting what they deem as the "brashness" of a
parent who, in their eyes, is over-eager to become an accepted
member of the team. How often does one hear members of staff
warned about a particular parent who "will take the whole
place over given half a chance!" Perhaps the best initial

treatment will be accorded when the parent is seen as a welcome guest, but not yet a member of the family. The first
steps in the intervention with the child and family must take
into account that the multiply disabled child has effectively
undermined the foundations upon which his own progress would
normally depend. We take for granted in therapy that progress
with such children will be dependent upon family support.
However, the family with a disabled child is potentially a
disabled family and, hence, the capacity for normal family
relationships may well be disastrously threatened. As a
result, the capacity for support in therapy may be severely
modified. For instance, one often sees parents who are
successful in business and general social activity, but who
have lost confidence with their own disabled child to such an
extent that they find difficulty dressing him in public. They
make simple errors in buttoning a coat or tying shoe laces,
and unless they are helped unobtrusively, may well flee from
the waiting room with the child, looking for a quiet corner
to reorganize themselves in privacy and free from scrutiny.

The first practical step in intervention cannot but be
another interview. Because of the parents' past interview
experience, it is necessary to plan the first interview with
great care. Such written material as exists should have been
collected into one file and current knowledge summarized.
Whoever is going to have first stage responsibility for the
child's investigations should also be available. This can be
achieved in a variety of ways but should begin when the
parents and child enter the waiting room.

The waiting room gives the parents their first impression
of the programme they are joining. The attitudes of all members of staff are particularly important. The diagnostic
team needs the support of a variety of workers. Clerical
staff, receptionists, nursing auxiliaries, orderlies, transport workers, porters, may not see themselves as part of the
diagnostic process. Though they may not be directly involved
in diagnosis, they are an important part of the diagnostic
team. The extent to which a team spirit is fostered will have
a profound effect upon intervention strategies. The interest
of all members of staff should be encouraged by informal
dissemination of information about techniques of management
relevant to the children within the programme. Steps of progress, the role of the centre and its place in the whole
therapeutic regime, can be discussed over coffee breaks.
Positive steps should be taken to create a warm, friendly,

collaborative environment. The maintenance of a high level
of staff morale is essential.

     Parents should have their first interview with the per-
son who will have ultimate responsibility for the child's
early care. By this we mean that parents should be able to
meet the Director or Physician in charge <u>first</u>. It should be
clear that he should have enough time to peruse background
information although the initial interview is designed to
carry preliminary investigations slightly further forward.
The main concern is to establish working relationships with
the parents and to explain in comprehensible terms the programme of investigations which are planned. It has become
increasingly clear that parents are often alienated by a
situation in which it is obvious that the doctor has not had
time to study the case notes in detail. Parents writing
accounts of their experiences claim that questions already
answered in the notes are repeated regularly by each new
interviewer, almost as though previous interviews (and, by
implication, previous interviewers) have been discounted. It
cannot be stressed too strongly that the interviewer should
have the time and ability to summarize the collected information for the parents and to check its accuracy with them,
noting those areas which have been left for further investigation or which the current interviewer planned to reveal. This
interview should be designed to develop a bond between the
parents and the interviewer. The foundations of the therapeutic process should be laid at this point. The parents should
feel that there is genuine interest in the child and in the
elucidation of the problems. They should also feel that
there has been time for the doctor to study the case in
advance, to identify areas requiring further investigation
and to have the investigative routine planned ahead. Parents
should not only know what is planned, but also what purpose
each investigation serves and its relevance to the child at
the current stage of his relationship with the assessment
process. In many centres we have visited, the clinical
investigations of the child's residual functions do not take
place until both parents and child have visited the centre a
number of times and have had time to settle in. They require
the visits to gather their own quantum of new or revised
information, and for the child to relax in the new environment
and to get used to the few new contacts to which he has been
exposed. The medical investigation in such centres takes
place after the child has spent time with the therapeutic
team, particularly with the psychologist, the teacher-
therapist and the nurse or house parent.

We feel that the introductory interview with the team-
leader, though of the utmost importance, should be seen by
all to be introductory. However, this does not mean that the
interview is _merely_ introductory and can, therefore, be
delegated to a junior assistant. The parents should feel
that the doctor responsible for the child's investigations
and for signing the final report is the first person they
meet and that they will then be introduced to the member of
staff who will carry out the next stage of investigations or
therapy. In a recent visit to an assessment centre, we saw
a large board in the interview room on which the name, role
and photograph of each member of staff was displayed. We saw
the physician in charge get up from time to time to point to
the name and picture of the person who would be involved at
each level of investigation. We gained the impression that
the parents were reassured by evidence of pre-planning, and
impressed by the extent to which they themselves were being
considered and prepared for a new form of involvement in
their child's assessment.

     Later in this chapter we will be discussing parent
counselling and will deal in detail with the planned role
for each parent. At this stage, we would emphasize that the
early interviews and early stages of work with the child will
function best if both parents are present. History taking,
interview of and by parents, accuracy of parental recall,
inter-parental relationships, are all helped if both parents
are present. If husband and wife are both present in the
first interview, both are in a position to remind themselves
or each other of questions they have been waiting (sometimes
months) to ask. All too often the preliminary interview can
be such an ordeal for the mother if she is not accompanied by
her husband, that she has difficulty in remembering what
occurred. Domestic tension is often heightened when the
father seeks further information or begins to ask a series of
questions which mother suspects are sometimes designed more
to emphasize the father's opinion of maternal inadequacy than
to seek information for its own sake. Where the husband
cannot be present, it is often helpful to provide a brief,
simple leaflet outlining the short term programme and explaining that the long term programme will be developed in co-
operation with the parents, when the results of current
investigations are collated and discussed by all concerned.
We see the involvement of the father to be so important,
however, that every possible step should be taken to facilitate it. Arrangements with social services, social security,

and voluntary transport services should ideally be of such an
order that they can be provided as routine with the minimum
of fuss.

    In discussing a severely retarded child's current level
of skills with parents, we have noticed that those who are
not accurate in their descriptions may be divided into two
main groups. The first group of parents tend to be over-
pessimistic and the second to be over-optimistic. For
example, when asked about her child's speech, one mother told
us that the child "spoke perfectly". When pressed, she
amended the statement slightly by saying, "She just talks like
anyone else". In a sense she was right. The child echoed
everything she heard. In the strict sense, her speech was
perfect; but she had no spontaneous spoken language and needed
a very considerable amount of speech therapists' time before
any spontaneous spoken language began to develop.

    We have found that the pessimistic group can be helped
by being reminded of the skills the child actually has. One
deeply distressed mother brought a blind, severely hearing
impaired, non-ambulant, severely subnormal child to us and,
at first, stated flatly that the child could "do nothing".
After a brief period of familiarization, the child, in fact,
developed strategies of identification and within an hour or
two of the commencement of our first meeting, had devised a
tactile/olfactory identification system which worked very
well indeed. At first the mother was not prepared to accept
this as a learning strategy. It was clear that her attitude
toward the child was such that any signs of potential were
almost oppressive in their significance.

    For many reasons, therefore, the information collected
in the initial interview cannot be regarded as a basis for
accurate diagnostic statements. We feel that the behavioural
skills of such children need prolonged interaction with
experienced workers before accurate profiles can emerge. In
the teams which we have visited, such interaction may occur
between the teacher/therapist and family, or between the
psychologist and family. Where we have seen the best results,
however, has usually been when the teacher, nurse and psychologist form a team. In these circumstances, the group
spokesman is introduced to the parents and it is at this
stage that the active intervention programme begins.

    The notion of Diagnostic Therapy and the structure of
the diagnostic procedures will be discussed later.

Hence, at this stage, we are concentrating on the strategies
involved in developing a diagnostic process. So far we have
seen the emphasis on parental involvement, and acceptance,
and the importance of the presence of both parents together
in the early stages and subsequently at different times,
depending on the topic under discussion or the general convenience of the family. The foundation has been laid for an
interaction in which the parents do the questioning, the
parents volunteer information, the parents begin to acquire
specialized observation skills, and the parents act as their
own evaluators. With luck (and careful planning) a relationship between parents and team will emerge in which the parents
will feel free to bring to light any problem, question or
other threat to equanimity. They will feel that their concerns are an accepted factor in the total group's concern for
anything likely to affect the child's continued progress.

The spokesman for the diagnostic-therapy team may begin
by pointing out that the child is at the centre of the new
group's concern and that the role of the group, in the short
term, will be to plan a system by means of which an accurate
picture of the child's daily function can be collected. If
the doctor in charge has not already done so, the spokesman
will point out that the duration of diagnostic therapy is
short-term - perhaps no more than a week - and the whole
course of that week will be outlined in broad detail. For
instance, if the Unit has an observation apartment, the
parents will know that they are to move in for a certain
period. They may not know, however, that the team see the
settling-in period as potentially disturbing for the child
and that during this period, the family may be left with
little or no contact with staff. They should be advised in
advance to bring domestic mending, knitting, reading or
hobby materials. Similarly, they may not expect to be
involved in observation or "event-counting" from the moment
they enter the apartment.

Where residential facilities do not exist, the duration
of the intervention period will still be explained and event-
counting, which is appropriate to travelling from home and
entering a new environment, will begin. Parents will learn
(if they do not already know) that positive or negative
emotional behaviour can be identified as indices of observation and learning. They will also learn to describe and,
hence to observe with relative objectivity. For instance,
such expressions as, "He enjoyed that" will ultimately be

presented as, "You can tell he enjoyed that because he
always ... (e.g., bounces up and down, breathes deeply, claps,
grinds his teeth, stops head banging), when he is happy".
Behaviour will then be seen as an index of emotional or
intellectual state. It will be collected within such categories and organized for description and codification. From
this, parents will learn to see the value of an itemized
description or diary of a day's progress and to see its
relevance to behaviour at home. From such a comparison, it
should be easy to construct a picture of the normal pattern
of daily management at home and to identify such skills as
the child may have. In Appendix I (at the end of this
Chapter), we have presented an observation schedule which
summarizes the kind of information that parents can be
encouraged to contribute. This should never be presented in
the form of a questionnaire, but separate items can be discussed and selected for scrutiny. At first, some parents
may not see that selective display of affection is an index
of cognitive function. If they begin to list events which
illustrate emotional relationships, comprehension, or co-
operation, it will become apparent to them that their first
attempts are more likely to represent the quality of their
own observation skills than the child's skills or capacities.
Suppose, for instance, we consider some such simple factor
as feeding. By the time the parents have identified likes
and dislikes, preference for sweet or savoury, solid, semi-
solid, mashed or liquid foods, they will have begun to see
that the child cannot express these preferences without some
mechanisms of selection or rejection.

One of the more interesting aspects of a residential
programme may be noted in the extent to which parental predictions of dietary predilection are confirmed or contra-
dicted. Children may have developed dietary routines which
represent parental preferences (convenience, habit, dietetic
theory, advice which may have been relevant at the time but
no longer relates to the conditions upon which it was first
given). For example, recently we were faced with a 12 year
old child who had been fed liquidized foods all her life.
Though herculean efforts were required, the child was trained
in a period of three weeks to accept, masticate, swallow,
absorb and eliminate solids. In fact, our breakthrough to
communication with this child occurred when she developed a
passion for pickles and began to display her own patterns of
selection, identification, request and rejection.

The same kind of thinking can be applied to such factors
as sleep patterns, acquiescence in bathing, toiletting,
dressing and the like. Once we begin to identify consistency
in behaviour, even stereotypics can be used as sources of
information about sensory function. A child will not use
visual flicker if there is not some visual sensation. Even
if there is only a primitive relation between central and
peripheral vision, such a fact is worthy of note and also
unites the parent and therapist in a constructive approach to
an apparently negative phenomenon. The same may be said of
tapping, spinning, rocking or head banging. These would be
unlikely to occur if they did not stimulate some proprioceptive function.

A child who has been regarded by his parents as almost
totally inert may be seen to make choices - no matter how
minimal; to be excited or calmed by certain events or circumstances. The same child may indulge in spontaneous behaviour.
Even bizarre behaviour may have a relevance if it is seen to
be provoked by certain events or patterns of circumstances.
Many dismissive or "throw away" statements by parents or
therapists are made because the significance of the stimulus-
response arc has not been identified. How often one hears
such statements as, "He always does that when ...". The
parent then attempts to minimize the effect of the precipitating factor and is so concerned to preserve equanimity that
the essential link between cause and effect has been missed.
Careful listing of all patterns of behaviour forms a basis
for discussion with the team in which certain cognitive and
sensory factors may be identified. Once such clarifications
have emerged, a basis for diagnostic therapy may be created.
At the same time, evidence of sensory function can be
communicated to the diagnostic specialists who are waiting
to begin their evaluation of inter-sensory organization and,
hence, carry-over to long-term therapy, which is basic to
educational provision.

As the behaviour patterns are recorded and structures
begin to emerge, the team may be in a position to suggest an
area of investigation and to outline a strategy of therapy in
a brief, succinct form. Though it is essential to give
enough information to maintain group collaboration, patterns
of information should be confined to the relevant minima.
Hypotheses, general theorizing, long-winded descriptions of
the extent to which such approaches have or have not succeeded
with other children, are irrelevant at this stage. The main
aim of the programme in its early stages should be the

development of patterns of cooperation, the elucidation of
assets, the development of observation and recording skills,
and a rebuilding of confidence.

During this period, the experienced counsellor will be
alert to dynamic shifts in the roles of various members of
the team. There will be times when one or other member will
expect to lead. The parents, in particular, will need to
feel secure in testing their relationships with one another
and with other members of the group. It is wise, therefore,
to ensure that there is access to an experienced counsellor.
This can be the psychologist, of course, but it need not
necessarily be so. Many psychometricians or educational
psychologists find themselves thrust into counselling roles
for which their training is less than adequate. It is
necessary for any diagnostic team to be aware of its limitations as well as its strengths.

As cooperation and mutual trust develop, new or renewed
coping mechanisms can be developed, management of such situations as bathing, handling, dressing, feeding, sleeping, and
communication can be discussed, and strategies for tentative
experiments can be devised. Parents and child can be prepared for a more intensive pattern of investigation. For
instance, short visits to the centre can be extended to
include a meal, then possibly a meal and one sleep, followed
by a one night stay with parents and eventual placement for a
week.

Such a programme has a beguiling simplicity in description, but may well represent a challenge to a long-standing
system of parental control. The parents, too, will find the
domestic problems of family re-organization difficult. At
the least, such problems will provide good reasons for hesi-
tancy and procrastination. When such reasons are advanced,
it is difficult, without a social worker's advice, to assess
the extent to which barriers are realistic or are rationaliza-
tions. Other members of the family need to be considered.
All too often other siblings have had to accept subordinate
family roles and such difficulties as broken sleep, family
tension, the interruption of schooling and embarrassment with
their school friends. Now they may need to be prepared for
coming into an assessment centre in close proximity to groups
of children with severe disabilities. Other relatives,
particularly grandparents, need to be considered. Traumatized
by the family tragedy, they may see the move to an assessment

centre as a public seal upon a private tragedy. This is particularly the case when the assessment centre is part of, or
shares the same address as a mental subnormality hospital.

Once the family is settled into the programme, it is
wise to arrange for all the major medico-psychological
investigations of function to occur, as well as the normal
paediatric investigations. The state of visual, auditory
and neuromotor integrity and integration will be required.
This is a potentially traumatic period. Every possible step
should be taken to smooth the paths to specialist clinics.
Ideally, the family should be quartered in the assessment
centre and investigations should be carried out in an environment in which the child has learned to feel secure. We must,
however, face facts. Many specialist investigations require
specialist environments, equipment and/or teams which cannot
be transplanted from their normal working centres. With good
will and careful pre-planning, transport, escorts and special
time-tabling are all relatively easy to organize. Yet all too
often snags occur. Children arrive at out-patient centres
late or hurried into a state of stress. Waiting lists or
waiting conditions which are just (and only just) tolerable
for children without such severe and multiple disabilities,
are totally unacceptable for the children in our special
group. Even if parents and children are placed in day-rooms
apart from the rest of the out-patient population, there is
a danger that departmental work loads will develop pressures
on all concerned which may make full, complete and stress-
free investigation difficult, almost to the verge of
impossibility.

Specialist investigations will be incomplete without
concise, up-to-date information on the recent diagnostic
regime. Clerical services are often stretched unbearably in
trying to prepare summaries for circulation. The weight and
quantity of paperwork accompanying each child may be too much
for the busy specialist to absorb in the time available.
Parents find themselves in danger of reverting to their
earlier role of passive receptivity, or if they find that
such a role is no longer possible, there is a danger of being
classified as "difficult" or "demanding". During all this
time, the family is still part of the assessment centre's
programme. Trials of diagnostic therapy are still in progress.
Each specialist visit may be discussed in depth in order to
extract information about the child's reactions to the test
situation. Eventually, the specialist reports come to hand.

With luck, not too much time has passed. The medical director
summarizes the reports from his own diagnostic team and also
from his specialist colleagues. His own experience should
lead him to the presentation of a balanced picture of what
the experts have discovered and what he is able to suggest,
in cooperation with his team, for long term care.

    At the end of all this, ideal placement waits upon
administrative process. Vacancies may or may not exist in
special centres. Placement may be speedy or delayed. Parents
are consulted about their preparedness to accept placement
in the environment recommended by the diagnostic team. Now
is the time for the diagnostic therapy to bear fruit. The
summaries of investigations have gone to the Community
Physician and to the Education Officer responsible for the
domiciliary care of such children. How much of this reaches
the teachers? The purpose of diagnosis is therapy. Unless
the diagnostic process leads naturally to a planned and well
informed therapeutic education, much of our intervention
strategy has been wasted. Under ideal circumstances, case
conferences will inform all concerned of the child's assets
as well as deficits. The clinical condition will be
explained. The effects of any medication will be described,
as well as its purpose. From all this, an outline programme
for therapy and education will be developed. Regional
advisers, visiting teachers, social workers, school nurses
and teaching staff will begin the complex and slow process
of creating an educational programme based on the child's
known skills.

    We will deal, later on, with the patterns of diagnostic
therapy in greater detail. This section has been designed
to illustrate that the parent can be absorbed into the
diagnostic team; that such absorption can be supportive and
therapeutic; that skilled observation can be developed; and
that the pattern of coordination is not only feasible, but
essential. So much of the success of classifying in diagnostic centres depends on the smooth running of a wide variety
of social and administrative procedures, that intervention
strategies must be planned with these factors in mind. We
should all be aware that rebuilding family confidence and
encouraging parents to involve themselves in early therapy
may not only be a waste of time, but also a potential source
of stress, unless they are carried through into the school
years.

III.   Principles and Practices of
       Diagnosis of Function in
       Multiply Disabled Infants

(1) Principles

In the care of multiply disabled children, diagnosis is
not a "once and for all" procedure. In particular, the fact
that specific objective measures of acuity have given certain
amounts of information, may or may not be significant. The
relevance of such information to present function, or indeed
to long-term prognosis, is doubtful in the extreme. Only
where there is a near total absence of sensory function as
measured by "objective" criteria, can we make confident
assertions about levels of future sensory or intersensory
function. Such terms as auditory training, audio-cognitive
function, auditory learning, auditory memory, would be meaningless if we were not implicitly stating that there is a
significant difference between acuity and function. Hence,
therapy and diagnosis are linked in a continuous process of
assessment, training, parent counselling, more assessment,
the development of new training procedures and equipment for
the whole of the infant's trainable life-span. Therapy and
diagnosis are inextricably linked. Diagnosis is often therapeutic and therapy with multiply disabled children is
inescapably diagnostic. As far as possible, however, diagnosis should be as complete and accurate as can be managed for
the following reasons:

(a)   Though it is more convenient for the diagnosis to be
concentrated in one centre or at one period of time early in
the child's life, therapy, too, may begin there but rapidly
shifts to the home.

(b)   The parents have needs. They need to know that
their suspicions are well founded, that the presenting condition is of a certain type and also of a certain severity.
Subsequently, they need to know the consequences of the condition, the extent to which they are likely to be able to
help and the course that therapy is likely to take.

(c)   A clear and accurate diagnosis is essential for the
initiation of relevant therapy. Much time can be lost in
experimental or, indeed misplaced therapy, when diagnoses
have been unclear, incomplete or imprecise.

(d) At the same time, therapy itself should be seen to
have a diagnostic significance. In the unit in which we work,
we look for a constant dialogue between clinicians, therapists and teachers, so that therapeutic and educational information can be added to the original diagnostic statements,
either as a basis for confirmation or as necessary for its
amendment.

(e) From the foregoing, it should be clear that though
it is essential for the diagnostician (who may well be the
therapist!) to have confidence in his diagnostic skills,
there is no room for arrogance. There are such things as
faulty and incomplete diagnoses. There are spontaneous
changes in the course of disorders which merit continuing
supervision and amendment of the original diagnosis. First
symptoms may not be the only conditions which change. The
emotional or family aspects of a disability may deteriorate.
The diagnostic services may be called in again for advice
or new therapeutic approaches. For this reason, it is
obvious that in cases of multiple handicap, there is need for
a multidisciplinary approach. Each speciality needs to
remember all the other diagnostic and therapeutic facilities,
and to so arrange its care for the child that the maximum of
information is obtained with a minimum of trauma to child and
family. In the end, the diagnostic team may have to help
educators and therapists to develop short term and long term
aims, and as a basis for realistic plans for the future,
advise the parents concerning the development of a clear
picture of the child's educational assets and deficits.

When we consider multiply disabled children, we are in
danger of assuming that they form a unique group in which
the central problem is one of intellectual deficits. This is
not necessarily the case. We should guard against the dangers of "labelling" children in such a way that levels of
educational expectation are lowered. Or, even more particularly, that the child is debarred from further diagnosis by
the assumption that apparent perceptual problems are results
of conceptual deficits rather than disorders of sensory,
sensory motor or inter-sensory function.

Each sensory deficit is a potential source of further
educational hazard, but the disastrous effects of multi-
sensory deficits cannot be over-emphasized. Bad as the above
facts may be, they are appreciably worse if they are either
misdiagnosed or undiagnosed. We may begin, therefore, by

asking ourselves the primary question: "How many severely
educationally sub-normal children are, in fact, not suffering
from impairments of intelligence, but from undiagnosed sensory
deficits which have led to misdiagnosis? The answer to this
is probably "very few, if any". A second question follows
logically: How many severely educationally sub-normal children (ESN) are exposed to an additional source of retardation
due to undiagnosed or misdiagnosed sensory deficits? Lest it
should be thought that such questions are too simplistic, can
we consider one more. How many ESN children, though not
affected by primary sensory deficits, have specific intersensory defects which might seriously interfere with cognitive
development? We now accept that auditory responsivity in
infants under the age of 6 months is likely to be modified
by stimuli which involve other senses. It follows, therefore,
that intersensory organization is either a learned skill or
is dependent on the maturation of intersensory association
processes and, hence, is vulnerable either to learning failure or to intersensory pathologies. To a very considerable
extent, our diagnostic approach to ESN children has, in the
past, been concerned with "intelligence" which has been
tested by materials that require intersensory organization.
In the past, we have all been critical of the naivety of those
who have used language-saturated tests of intelligence with
children who are hearing impaired and who suffer from language
failures. But such testing still goes on. Indeed, it would
be difficult to think of any so-called non-verbal tests which
would not be affected by severe language deficits. Is it not
time now for us to draw attention to a fact that every psychologist will accept immediately in theory? That is the likli-
hood that failures of sensory integration will lead to low
scores on intelligence tests. One does not want to re-tread
the weary pathways of earlier discussions concerning the
validity of intelligence tests, but we all need to remind
ourselves that the designation Educational Sub-Normality is,
at least in part, dependent upon some form of intelligence
test. If sensory deficits or intersensory pathologies have
not been diagnosed, how confident can we be of the accuracy
of the primary diagnosis. At the simplest level, detection
of an auditory deficit in a so-called ESN child may lead to
a re-classification in terms of educational potential and,
therefore, in educational placement and more importantly, in
educational "labelling". Such re-classification has led to
several older children known to these authors being removed
from hospital supervision and placed in schools for deaf or
blind children.

The problem does not stop at the level of intersensory function or single-sense acuity. Many of our patients are affected by problems of sensory-motor or loco-motor malfunctions. In recent years, much of the early educational work with cerebral palsied children has reinforced our recognition of the importance of early and accurate diagnosis as a basis for planned remediation. There is no doubt that sensory, sensory-motor and neuromotor malfunctions can be the bases of intellectual delay, and in their severest categories, can severely inhibit or even preclude learning. But do we pursue this argument to its logical conclusion? To what extent do we agree that minor degrees of sensory, sensory-motor or neuromotor deficits can be significant potential educational hazards for our multiply disabled population? Before considering this, we may remind ourselves that in older children, minute degrees of hearing impairment (Ling, 1958) lead to major modification of auditory attention or listening (Murphy, 1969). What happens to the very young child who has problems of attention focus exacerbated by failures of listening? Speech and spoken language will be delayed. Environmental observation, basic to pre-linguistic conceptualization (Furth, 1966) will be modified, and if we add to these factors minor degrees of incoordination, we now see the emergence of the major sequelae of retardation: impaired language, impaired conceptualization, impaired attention focus and impaired neuromotor coordination.

Lest it should be though that we are over-stating our case, let us emphasize that we do not think that educational subnormality is commonly caused by the factors outlined above. The point we wish to make is more direct and more amenable to therapy. Simply, some children need not be categorized as ESN's if we knew more about their sensory, sensory-motor or neuromotor function. Since current research places between 10 and 15% ESN children at auditory hazard, we may surely ask ourselves if there are not at least 30% - possibly more - of our ESN population who have undetected (and, therefore, untreated) secondary deficits or learning hazards. We are also concerned with a symptomatology which resembles mental retardation though based on other deficits. How many children in our specialized institutions have developed problems of learning, of self-image, of confidence, of frustration which represent major hazards to normal intellectual function, because we have failed in differential diagnosis? For how many of our slow learners have our therapeutic and educational goal gradients been unnecessarily restricted by diagnostic

errors? Return to our earlier comments about cerebral
palsied children. Surely, the most important lessons we can
learn from the education of such children is the need for the
establishment of accurate learning targets and the rapidity
with which their educational goal gradients have improved in
the course of the last two decades. Diagnosis of function
stems from therapeutic progress. Without that, prognostic
statements are impossible. Hence, prognosis and therapeutic
programs demand the early initiation of therapy.

     Under the community health program in the United Kingdom,
there is increasing opportunity for full investigation of
sensory or additional disabilities in children who have been
identified as multiply disabled. We are faced, however, by
two major problems. The first relates to the phenomenon of
observer bias on the part of the diagnostician. It is only
too easy to assume that minor sensory disabilities seen in
the child who has already been identified as underfunctioning,
stem from the primary condition, and to accept as normal,
degrees of sensory deficit which would give rise to concern
in children of normal intelligence. The second problem is
more difficult. Training of medical officers in recent years
has produced a number of excellent diagnosticians. It has
also produced, in some cases, an undue confidence in the
accuracy of diagnosis and perhaps, more importantly, the
permanence of any diagnosed condition, be it normal or
abnormal. Those of us who work in the field of audiology
know that in certain young children, particularly in residential establishments, 40 dB fluctuations of threshold of hearing can and do occur from day to day. To the paediatrician,
the notion of fluctuation of metabolic state is only too well
known. Certain psychiatrists are now relating emotional
state in some children to metabolic or allergic variations.
Yet, the study of metabolic state in multiply disabled children tends to be confined to questions of growth and feeding
habits.

     As diagnostic skill improves, the identification of
transitory and minimally severe modifications of function will
become more common. New criteria of attention focus, auto-
distraction and hyper-activity will be developed. There
should, therefore, be a build-up of children requiring special
remedial education. Are we prepared for it? Have we
specialist teachers and specialist schools for such children?
Though the administrator might quite rightly boast of our
specialized educational facilities in the United Kingdom, we

we cannot deny that in the preparation of specialist remedial
teachers and in the creation of specialized educational
centres for multiply disabled children, we are still "whistl-
ing in the dark". Not to put too fine a point on it, we have
almost no specialized training facilities for teachers of
multiply handicapped children. Indeed, if we look into our
special school populations, not only have we not got the
specialist teachers for such children, but according to Ives
(1974), we have not even identified them within our current
provisions for hearing impaired children. If his surveys of
deaf children are accurate, there is no doubt that a high
proportion of children educated by Teachers of the Deaf are
suffering from misdiagnosed additional sensory or emotional
deficits which are potentially harmful to educational success.

One definition (Butterworth) of diagnosis is "The art of
applying scientific methods to the elucidation of the problems
presented by a sick person". That definition also states
that diagnosis forms "a sure basis for the treatment and prognosis of the individual patient". Treatment is described as
"The management of the patient condition" and is "designed to
ameliorate or to prevent deterioration". Surely, then, our
own aim with our multiply disabled children should be to
reach, as early as possible, a clear knowledge of their
individual problems as a basis for current educational treatment and the creation of satisfactory goal-gradients based on
reliable educational prognoses. The twin aims of early
diagnosis will be amelioration and the prevention of deterioration. In either case, we should recognize that early
amelioration and/or prevention of deterioration is likely to
present new patterns of needs for educational management.
Though the current financial climate may seem to be against
such new provisions, socially, financially and ethically we
cannot afford to neglect any opportunity of fulfilling our
responsibility for optimizing the growth of every child with
disabilities towards increased independence.

In a paper about intelligence testing for infants presented to the 1976 N.I.H. Conference on "Early Behavioural
Assessment of the Communicative and Cognitive Abilities of
the Developmentally Disabled," Horowitz and Dunn stressed the
importance of a supportive and stimulating environment. It
seems obvious to us that to simply label a child as multiply
disabled and then to return him to the parents without considerable guidance and support is unlikely to produce the kind
of supportive educational relationships that the whole family

need in order to optimize prognosis. Hence, our therapeutic
regime does not begin with the child, but with the parents,
and the teachers who will have responsibility for care. The
same emphasis should occur for the multiply disabled child as
for blind or deaf children. Just as we have domiciliary
teachers working with the hearing impaired or blind child
from the moment of diagnosis (i.e., well before the first
year of age), so should we have access to parent guidance and
educational support for the multiply disabled child from the
moment of identification. Optimization of early steps in
learning should lead to increased confidence on the part of
parent and child. The tension, stress and anxiety which tend
to accompany early steps in the management of any child with
a disability should be ameliorated as quickly as possible.
Sensible growth predictions in the cognitive areas should, in
turn, lead to accurate prognostications which, in turn,
should facilitate positive reinforcement for the child,
parent and teacher. Even the briefest contact with children
affected by learning disabilities shows the teacher and
therapist how rapidly the positive or negative effects of
satisfactory or unsatisfactory progress affect not only the
child, but all concerned. The teacher and therapist are at
least as vulnerable as the parents to negative reinforcement.
It is important, therefore, that teachers should be helped to
identify their own vulnerability to ensure that satisfactory
progress in a carefully planned programme of remedial education should: (1) occur as soon as possible; (2) be communicated to all concerned from the first moment that it can be
confidently identified. We need the following:

(a)   A short-term programme designed for the earliest
identification (and amelioration where possible) of sensory,
sensory motor and neuromotor deficits.

(b)   A long-term diagnostic programme designed to identify and monitor the existence of, and fluctuations in,
secondary sources of educational deficit in multiply disabled
children.

(c)   Arising from (a), and as a part of (b), the development of improved techniques for identifying and evaluating
the educational significance of minimal deficits of sensory,
sensory motor and neuromotor function.

(d)   The development, where necessary, of specialized
prosthetic devices (hearing aids, spectacles, aids to neuromotor function) designed specifically for use with multiply

disabled children.

(e)   Improved tests or observational schedules which
will increase our diagnostic skills.

(f)   Improved training programmes for the teachers of
multiply impaired children.

(g)   Improved educational facilities commencing in the
recognition that the parent is the logical child educator.
In our role as the diagnosticians and therapists or teachers,
we must see the rights and responsibilities of the parents as
central to our programme; our efforts, though aimed at the
eventual well-being of the child, should begin with the
parents as primary objectives.

IV.   Therapy as the First Stage
in Education

The section which follows is designed specifically to
deal with infants who are affected by severe to profound
multiple disabilities. It stresses that sensory information
may be separated into two components which, in the normal
infant, are seen as emergent and interdependent functions of
the near and distance receptors. Because many multiply disabled infants are temporarily "locked on" to the near receptors, the strategies we present combine usage of the near
receptors in the early stages (in particular, the tactile
and vibro tactile systems), with neuromotor activity designed
to encourage cognition and, thus, provide a foundation for
learning via the residua of the distance receptors. The early
stages of experience begin with the near receptors. In those
cases where there is modification of distance receptor function, there is often a delay in the usage of that particular
sense. Thus, the young deaf infant tends to be hypervisual,
while the infant with audio-visual problems tends to be hyper-
tactile. Therapy walks the tight-rope between developing any
presented function as a basis for cognition on the one hand,
and the possible discouragement of alternative sensory function on the other. Just as some deaf educators have suggested
that visual inputs should be masked during auditory training
to encourage greater reliance on audition, so the teacher/
therapist has to decide at what stage and in what manner
tactile information sources will be replaced by more direct

usage of the audio-visual residua. Ultimately, the plan will
be to optimize the use of all (or any) senses as sources of
learning. We are not thinking, therefore, of auditory or
visual acuity or sensitivity, but of audio-or-visuo-cognitive
function. This, obviously, will be based on developing cognitive skill. We now have had sufficient experience with
older children to know that when cognition reaches certain
functional levels, peripheral auditory or visual sensitivity
appears to markedly improve. Just as listening demands hearing, attending and cognition, so all other sensory learning
is dependent on attending and cognition as well as peripheral
sensitivity.

The Initiation of Therapy

     The major problem in establishing therapeutic goals
stems from the current inadequacy of assessment of function.
Accurate assessment of children with multiple disabilities is
extremely difficult in the first eighteen months of life.
Additional sensory, sensory motor or neuromotor malfunctions
are often present in varying combinations to confound the
problem of differential diagnosis. In the initial assessment,
for example, the resulting information about visual or auditory function can rarely be regarded as complete and final.
On the one hand, the child may be suffering from a degenerat-
ing condition. On the other hand, the child may have much
better visual potential than the initial assessment suggests.
The child's real level of visual acuity can be misdiagnosed
for the following reasons:

(1)   short attention span

(2)   poor emotional rapport (related often to a lack of
      socialization skills)

(3)   cognitive deficiencies; (memory impairments or lack of
      knowledge of the function and use of objects in the
      environment)

(4)   lack of eye contact

     As the child's attention span increases and as he
becomes a much more predictable and successful manipulator
of his environment, he often demonstrates that his vision is
much better than was originally thought. For example, when
the child learns to crawl, the directions in which he crawls

or the objects he seeks may demonstrate that he can see large
objects in his environment. Also, when he learns to finger
feed, he may find crumbs visually without feeling for traces
of food with his fingers, showing that he can see relatively
small objects. The educational process helps to clarify and
define more accurately those assets and deficits which had
originally been identified by the diagnostic strategies of
the medical and paramedical members of the team. In that
sense, therapy is diagnostic.

The original diagnosis has been arrived at mainly through
the use of a medical model. In subsequent assessments, the
educational model becomes more and more prominent. Its
emphasis is related more directly to the purposive and cognitive characteristics of the child. Before education and
therapy begin, the child's behaviours are too often, to say
the least, chaotic. There are few meaningful patterns of
behaviour through which they can relate to their immediate
environment, be it animate or inanimate. They often engage
themselves in bizarre and repetitive behaviours which we
refer to as stereotypics. These patterns of behaviour become
so ingrained that it is often difficult to penetrate through
them to the child. The problem of arousing the children to
an awareness of something outside themselves is also con-
founded by the five factors mentioned earlier, which may
concurrently lead to a misdiagnosis. These factors tend to
be common to the population considered in this paper. However, there is a great deal of variance in the amount of
spontaneous activity from child to child within that population. It should be remembered that spontaneous activity may
be self-informing. In some children it may be stereotypic
and preclude the development of self-informing strategies.

Knowledge is conveyed to us through our senses. These
can be divided into three groupings: distance, near and the
internal. The distance senses are the visual, auditory and
olfactory. The near senses involve touch, taste, temperature,
pressure and vibration. The internal senses incorporate the
neuromuscular information derived from posture and movement,
activity of internal organs and possibly hormonal influences.
Therefore, one can define the near and internal sense modalities as those which receive their impulses by direct stimulation. The distance senses require a transmission medium
through which the appropriate energy impulses can pass to
reach them.

Vision and hearing allow us to create a picture of the world in which we live. Visual information helps us to understand the function of the space around us and how the animate and inanimate relate in that space. Hearing has first an alerting and scanning function. However, at a much more sophisticated level, it allows us not only to categorize our world and organize our thoughts through language, but also to communicate at the symbolic level.

Hearing and vision will be disastrously thwarted without supporting information from the near and internal senses, which have a structuring function on the global images from the two distance senses. Such information helps to complete a much more meaningful picture.

It is obvious from the previous discussion that if a child is to develop a complete concept of an object, he must at first have direct contact with this object. This is often not possible unless he is able to coordinate these sensory inputs and develop control over his neuromotor functions. Hence, in the normal course of events, in the first few weeks of a child's life, most of the information about his world is perceived through his near senses. Then, as his motor skills mature and develop, the distance sense modalities make greater and greater contributions to his establishment of the normal cognitive structures as we know them.

Therefore, the severely multiply disabled child, with or without losses of either visual or auditory acuity, will have extreme difficulty in creating order or meaning out of an agglomeration of disrupted sensory impressions. One finds many infants in this category who, even though their sense organs are not impaired, make little use of the information which is conveyed by these senses. Many of them live in an infantile bipolar world of pleasure/displeasure which is often focused on their basic needs and involves only the near and internal senses. In an attempt to make order out of chaos, they indulge in spontaneous, undirected, repetitive behaviour which has been discussed previously. Such manneristic behaviour can involve them for long periods at a time. These mannerisms may not only be a substitute for, but may well be a barrier to the development of basic cognitive structures.

Severe lack of purposeful activity in multiply disabled children poses a threat to the spontaneous development of motor function which we take for granted in unimpaired children. To begin on the long road of conceptual development, we

must start by creating a foundation of meaningful motor
experience for them.

Therefore, diagnosis and assessment of the early behaviours that the children display begins with broad categories,
examples of which are given below:

1. Activity versus passivity.

2. Voluntary versus involuntary motor activity.

3. Voluntary versus involuntary passivity.

4. Voluntary constructive versus voluntary unconstructive
    activity.

5. Gross versus fine motor activity.

6. Purposive versus non-purposive gross motor control.

7. Purposive versus non-purposive fine motor control.

Though we have referred several times to the problem of
hyperactivity and stereotypy, the problems of passivity are
no less severe. Often the activity of an infant can be
channelized by selective reinforcement. At the same time,
the lethargic, inactive child may need constant stimulation
and intervention by his family or teacher to maintain some
semblance of exploratory behaviour.

The task of early education is to create purposeful
sensory motor activity in both the gross and fine motor areas.
Where the children display an abundance of spontaneous but
often undirected activity, however, the creation of purposive
motor activities alone is not the total answer. If we were
fortunate enough to replace all non-purposive with purposive
activity, obviously management problems would still arise.
Therefore, in order to reduce the overall level of activity,
whether it is purposive or non-purposive, inhibitory processes
also need to be developed. On the other hand, where children
display activity which is rarely spontaneous and usually
undirected, we attempt to promote purposeful and constructive
actions.

Figure 1 summarizes our early educational model for the
teaching of meaningful motor patterns which will form the

basis of necessary skills for everyday life and communication.

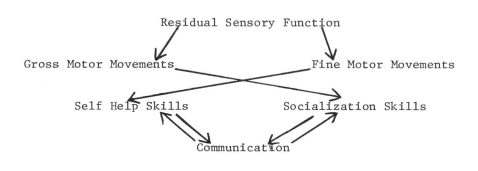

FIGURE 1: An Educational Model Based on the Creation and
Exploitation of Meaningful Motor Patterns

We have developed The M.B. First Stage Graded Progress
Chart (see Appendix I, this chapter), to assess the five
areas mentioned in the above model. Such a chart is to
identify and record the child's initial functions and then to
select realistic goals for future training. As the gross
motor and fine motor areas form the base of our model, we
shall elaborate on those areas first. This allows us to
isolate the initial assets of the child and then to select
realistic goals for the future. For example, a child may be
able to roll from front to back, but not from back to front.
Therefore, "rolling from back to front" is likely to be this
child's immediate future goal in the gross motor area.

The chart allows us to record all gross loco-motor function and to categorize it as constructive or unconstructive
behaviour. The point we wish to emphasize at this stage is
that all gross motor function should be recorded. When constructive versus unconstructive classifications are made, it
is easy to determine those patterns of behaviour which require
encouragement and those which are unproductive and, hence, to
be discouraged. As a guide to categorization, we suggest that

gross motor functions which are used to facilitate some other
perceptual function should be categorized as "constructive".
For instance, the child who crawls aimlessly would have his
crawling behaviour categorized as unconstructive. If, however, he crept towards a pattern of light or an object on the
floor, we would describe it as constructive.

Fine motor functions are assessed and recorded in a
similar manner. At the most primitive level, the manipulative skills of the hands allow the child to explore his
environment for its sensory qualities. For example, the
child may pick up an object to smell, tap, mouth, look at or
feel. Hopefully, the processing of such sensory motor inputs
will eventually lead not only to his discrimination of these
sensory inputs, but will be extended to the beginnings of
concept development. Therefore, such aspects are included at
the end of the fine motor chart.

As indicated by the model presented in Figure 1, motor
movements are necessary for the development of self-help
skills. For example, for a child to drink from a container,
he must be able to grasp it using palmar grasp and then lift
it to his mouth by bending his elbow. At a much more sophisticated level, he can use a pincer action to finger feed.
Similarly, all self-help skills can be viewed as constructive
use of fine and/or gross motor movements. The main areas
assessed here are drinking and feeding. All areas have three
columns for recording purposes; this allows us to indicate
whether the child only completes the skill with help, whether
he attempts it alone, or whether he completes it unaided.

The socialization chart is divided into two areas: self
concept and environmental interaction. The socialization
skills that are involved here promote interaction by their
very nature. Therefore, this area is critical to communication.

As indicated in Figure 1, self-help and socialization
skills promote the development of communication. The necessary prerequisites listed in the communication charts stress
this fact. However, as communication develops, it also
enhances the acquisition of skills in the self-help and
socialization areas. The communication charts are designed
for pre-syntactical behaviour.

To score the children's assets on the charts, a tick is
placed in the appropriate box. As with any form of continuing assessment, goals should be regularly reviewed, care

being taken to observe and record any information with regard
to the educational progress which may refine the diagnostic
information from the medical model.

V. Sensory and Intersensory Function
as a Basis for Communication

For all children wearing hearing aids, voicing conveys
tactile information derived from the very effort of voicing
(cranial thoracic or laryngeal proprioceptive functions), and
also from the sound of the voice setting the ear mold into
resonance before the signal reaches the cochlea. Every hearing aid wearer, therefore, receives bimodal (i.e., auditory
and tactile) stimuli from his own voicing. In responding to
the voice of others (unless he is held by the person presenting such stimuli), the tactile inputs are restricted, in the
main, to the outer ear. That is, the other proprioceptive
cues are absent. Thus, the infant has to learn to identify
the presence of voices other than his own by both the absence
of proprioceptive inputs and by pitch differentiation (in the
case of adult voices). The multiply disabled infant, however,
may be neither intellectually nor experientially capable of
making such judgments. Hence, additional information of a
tactile nature has to be supplied. This, too, should be
designed to present stimuli to the cochlea and to the cranium
simultaneously, and, in addition, to amplify proprioceptive
inputs. By means of the equipment described below, the child
is encouraged not only to search and to move in space, but
also to make judgments as a basis for the acquisition of
skill in judgment making.

Non-purposive voicing leads, in normal circumstances, to
purposive voicing. One of the early components of any form
of planned auditory stimulation of hearing impaired infants
is the maintenance of voicing, so that this may be used pur-
posively and also so that the child can learn to discriminate
between his own voice and that of others. Identification of
these differences is added to the visual, gustatory and
tactile components of need satisfaction by others, so that
the notion of demanding and environmental manipulation can
emerge. If we accept that early signalling is used, in the
main, for achieving need satisfactions, we again postulate
that the infant is capable of deriving such conclusions from

events. The cognitive skills required for such behaviour may
be of very low order in the multiply disabled infant. Hence,
both the time scale and the amplification of multi-sensory
inputs require complex judgments and careful observation as
the child matures. We have adopted the principle at the
early stages of therapy that discrimination between self-
initiated stimuli and environmentally initiated stimuli will
take time. Every step must be taken to assist these discrim-
inations in order that needs or wants will, in fact, be
signalled in such a way that meeting those needs will reinforce signalling and, thus, form the basis for a primitive
communication modality.

     In our earlier sections we have stressed the need for
developed cognitive manipulation of sensory inputs. Working
with older children, we have seen that the tactile components
described below can be "faded" in order to encourage the more
"normal" processes of auditory monitoring. However, we have
also discovered that, though specific signals can be generalized from the tactile to the auditory, in many cases the
development of new generalizations must begin again at the
tactile level. For our infant population we retain the
tactile inputs as an integral part of sensory learning so
that incidental auditory generalization may be derived concurrently from the tactile modality.

     Other papers in this text deal with the use of communica-
tion as a reinforcer of signalling and also of the effect on
a household of the infant's use of signalling systems. For
the parents of multiply disabled children, any point of
contact with the child that indicates a realization of parental presence and role is avidly awaited. The encouragement
of such communication structures is not only of inestimable
value to the child but, from a parental point of view, is
essential to bonding and to encouraging continued stimulation
by the parents. In dealing with older children, much of our
effort is directed towards recreation of bonding and facilitation of pleasure and pride in communication, especially where
such structures have lapsed due to faulty or inadequate
therapy and counselling. For the sake of the child and the
family as an entity, we cannot sufficiently stress the need
to evoke satisfactions derived from simple communication and
the capacity to signal and to identify needs or wants.

The same comments apply to the notion of exploration and curiosity. The <u>what</u> and the <u>why</u> of objects outside ourselves can only be derived from the capacity to identify <u>that</u> objects exist outside and independently of ourselves. Hence, exploration of the environment is another essential aspect of sensory and sensory-motor learning. Just as we say that to teach language to deaf children is impossible without a purpose and function for that language, so for the multiply disabled child. Cognition requires a purpose before functioning can be encouraged. How, then, is the child to be presented with a series of stimuli which can be "tied " to objects, activities or events, in such a way that there is encouragement to examine them and find structures in their investigation that can be coded and used as a basis for identification?

In our early work with older children, we used massive vibro-tactile inputs to encourage conforming behaviour as a basis for primitive learning. In the last year we have found that objects can be given a tactile identity which is not simply related to weight, heat or texture. As will be seen below, the hand-held vibrator unit can be applied to a number of objects in order to attract exploration (see Figure 1). When exploration occurs, the vibro-tactile components are removed and the identification process continues either in usage, or in further investigation (Figure 2). For instance an infant may be encouraged to grasp an object by vibro-tactile stimulation, but having grasped it, will be allowed to investigate it by the handling, mouthing and smelling processes typical of his stage of development. Other events such as the approach of others may be related to need satisfactions when vibro-tactile inputs are added to olfactory inputs as a preliminary to feeding or social contact.

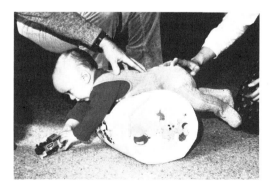

Figure 1.   Illustration of the use of vibro-tactile inputs from four (4) pressure switches embodied in the periphery of an inflatable ''crawler.''

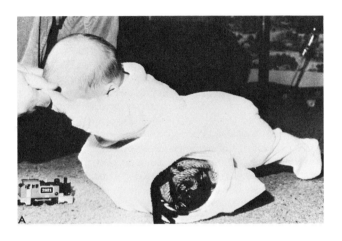

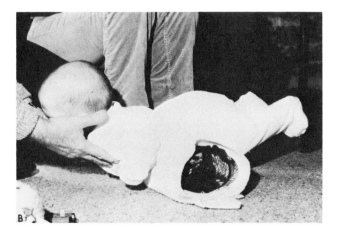

Figure 2. Illustration of the extended use of behavioural patterns originally learned through vibro-tactile inputs and the extended use of vibro-tactile techniques to encourage the growth and development of exploration and experience. (A) abdominal support; (B) encouragement of crawling; (C) (right page) reach-grasp after crawling; (D) (right page) ''Eureka!'' an infant shows triumph after vibro-tactile reinforcement in the search for a toy which emits vibro-tactile signals.

408

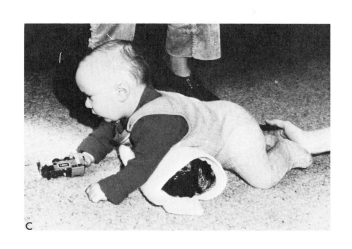

C

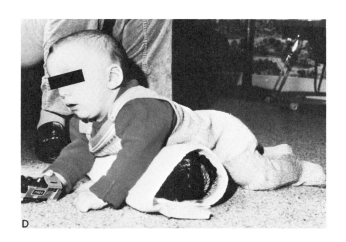

D

409

As will be seen from the following illustrations, the equipment ranges from head-worn devices through a hand-held unit, to larger devices which are environmentally informative or encourage environmental investigation. The head-worn devices began as a simple body-worn aid, which drove a bone conductor as well as a receiver system (Figure 3). Instead of the usual spring head clips for the bone conductor, a simple head-band of elasticized material was made, which held both receiver and bone-conductor securely in place. Technological progress has facilitated the use of head-worn aids, one driving an "in the ear" receiver and the other a bone conductor, each held by the head band. The device does not include chin straps, but we have found that these are easily added to the head band and, in any case, are not needed after the first few days of therapy.

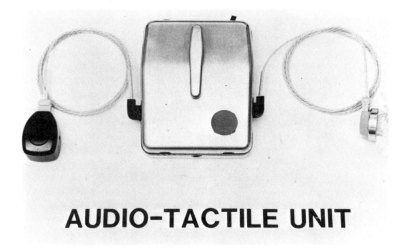

Figure 3.   Hearing aid used to drive a bone conductor and an air conductor.

The hand-held vibrator unit (Figure 4) is essentially the same as the remainder of the equipment described below in that it consists of a simple electric motor, the axle of which carries an eccentric weighting system. This causes a modification of rotation which is carried via the axle to the bearings, and from this to a probe tip which can be applied directly to the infant or to objects as required. A simple power control permits changes of speed of rotation. This, in turn, leads to modification of frequency and intensity but will not, however, permit independent presentation of either.

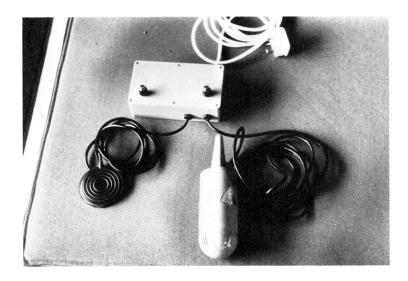

Figure 4.   Hand-held vibro-tactile unit and control system.

The original hearing aid equipment included a balance
switch which permitted a shift from tactile to auditory
dominance. In two post-aural aids this is achieved by
independent adjustments of the controls on each individual
aid. The head-worn equipment permits continuous monitoring
of events, including the wearer's voice and those of others,
both in terms of audio-tactile and auditory information. The
other tactile units are not so specific and serve, by rhythmic
variation, to alert the infant to external events, to encourage investigation and, perhaps most importantly, to control,
by the experimenter, of reinforcement strategies. In this
sense, the units which are not worn on the head should be
seen as limited to bi-stratal and non-syntactic information
systems. These encourage learning and communication, but do
not provide the tri-stratal information basic to patterns of
semantic or (at a later date) syntactical linguistic con-
structs. The cognitive elements which underlie bi-stratal
learning are presented, of course, so that the child can
relate cause and effect to other sensory inputs associated
with the satisfaction of needs and wants. Encapsulating
these in language structures depends on both the audio-
tactile tri-stratal devices worn on the head and the quality
of training.

The principle of the hand-held vibrator has been adapted
to the design of two types of vibrating tables, a stimulating
platform, a walk-way and a crawl-way. The two tables differ
considerably in the information they supply and the cognitive
demands they make on the child. The simplest device is a
single unit clamped below a table so that the child may be
given quite powerful stimuli. Such stimulae have wide uses.
For instance, the young infant may lie on the table or be
seated on it, or, when the child is able to sit in a chair,
the table may be juxtaposed so that manual manipulative skills
can be taught. For example, palmar grasp can be encouraged
in early feeding training. This leads to manipulation of a
spoon or beaker.

A more complex series of four vibro-devices are adapted
to lie inside the tray on the infant's chair, and provide
facilities for dividing the area of the table into four potential information sources. With these, the more intelligent
child can be taught to identify the difference between near
and far, left and right, or such combinations as may be
required. Small vibro units are driven by these four areas
and may be attached to the wrists or the feet by means of
velcro bands. We have found that the normal woolly garments
worn by infants in the United Kingdom permit the leads to be
run down the sleeves or down the legs of rompers so that the
process of "plugging the infant in" is simply a matter of
inserting a four point plug into a socket located under the
table top.

The stimulation platform (Figure 5A) has proven invaluable in developing gross locomotor function. Crawling,
standing, balancing and rolling are all encouraged when the
child feels the vibrations through those parts of the body
in contact with the platform. Where the infant is not yet
ready for mobility training, the vibrations felt through the
whole body are potent sources of pleasure and often of
muscle relaxation or of increased blood flow. Larger areas
may be created by linking a number of platforms. These may
then be used for group work, or to form longer pathways to
develop exploratory behaviour.

Experience with the longer pathways led us to develop a
novel switching system. The original devices required external switching and effectively tied the operator to the infant.
Our more recent developments encourage purposive behaviour
by the incorporation of a complex electronic self-switching
system. Under the soft waterproof covering of the platform

modules, twelve pressure switches (Figure 5B) are connected
to an electronic memory. This memory is linked to progression
so that though each switch is, in fact, activated by the
infant's movements, each will only switch when a complete
series has been triggered. Thus, no switch in the series one
to twelve may be reactivated until the twelfth switch has
been depressed. Progression forward from any point in the
series to the next will lead to stimulation. Remaining on
one point for more than three seconds, or moving back from
that point to the switch before it will not be rewarded. The
typical squatting or rocking of many multiply disabled children is not reinforced and the parent/therapist is left free
to guide or direct the child without need for controlling the
reinforcement strategies.

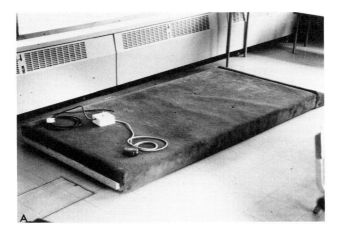

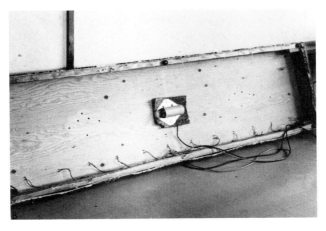

Figure 5. (A) Crawlway and controls ready for use. (B) Underside of crawlway with 2
pressure switches.

Other pieces of equipment (Figure 6) are now being built
to aid the development of more sophisticated skills. A proto-
type ultra-sound scanner used with blind children to provide
auditory cues about the environment is in the process of
modification to provide audio-tactile inputs.

To encourage developing communication systems, we have
devised a simple set of notes which we provide for parents/
therapists. These are given to the parents to reinforce the
information acquired during counselling and training sessions.
A brief excerpt is included below.

                 Extract From Notes to Parent/Therapist

One could cite many more examples but it should be clear
that the sign has its origins in the physical and verbal
prompts which trigger a specific meaningful behaviour pattern.
Hopefully, the sign will become less related to the specific
motor activity within the context in which it has been learned
and will eventually relate to all contexts. To this point,
the signs have been utilizing, in the main, the tactile modality. Now the sign is shaped into a more abstract entity.

In the main, because the tactile modality is limited in
space, its use compels physical contact with the child. Therefore, except in extreme circumstances (with the deaf-blind
child, or the deaf child who is also a visual avoider) one
would select either the tactile or auditory modality. The
auditory modality is preferable in that it is used by most
people in the culture. In these circumstances, make the
transition from physical and verbal prompts presented simultaneously, to verbal prompts alone. If this is impossible
because the child has a hearing loss or brain damage or
avoids auditory stimuli, try, using the visual modality, to
shape a more abstract visual sign from the tactile sign. Some
examples of this are as follows:

(i) Tactile to tactile: Prompt the child to lift the
     cup by actually placing your hand over his while he
     holds the cup in a gross pincer grasp and lift.
     Place the cup back on the table. The child will
     gradually, then, learn to pick up the cup and drink.
     Increase the abstraction of the sign by placing your
     hand over the child's, shaping it into the same
     configuration as previously, but without the cup
     actually being held. Encourage lifting movement.

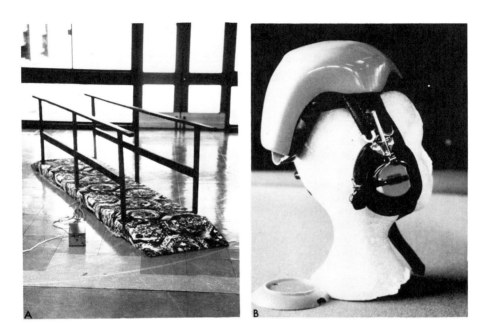

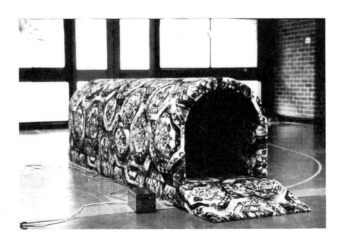

Figure 6. Additional equipment is being developed to stimulate development. These include: (A) walkway with support rails and 12 pressure switches; (B) audio-tactile helmet for use by older children; (C) a tunnel crawlway with 12 pressure switches.

Gradually the child will learn to reach out for the
cup when the sign has been completed.

(ii)   Tactile to auditory: First, using physical and
       verbal prompts simultaneously, encourage the child
       to stand in a similar manner to that previously
       described. Then gradually fade the lifting action
       until the child stands for the verbal prompt alone.

(iii) Tactile to visual: After establishing the tactile
       sign of taking his hands and rubbing them together
       for wash, let his hands go while he is still rubbing
       and rub your own hands. The child will eventually
       learn to respond to the sign "wash" when the adult
       rubs his own hands together. (More sophisticated
       shifts are sometimes developed. A blind, hearing
       impaired child, for example, may undergo the
       following sensory shifts: the tactile to the vibro-
       tactile to the auditory).

       At this stage the tempero-spatial situation (i.e.,
       the situation in time and space) in which the sign
       occurs is essential. As soon as a level is
       reached in which hearing the tinkle of the spoon
       without actually seeing the food causes the child
       to stop and wait expectantly for the food, communi-
       cation has passed on to another level. (This is
       an extension of the initial example in the present
       section). Such a specialized version of a sign is
       called a signal. The information is conveyed to
       the child without the food being actually present.
       In other words, the signal is free from tempero-
       spatial relationships.

To help clarify that a signal is tempero-spatially free,
suppose that the signal "toilet" has been presented to the
child in a room not remotely connected to the toilet. If the
child then goes through to use the toilet, the signal has
been established and is, of course, tempero-spatially free.

    The next stage in the hierarchy occurs when the child
uses the sign to signal needs. We must remember that the
sign can be vocal or gestural. Expressive function begins to
develop now from the receptive function which began earlier.
In other words, comprehension of language precedes expression.
As with so many laws of nature, absorption precedes production.

Enough has been said about behaviour modification to
show that the child can be trained to imitate a vocal or
neuro-motor gesture which will relate to one of his needs.
At first, imitation will simply be a compliance with the
training procedure and, as such, will have no symbolic
function. However, once the child has developed the conceptual relationship between the gesture in which he is being
trained and the satisfaction of his needs, we see the emergence of the symbol. Hence, our first steps in behaviour
modification as a basis for communication consist of training
the child to make the gesture or vocalization, and then
facilitating the development of the concept that the gesture
has a specific symbolic value. It should be clear that conceptual skills are essential prerequisites for the development of symbolization. The following quotation probably
best sums up the progression of the communicative process
from sign to signal to symbol and ultimately, to language:

> "The spoken word, at first a sign because it
> reached the child embedded in a situation,
> becomes a signal as he hears it in the absence
> of the situation; becomes a symbol as he, him-
> ·self, utters it with some direction of his
> attention towards the situation; becomes
> linguistic as it is bound into a system of
> relationships, syntactic and semantic (Lewis,
> 1968)."

This system of relationships is usually referred to as the
syntactical component. Therefore, it is obvious at this
stage that there are three components: the sensory, the
syntactical and the semantic. One has made the transition
at this stage from a bi-stratal to a tri-stratal system.
In other words, one now finds language being used in the
communicative process and, hence, is capable of direction
both to the user and the recipient (Murphy, 1972). Some
children may never progress beyond the expression of needs,
wants or emotional state. Nevertheless, every effort must
be made to develop cognition to the stage where spontaneous
communication is developed, first out of emotional state.
This demands receptive skills on the part of the observer
and the ability to encourage the development and expression
of personality. Following this, the communication of events -
present, past and future - may well lead to the development
of a more mature language structure and, eventually, to the
development of formal communication skills, mime, gesture,
signs, pictorial presentation, drawing, or simple word

recognition in printed form. The significance of these for
parental satisfaction and social adequacy cannot be over-
estimated.

Conclusion

       In our discussions with parents, we talk of the three
"P's" of communication. Those are pleasure, pride and purpose.
The child enjoys voicing and usually the enjoyment is shared
by his audience. In multiply disabled children, parental
pride in such voicing, expressed by verbal or tactile responses, evokes pride in the child. Pleasure and pride combine to give purpose to the original non-purposive voicing.
As purpose emerges and specific responses occur, or needs
and wants are met, so purposive voicing is reinforced. Signalling begins, communication, though primitive, is developing
and pride and pleasure are increased. Pride is a precious
commodity in the case of multiply disabled children. Parents
are strongly encouraged not only to be proud of such events,
but to record them on progress charts and to show them to
therapists or to case conferences. In summarizing our contribution, the point we wish to stress is that, though
communication is vitally important as a source of information
interchange, its pleasure and pride components are essential.
Without these, the child will not develop, the parents will
not respond and communication will be stiltified. The social
competence of multiply disabled infants does not emerge
without considerable encouragement. We see communication as
an early step in social behaviour. We also see that such
communication is based on cognitive skills. Much of this
presentation has described our work in developing sensory
motor skills. This emphasis was deliberately designed to
relate early exploration to cognition and to the creation of
those cognitive skills which are basic to communication.

APPENDIX I *

The M.B. Stage 1 Graded Progress Chart.

NAME:....................... DATE:......................

Gross Motor Assessment:	Purposive	Non-purposive
(1) Primitive movements for sitting, crawling and walking		
(a) Lifts and holds head up when lying on back.		
(b) Lifts and holds head up when lying on front.		
(c) Etc.................		
(2) Hierarchy of essential skills for Sitting		
(a) Sits up with back support.		
(b) Sits up without back support.		
(c) Etc.................		
(3) Hierarchy of essential skills for Crawling		
(a) Takes weight on forearms.		
(b) Crawling position.		
(c) Etc.................		
(4) Hierarchy of essential skills for Standing		
(a) Stands up with human support.		
(b) Stands up with human support but without personal contact.		
(c) Etc.................		

* For more detailed explanation of this progress chart,
please contact the author of this paper. It is
considerably longer in each sub-section than it appears
here.

419

	Purposive	Non-purposive

(5) Hierarchy of essential skills for walking unaided.

   (a) Stepping reaction (putting one foot in front of other.)

   (b) Walking with human support.

   (c) Etc.................

(6) Hierarchy of essential skills for walking with Frame.

   (a) Stepping reaction (putting one foot in front of other.)

   (b) Walking with human support.

   (c) Etc.................

Fine Motor Assessment:

(1) The beginnings of fine motor movements.

   (a) Awareness of limbs and their movements and function.

   (b) Voluntary movements of hands or feet.

   (c) Etc.................

(2) Palmar Grasp (Closed Fist).

   (a) Grasps objects introduced to hand.

   (b) Grasps and holds objects.

   (c) Etc.................

	Constructive	Unconstructive

(3) Pincer grasp (finger thumb opposition).

    (a) Grasps objects introduced.

    (b) Grasps and holds objects.

    (c) Etc...................

(4) Explores objects for their characteristics.

    (a) Taste

    (b) Smell

    (c) Etc...................

(5) Has concept of, or ability to discriminate.

    (a) Taste

    (b) Smell

    (c) Etc...................

Self-Help Assessment:

	Completes with help	Attempts alone	Completes unaided

(1) Drinking

    (a) From bottle

    (b) From feeder cup

    (c) Etc...................

(2) Feeding

    (a) Accepts spoonful of food

    (b) Chews food

    (c) Etc...................

(3) Toileting

Bowels	Bladder

    (a) Cannot use toilet or potty

    (b) Sits on but does not use

    (c) Etc...................

421

Social Assessment:

(1) Self-Concept

    (a) Turns for people seen 1. Glances

                                2. Follows

    (b) Turns for touch   1. Glances

                                2. Follows

    (c) Etc............................

422

REFERENCES

Ball, T.S. in Itard, Sequin and Kephart (eds.) Sensory Education. A Learning Interpretation (Cleveland: Charles E. Merrill Pub. Co.), 1971.

Bailey, J. and Myerson, L. "Vibration as a reinforcer with the profoundly retarded child," Journal of Applied Behaviour Analysis 2:135 - 137, 1969.

Banham, K.M. "Measuring Emotional Motor Rehabilitation of Cerebral Palsied Infants and Young Children," Rehabilitation Literature 39:111 - 115, 1978.

Broadhead, G.D., Rarick, G.L. "Family Characteristics and Gross Motor Traits in Handicapped Children," Research Q 49:421 - 429, 1978.

Bruner, J. Sensory Deprivation (Cambridge: Harvard University Press), 1961.

Bruner, J. "The Growth of the Mind," in Davis, G.A. and Warren, T.F. (eds.) Psychology of Education (Boston: D.C. Heath and Co.), 1974.

Byrne, D.J. "Vibrator becomes a motivator for the multiply handicaped: Teaching and training," Journal of National Association of Teachers of the Mentally Handicapped 17: 137 - 139, 1979.

Casse, Robert M., Jr. "The professional's responsibility in aiding parental adjustment," Mental Retardation 6:49 - 51, 1968.

Chaney, M. and Kyshart, N.C. Motoric Aids to Perceptive Training (Cleveland, Ohio: Charles E. Merrill Pub Co.), 1968.

Clark, F.A., Shuer, J. "A clarification of sensory integrative therapy and its application to programming with retarded people," Mental Retardation 16:227 - 232, 1978.

Felsenthal, Helen, and Idwa, U. "The role of the school psychologist in counselling parents of the mentally retarded," Training School Bulletin 65:29 - 35, 1968.

Fitzgerald, M.D., Sitton, A.B. and McConnell, F. "Audiometric Developmental and Learning Characteristics of a group of rubella deaf children," _Journal of Speech and Hearing Disorders_ 35:218 - 228, 1970.

Gregory, S. _The Deaf Child and His Family_ (N.Y.: John Wiley), 1976.

Hardy, W.G. and Bordley, J.E. "Problems in the diagnosis and management of the Multiply Handicapped," _Archives of Otolaryngology_, 98:269 - 274, 1973.

Hischer, E. "Motor transfer in the presence of normal and subnormal intelligence - A paedigogic-empirical study of eight year old and eleven year old pupils," _International Journal of Rehabilitative Research_ 2:84 - 85, 1979.

Holt, K.S. "Assessment of handicap in childhood," _Child Care Health Development_ 5:151 - 162, 1979.

Hunt, J. McV. _Intelligence and Experience_ (New York: The Ronald Press Co.), 1961.

Itard, J.M.G. The Wild Boy of Aveyron, (trans) Humphrey G. and Humphrey M., 1907, (New York: Prentice Hall), 1962.

Johnson, D. Furth H. and Davey G. "Vibration and praise as reinforcers for mentally handicapped people," _Mental Retardation_ 16:339 - 342, 1978.

Kish, G.B. "Studies of Sensory Reinforcement," in Honig, W.K. (ed.) _Operant Behaviour: Areas of Research and Application_ (New York: Appleton - Century, Crofts), 1966.

Levarlet-Joye, H. "The Development of Motor Competency in Normal and Slightly Mentally Handicapped Children," _Pediatric Paedology_ 13:357 - 364, 1978.

Lewis, M.M. _Language, Thought and Personality in Infancy and Childhood_ (New York: Basic Books), 1963.

Loewe, A. "Just to have an undisturbed night's sleep again ...!" Multiply Handicapped Hearing Impaired Children (Kettering Institute), 1966.

Lundberg, A. Dissociated motor development – developmental
    patterns, Clinical characteristics, Causal factors and
    Outcome, with special reference to late walking children,"
    Neuropaediatrie 10:161 – 182, 1979.

McDowell, Richard L. "Parent counselling: The state of the
    art," Journal of Learning Disabilities 9:614 – 619, 1976.

Myerson, L., Kerr, N. and Michael, J. "Behaviour Modifica-
    tion in Rehabilitation," in Bijon, S. and Baer, D. (eds.)
    Experimental Analysis (New York: Appleton-Century,
    Crofts), 1967.

Miller, Nancy B. "Parents of children with neurological
    disorders: Concerns and counselling," Journal of Pediat-
    ric Psychology, 4:297 – 306, 1979.

Murphy, K.P. "Parent Guidance as an Attack on Handicap,"
    Paper presented to National Deaf Children's Society,
    London, 1974.

Murphy, K.P. "Development of Hearing in Babies," Child and
    Family 1:16 – 20, 1963.

Murphy, K.P. "Early Development of Auditory Function,"
    Paper presented to American Speech and Hearing Association,
    San Francisco, 1978.

Nickel, H. Entwiglungsphychogie des Kindes-Und Jugendarters.
    Band 1, Stuttgart, 1975.

Palfrey, J.S., Mervis, R.C., and Butler, J.A. "New direc-
    tions in the evaluation and education of handicapped
    children," New England Journal of Medicine 15:819 – 824,
    1978.

Ramsey, Glenn V. "Review of group methods with parents of
    the mentally retarded," American Journal of Mental
    Deficiency 5:857 – 863, 1967.

Rehagan, N.J. and Thelen, M.H. "Vibration as positive
    reinforcement for retarded children," Journal of Abnormal
    Psychology 80:162 – 167, 1972.

Schact, E.G. Metamorphosis (New York: Basic Books), 1959.

Schopler, E. "Visual versus tactual preference in normal and
  schizophrenic children," Journal of Abnormal Psychology
  71:108 - 114, 1966.

Seguin, E. Idiocy and its Treatment by the Physiological
  Method (New York: Teachers College, Columbia University),
  1907.
Sherington, C.S. The Integrative Action of the Nervous
  System (London: Cambridge University Press), 1906.

Stayton, S.E. "Multi modality responding as a function of
  mental age and retardation," Journal of Perceptual and
  Motor Skills 33:1122, 1971.

Sternlight, Manny "Parent counselling in an experimental
  rehabilitation center," Journal of Rehabilitation 35:15 -
  16, 1969.

Strauss, A.A. and Kephart, N.C. Psychopathology and Education of the Brain Injured Child, Volume II (New York:
  Grune and Stratton), 1955.

Taylor, I. Neurological Mechanisms of Hearing and Speech in
  Children (Manchester: University Press), 1964.

Temple, I.G. "A Test Battery to Assess Intrasensory and
  Intersensory Development of Young Children," Percept. Mat.
  Skills 48:643 - 659, 1979.

Vernon, M. "Multiply Handicapped Deaf Children, Medical,
  Educational and Psychological Considerations," Council of
  Exceptional Children Monograph, 1969.

Wenzel, D. "The development of the parachute reaction: A
  visuo-vestibular response," Neuropaediatrie 9:351 - 359,
  1978.

THE EFFECTS OF NEW UNITED STATES LEGISLATION ON SERVICES TO VERY YOUNG HEARING-IMPAIRED CHILDREN AND THEIR FAMILIES

Linda W. Nober
Westfield State College, Westfield, Massachusetts

Professionals involved with services to hearing-impaired children in countries other than the United States may be surprised to learn about the service delivery system to children, birth to 3 years,* within that country. Leaders from the United States may describe particular service delivery models, but the critical issue is the lack of a uniform system which is consistent from one community to another. Very young children (birth to 3 years) are not exposed to a universal maternal-child health care system, and the problems of early identification of hearing impairment are but one measure of the health and educational problems faced by our citizens. A review of services available in other countries presents a wealth of information, notably that many countries with social-welfare systems for early identification of all handicaps surpass the efforts and types of services available in the United States. However, early identification and intervention have been determined by the Congress to be a national priority as a vehicle to upgrade services to all handicapped children. The plan encompasses many of the most desirable tenets of programs well established in other countries and at the same time, establishes, internationally, some unique incentives and components of interest to special educators.

This paper describes current service delivery systems to very young hearing-impaired children in the United States and identifies exemplary models of early intervention affected by the newest federal legislation. In addition, those components of legislation are described which portend the greatest international impact on practitioners.

---

* Ages are described according to U.S. government groupings:
  Birth to 3 years;
  Very young children;
  Three to 5 years;
  Preschool age children

Current Service Delivery Systems
in the United States

A.   Administrative Location

       Traditionally, programs serving very young hearing-
impaired children are provided by schools for the deaf,
state mental health or public health facilities, medical
centers, or university settings (Cox and Lloyd, 1976).
Early identification by multidisciplinary medical and support
staff teams enable families to enroll in Parent-Infant
training so that aural habilitation and language acquisition
training can be initiated at the earliest developmental
stages.   The diagnostic/identification team is responsible
for referral and continued audiologic-otologic management
during these years (Northern and Downs, 1974).   A variety of
program descriptions which trace screening, diagnosis, and
rehabilitation protocols have been presented as part of these
conferences (Mencher, 1976; Gerber and Mencher, 1978).

       Handicapping conditions such as hearing impairment,
involve many agencies which attempt to interact on behalf of
an individual child.   For example, in Massachusetts, a child
of 1 year, identified via a school for the deaf diagnostic
center upon referral of a pediatrician, would be able to have
the cost of diagnostic services paid by the Department of
Public Health; may have purchase of personal hearing aids
funded through the Massachusetts Rehabilitation Commission;
and, may have Parent-Infant training programs coordinated
by a center jointly funded by the Departments of Public
Health and Mental Health, but provided in part at the school
for the deaf.   Within the year following diagnosis of the
hearing impairment, all these agencies would be faced with
coordinating their programs with those of the school district
in which the child resides.

       This sample description may vary from state to state,
but similar procedures are found nationwide.   The most significant trend nationally has been the inter-relationship
among educational agencies and human service agencies of a
state.   This process becomes more complex, even cumbersome,
when other dimensions are present in the profile of the child,
such as: fluctuating hearing loss, bicultural/bilingual
families, and additional handicapping conditions.   The
administrative location of an early intervention program may
affect its adequacy, due to a continued need for referrals

to other centers where the primary expertise is not management of the hearing impairment. As the etiologic bases of
hearing impairment changes with each resulting condition,
more complex program delivery for families must become more
comprehensive.

B. Exemplary Models of Services
    to Very Young Children

     One federal agency in the United States is responsible
for most of the design, coordination, and evaluation of
services to handicapped children, that being the Bureau of
Education for the Handicapped (a division in the Department
of Education). Their efforts to upgrade services to handicapped children involve collation of technical information
as well as qualitative program assistance through monies
which are allocated nationwide. The Bureau of Education for
the Handicapped compiles data which individual state or
private agencies can assess for assistance in designing
programs for handicapped children. A priority of the Bureau
has been to help several state and private centers develop
and evaluate innovative programs for the very young handicapped children. These programs are funded via the Bureau's
Division of Innovation and Research and are available to both
rural and urban communities. Generally, the funded programs
provide comprehensive services to families with children with
a range of handicapping conditions, classified according to
severity rather than category of handicap. Due to the historic trend in services to hearing impaired children who have
traditionally been segregated by category and provided for in
segregated facilities, there exists a dichotomy within the
fields of early childhood/special education/education of the
deaf, regarding the level and degree of handicap which can
be absorbed by cross categorical programs. One of the goals
of the Bureau of Education for the Handicapped demonstration
projects has been to provide staff with expertise in areas
which clearly overlap the handicapping conditions found within low-incidence* groups. Significant progress has occurred

---

*   Low incidence includes:
    Hearing impaired
    Visually impaired
    Multiply handicapped, as opposed to high incidence (within
    the 12% total) such as mental retardation, learning dis-
    abilities, and speech impaired (Sontag, 1977).

in the development of materials designed to be used with
parents and siblings of the handicapped.

Educators of the deaf, who have distinguished themselves
in developing programs for very young hearing-impaired children, feel strongly about segregating their children from
handicapped with different disabilities. The literature
includes many descriptions of integrated nursery school programs for hearing-impaired children (integrated with non-
handicapped children). However, the national exemplary programs for very young handicapped children tend to provide
language intervention, related services, and parent training
for groups of handicapped children with differing handicaps
(Graham, 1976). Additional research is needed in this area
of program design, especially regarding hearing-impaired
children who display additional handicaps (Lowell and Lowell,
1978). One alternative used in some early intervention programs is differential staffing in order to meet the special
needs of the hearing impaired in a cross-categorical program;
i.e., educator of the deaf along with consultative audiologic,
otologic, pediatric, and speech and language services.

Some states have designed regional area agencies to provide services to all very young handicapped children. Staffing of these regional centers includes, among others, educational audiologists, speech clinicians, early childhood
specialists, and family guidance social workers. An established team of professionals is available throughout the
region to assist families with management of their handicapped
children throughout identification, assessment, and placement
facets of the child's educational life, birth to 21 years.
The same personnel work with the family until vocational
training occurs. When necessary, the team works with medical
and related service providers. The professionals have direct
contact with the school districts in the region. This model
(particularly well defined in Iowa) assists families of
hearing-impaired children and multi-handicapped children. A
consistent case manager is known to the family and to the
other professionals who may be called upon to assess the
child's needs at a particular developmental stage. Direct
articulation with the local school districts is possible and
the inter-agency funding resources necessary to support the
child and family are established centrally.

The United States government requires differentiation
between the hard of hearing and deaf categories of hearing
impairment. Hard of hearing children are not solely

classified by dB thresholds, but rather according to behavioural criteria for speech and language proficiency and the
need for special educational placement for academic achievement. Typically, hard of hearing children are served via
local schools, public or private nursery schools, and regular
class placements with support services. Deaf children require
special class placements, special educational services, etc.
There is a growing effort to recognize the various educational assessment and direct service needs of the hard of hearing
child and to identify all hearing impaired children geneti-
cally. In effect, an awareness of the inadequacy of services
to hard of hearing children is addressed by using the inclusive term "hearing impaired" (Davis, 1977; Ross and Nober,
1980).

     According to the available data on educational placement
of handicapped children, preschool (3 - 5 years) hearing
impaired children are served in various educational environments: 22% in regular school programs, 55% in separate
classes for the hearing impaired, and 20% in separate school
facilities for the hearing impaired (Report to Congress,
1979). These data, obtained for the 1976 - 1977 school year,
indicate differences with educational environments of children with other handicaps. It is explained as an extension
of the historic leadership factors of education of the deaf
(Report to Congress, 1979). This perspective is consonant
with other countries' services to the hearing impaired in
contrast to other handicapping conditions.

C.   Concerns of Parents and
     Early Identification Programs

     The formidable responsibilities of early intervention
programs to parents of hearing impaired children have been
described by many authors (Northcott, 1976; Murphy, 1979).
It is significant that services to very young children are
new (relatively) in the United States and are not universal
(Northern and Downs, 1974). Parents often feel strongly
dependent on the personnel and philosophy of the center
which initially diagnosed a problem and assisted them with
programs for themselves and their children. An impressive
description of the behaviour of audiologists in relation to
diagnosis is presented by Jersch and Amon (Northern and Downs,
1974).

While many professionals describe parents who reject the diagnosis of hearing impairment and seek alternate opinions regularly, I believe this need for parents to seek confirmation and validation of the handicapping condition is appropriate behaviour for the family. Each professional may add to the family's awareness and additional counsel may assist the family in their search for better educational opportunities for their children (Northern and Downs, 1974). The burdens of learning about the consequences of hearing impairment fall on the parents. Programs for very young hearing impaired children may not provide adequate information to parents who may have different expectations, cultural background, or abilities to act as trainers for their young children. The elitism issue of professionals dealing with parents of handicapped children is one which has not changed, even with all of our information.

New United States Legislation

A. Components of Education for
    All Handicapped Children's Act

The Education of All Handicapped Children's Act, (United States Public Law 94-142), and many state laws enacted in the early 1970's, attempted to alter the service delivery system to special needs children. As a culminating piece of legislation, technical assistance and federal funds were made available to states and territories so that previous discriminatory practices toward handicapped children would be eliminated and prevented in the future. Indeed, civil rights of handicapped children, youth, and adults are guaranteed. The concept of "Education as an equalizer," a basic tenet of the American democratic system, has been affirmed in legislation (Weintraub and Abeson, 1976).

Several components of the federal legislation are important to the service delivery system for hearing impaired children, ages 3 - 21 years.

1. The Local Education Agency (LEA) (i.e., the local school district) within the individual state is deemed the appropriate agency to determine identification, assessment, and placement of all handicapped children. The State Education Agency (SEA) monitors the functions of

the Local Education Agencies and collates and reports
information on services to the handicapped directly to
the Commissioner of Education via the United States
Department of Education, Bureau of Education for the
Handicapped (Ballard, 1977).

2. Each child identified as handicapped will have an Individualized Education Program (IEP) prepared by a team of
parents and professionals. This IEP will include general
goals and specific objectives to be attained by the child
within a one year time frame. The IEP must be reviewed
annually to determine appropriateness of services for
the child (Torres, 1977). Special educational and related
services the child will receive during the year must be
delineated in the IEP.

3. The Education of All Handicapped Children's Act states
that all handicapped children, ages 3 - 21, shall be
eligible for services to meet their individual special
educational needs at no cost to parents. In order to
effect this aspect of the federal law for preschool
children (ages 3 - 5), a financial incentive was incorporated into the funding formula by Congress. In effect,
it provides additional monies for each preschool handicapped child identified and served by the school district.
Early intervention was considered a significant priority.
To defray additional costs, local Head Start programs,
integrated public and private nursery schools, and new
programs within school districts were designated as
appropriate providers of services to preschool handicapped
children (Ballard, 1977). Although public education for
non-handicapped, preschool children is not mandated by
federal law, the importance of early identification and
intervention for handicapped preschool children is clearly
incorporated into the legislation.

B. Relationship of Legislation to
    Birth to Three Year Age Group

These few components of federal and state legislation
have a direct relationship to those institutions and agencies
involved in programs for hearing impaired children, from
birth to 3 years. To date, the Education of All Handicapped
Children's Act guarantees services to hearing impaired children after they reach their third birthday. Many states
currently provide programs to children, birth to 21 years, an

extension of the federal mandate (Abeson and Ballard, 1976).
The White House Conference on Handicapped Individuals (1977)
included recommendations from the Education subgroup advocating extending the age range of services downward (White House
Conference Summary, 1978). Organizations involved with
handicapped children and youth have testified before Congress
in support of extending the age range to birth (Alexander
Graham Bell Association for the Deaf, Council for Exceptional
Children, American Speech-Language-Hearing Association).
Indeed, advocacy groups which represent hearing impaired
individuals have been most effective in previous lobbying
efforts to upgrade services to the handicapped (Northcott,
1973; 1980).

C. New Requirements for Early
    Intervention Programs

     Since there is direct referral between programs serving
hearing impaired children ages birth - 3, and those serving
children 3 - 21 years, it is important for programs dealing
with the youngest handicapped children to be knowledgeable
about all requirements of federal law (Northcott, 1976). The
components of state and federal legislation have a direct
relationship to the program design of early intervention
services for hearing impaired children. Some of the outstanding requirements are:

1. To report all children identified as handicapped to the
    school district in which the family resides before the
    children have reached their third birthday.

2. To identify an appropriate liaison person from the early
    intervention setting to work cooperatively with the state
    education department and the local school districts.

3. To establish workable interagency relationships with
    human service agencies in the region.

4. To facilitate parent choice in determining "appropriate-
    ness" of programs rather than promoting self serving
    needs for enrollments.

5. To establish a relationship with local school districts
    so that personnel from the early intervention setting are
    invited to act as advocates for children entering into a
    new educational setting. In effect, to be invited to the
    local school district IEP meeting.

6. To provide appropriate "Related Services" for those
    hearing impaired children as needed; such as, special
    transportation, physical therapy, occupational therapy,
    movement education, and other services (Ballard, 1977).
    If the range of etiologies which result in hearing
    impairment also result in multiple handicaps, integrated
    interventions with other specialists will be necessary
    during infancy (Graham, 1976; Lowell, 1978). Children
    with multiple handicaps may not be good candidates for
    Parent-Infant programs located at schools for deaf where
    related services necessary for other handicaps are less
    available.

7. To gain expertise in developing IEPs for very young
    children consistent with parent views and concerns
    (Nober, 1978; Lowell, 1979; McGee, 1979). Perhaps local
    school districts and schools for the deaf are better
    prepared to meet this requirement than personnel from
    health related agencies.

    A critical issue for programs serving very young hearing
impaired children involves the program's treatment and materials for parents regarding mode of communication for the
hearing impaired (Graham, 1976; Lowell and Lowell, 1978).
The apparent lack of descriptions of alternate communication
styles for hearing impaired children, youth, and adults, is
a continuing problem in education of the deaf. There is an
encampment attitude on the part of many programs which may
result in parent fears, or feelings of failure toward their
children if another mode of communication is introduced later
in life. This problem is not easily resolved. The need for
extensive and appropriate resources for parents of the hearing impaired has been overlooked. Early intervention programs should describe to parents the pros and cons of various
methods of teaching language to the hearing impaired and
presenting guidelines for selection of a communication mode
(Luterman, 1979).

D. Funding Sources for Handicapped
    Children

    Until the age range of the Education for All Handicapped
Children's Act is extended to birth, decisions about educational management of the hearing impaired child will need to
be made by early intervention programs and local school
districts when the child is about 2½ years old. Frequently,

decisions are made in consultation with other professionals
whose operational base is more medical/clinical than educational. Federal legislation which enables states to provide
this type of coordinated service to young children pre-dates
the Education of All Handicapped Children Act. In 1965, the
Elementary and Secondary School Act Amendment (known as
Public Law 89-313), Federal Assistance to State Operated and
Supported Schools for the Handicapped, was enacted (Lavor,
1976). A recent development (September, 1979) in the regulations governing P.L. 89-313 enables state departments of
education to divert educational funds to those public health
or mental health programs which serve very young children
who cannot be served by public schools. There is variance
among the states regarding the distribution and allocation
of education monies under P.L. 89-313, but in most communities, the agency providing services on a regional basis to
severely impaired children has maximized federal monies via
Social Security funds to dependent children, public welfare,
public health, mental health, and education funds. In effect,
the Education of All Handicapped Children's Act and the
revised regulations of other legislation are affecting early
intervention programs as the child reaches age 3. A legisla-
tive vehicle is in place for more severely handicapped children to attend segregated schools and have similar mechanisms
for the monitoring of programs.

Are Local Schools Ready
for Hearing Impaired Babies?

The issues raised in this paper reflect a growing list
of responsibilities and considerations which will be assumed
by personnel in early intervention programs for hearing
impaired children. These issues are:

1)   the components of federal legislation for 3 - 5 year olds;

2)   the interagency relationships;

3)   cross-categorical versus single handicap models of
     service;

4)   parent roles and guarantees.

As experience with new legislation expands, those professionals involved with early intervention programs for the
hearing impaired will have to design a set of guidelines so

that school districts will have professional input in their
decisions for individual children. Unless educators of the
deaf, audiologists, and speech clinicians can document the
special circumstances of early intervention programs which
are to serve a single category of handicap (hearing impairment), the school districts will follow the mandates of the
legislation and integrate hearing impaired children with
other handicapped children. Indeed, if the legislation age
range is extended downward to include children birth to 21
years, an extensive set of guidelines will be necessary.
Many models of service in countries other than the United
States include partial integration/partial single category
designs and may be appropriate to this low incidence handicap.

The most significant component of the United States
service delivery system should not be overlooked or under-
estimated; i.e., a written individualized educational program
for the child, determined by professionals and parents. Local
schools have had more experience with this component than have
segregated early intervention programs. As professionals, we
must become more adept at written documentation which includes
parent views in the same way local school personnel have
accomplished this function.

Families of very young hearing impaired children require
opportunities to meet and talk with adult hearing impaired
persons so that realistic educational planning for their
children can occur. Specialized centers for hearing impaired
children within established educational environments or
schools for the deaf may be best suited to fill this need,
rather than local schools. To date, this absence of consumer
counselling in schools for the deaf has not been addressed.

Each program attempting to provide multidisciplinary
services to very young hearing impaired children requires
established protocols for involvement of other specialists;
particularly special education, physical therapy, occupational therapy, and early childhood/special education so that
appropriate services are obtained for families in a facilitative manner. Individual families should not be required to
ferret out appropriate services or be denied those services,
but should have systematic and programmed referral and consultative contacts. Perhaps local school districts have had
to develop these related services more quickly than programs
for the hearing impaired preschool child. It is clear that
the mandates of the new legislation require alterations in
those programs we have deemed comprehensive, particularly
those located at schools for the deaf.

A review of personnel preparation programs reveals a
dearth of training to meet these changing responsibilities
in all fields relative to hearing impaired children (Northcott
1976). The American Speech-Language-Hearing Association,
the Council of Executives of the Deaf, special education,
community health, and other credentialing organizations do
not contain provisions or training competencies which would
reflect the needs of those individuals who will work with
very young hearing impaired children. The lack of consistency of regulations from state to state is a roadblock to
altering training mandates. The differences in service
delivery have resulted in on-the-job training by audiologists
and speech clinicians since, in many settings, they are
viewed by the agency as the most appropriate case managers
for a hearing impaired child (Ross and Nober, 1980).

These are significant problems for leaders in the field
to address. The exchange of information between professionals
may assist United States professionals in their efforts to
upgrade services to handicapped children via the new federal
legislation. Local schools can provide some answers to the
problems of educating very young hearing impaired children.
We need to define these parameters more effectively.

REFERENCES

Abeson, A. and Ballard, J. "State and Federal Policy for
    Exceptional Children" in Weintraub, F., Abeson, A.,
    Ballard, J. and LaVor, M. (eds.) Public Policy and the
    Education of Exceptional Children (Reston, Virginia:
    CEC), 1976.

Ballard, J. "Active Federal Education Laws for Exceptional
    Persons" in Weintraub, F., Abeson, A., Ballard, J., LaVor,
    M. (eds.) Public Policy and the Education of Exceptional
    Children (Reston, Virginia: CEC), 1976.

Ballard, J. P.L. 94-142 and Section 504 - Understanding
    What They Are and Are Not (Reston, Virginia: CEC), 1977.

Cox, B.P. and Lloyd, L. "Audiological Considerations" in
    Lloyd, L. (ed.) Communication Assessment and Intervention
    Strategies (Baltimore: University Park Press), 1976.

Davis, J. (ed.) Our Forgotten Children: Hard-of-Hearing Pupils in the Schools (Minneapolis: National Support Systems), 1977.

Gerber, S. and Mencher, G. (eds.) Early Diagnosis of Hearing Loss (New York: Grune & Stratton, Inc.), 1978.

Graham, L. "Language Programming and Intervention" in Lloyd, L. (ed.) Communication Assessment and Intervention Strategies (Baltimore: University Park Press), 1976.

LaVor, M. "Federal Legislation for Exceptional Persons: A History" in Weintraub, F., Abeson, A., Ballard, J., and LaVor, M. (eds.) Public Policy and the Education of Exceptional Children (Reston, Virginia: CEC), 1976.

Lowell, E.L. "Parent Infant Programs for Preschool Deaf Children: The Example of John Tracy Clinic" Volta Review 81:323 - 329, 1979.

Lowell, E.L. and Lowell, M.O. "Interaction of Assessment and Intervention" in Minifie, F. and Lloyd, L. (eds.) Communicative and Cognitive Abilities - Early Behavioural Assessment (Baltimore: University Park Press), 1978.

Mencher, G.T. (ed.) Early Identification of Hearing Loss (Basel: Karger) 1976.

McGee, D. "IEPs for Hearing Impaired Children: Information for Parents and Teachers" Volta Review 81:199 - 210, 1979.

Murphy, A. "The Families of Handicapped Children: Context for Disability" Volta Review 81:165 - 178, 1979.

Nober, L.W. "Developing Effective IEPs for the Hearing Impaired: Considerations and Issues" in Wiener, B. (ed.) Periscope: Views of the Individualized Educational Program (Reston, Virginia: CEC), 1978.

Northcott, W. The Hearing Impaired Child in a Regular Classroom: Preschool, Elementary and Secondary Years (Washington, D.C.: Alexander Graham Bell Association for the Deaf), 1973.

Northcott, W. "Mainstreaming the Preprimary Hearing Impaired 0-6: Practices, Progress, Problems" in Nix, G. (ed.) Mainstream Education for Hearing Impaired Children and Youth (New York: Grune & Stratton, Inc.), 1976.

Northcott, W. "On Behalf of Parents in the IEP Process" Volta Review 82:7 - 13, 1980.

Northern, J. and Downs, M. Hearing in Children (Baltimore: Williams and Wilkins Co.), 1974.

Report to Congress on the Implementation of P.L. 94-142: The Education for All Handicapped Children Act, HEW Publication No. (OE) 79-05003, U.S. Government Printing Office, Washington, D.C.: January, 1979.

Ross, M. and Nober, L. Educational Programming Considerations for Hard of Hearing Children (Minneapolis: Leadership Training Institute Press), 1980.

Torres, S. A Primer on Individualized Educational Programs for Handicapped Children (Reston, Virginia: CEC), 1977.

Sontag, E., Smith, S. and Sailor, W. "The Severely/ Profoundly Handicapped: Why Are They? Where Are They?" Journal of Special Education Vol II, 1977.

Weintraub, F. and Abeson, A. "New Educational Policies for the Handicapped: The Quiet Revolution" in Weintraub, F., Abeson, A., Ballard, J. and LaVor, M. (eds.) Public Policy and the Education of Exceptional Children (Reston, Virginia: CEC), 1976.

White House Conference of Handicapped Individuals, Summary, Final Report, Washington, D.C.: U.S. Government Printing Office, 1978.

EPILOGUE: THE WAY WE ARE

George T. Mencher
Nova Scotia Hearing and Speech Clinic, Halifax, Nova Scotia

In my prologue, I spoke of "The Way We Were"; that is, all the events and procedures which have brought us to this meeting. What we have heard in the last two days is "The Way We Are" - where we stand, where we agree, and where we disagree. I now have the awesome and somewhat dubious responsibility of trying to integrate what we have heard in the last two days; of trying to place it into some framework; of trying to highlight areas of agreement and disagreement; and, of course, of trying to focus our discussion to those areas where the recommendations of this conference can be definitive and meaningful.

There is no doubt, as Grace Harris pointed out in her keynote address, that each of our disciplines has demonstrated significant growth and improved capability in the area of early management of hearing loss. But gaps in our knowledge and in our interdisciplinary action are still present. Until those gaps are eliminated, progress and growth will be continually restricted. Miss Harris stressed that we have an obligation to encourage interdisciplinary action which is immediate and involves individual parent/child intervention as early as possible. Early management results in a child who is better prepared to function successfully in a communication centered world, and it does so at much less cost to the community than it costs not to do it.

Mrs. Downs also stressed interdisciplinary action. She suggested that it is only through a team approach to congenital deafness that necessary support and guidance is offered to the child and the parents. The initial diagnosis should be followed by ongoing monitoring and evaluation to determine the child's progress in his program, and to re-evaluate the original diagnosis, which may change with time.

Doctor Shea reminded us that the primary care physician is critical to the management team, and that family physicians need to be taught to be <u>AWARE</u> of the hearing impaired.

That is:

A - <u>aware</u> of at risk children and subtle signs suggesting
    hearing loss;

W - to know <u>what</u> to do to investigate suspect infants and
    what to do to preserve residual hearing;

A - to be <u>advocates</u> for development of facilities for assess-
    ment and habilitation;

R - to know <u>rehabilitation</u> facilities and to be able to pro-
    perly guide the patient and his family to appropriate
    programs; and, finally,

E - to be <u>empathetic</u> to the patient and the family.

    I should note in passing that the term "advocates"
which Doctor Shea used, seemed to appear as often in this
conference as any other concept.

    Dr. Robert Ruben presented the view of the otologist,
suggesting that otologic care include not only a complete
otorhinolaryngological examination, but evaluation of other
major organ systems as well (e.g., the CNS, or the Visual
system). Sometimes the otologist assumes the role of genetic
counsellor to the family; and, after the diagnosis of hearing
impairment, is responsible for monitoring for progression of
the hearing loss and for care of intermittent ear disease.

    Speaking of intermittent ear disease, Dr. Jerry Northern
suggested that the use of impedance measurements in infants
is still a very controversial issue, and that the final
answer is not within our grasp as more research is necessary.
However, in view of the fact that, of 3.5 million babies born
in the United States, about 70% will have otitis media with
effusion by age 3, impedance techniques must be improved so
as to reduce false negative errors. Doctor Northern recommended acoustic reflex as a valuable technique in the identification of deaf babies, in spite of all the difficulties
with impedance itself. He cautioned that the entire impedance battery should be used in complement and that no single
test stands alone. Doctor Brooks concurred. He also urged
early identification and management of middle ear disease and
intermittent hearing loss, so as to prevent learning disorders in otherwise normal children.

of all, the title of their paper, "Bilingualism: An Environment for the Deaf Infant", has to be one of the more controversial presented here today. The paper, of course, develops
a philosophic and pedagogic view that early management procedures which are truly total are the most appropriate. Key
to the address was an attempt to establish the linguistic
validity of American Sign Language, and a recommendation
regarding its usage in educational programming. Surely, this
controversy will occupy a great deal of our time within the
next few days, not to mention that it is a controversy which
has survived the centuries.

Doreen Pollock offered her view. She suggested that,
with the advent of modern hearing aids, the deaf infant of
today needs to spend very little time in a silent world. Our
expectations for deaf children must change as we put modern
technology to its optimal use, and as we study normal development. Limits should not be placed upon the infant at an early
age: he can develop the interrelated skills of audition,
speech and language following normal sequential stages. If
not, then we must look at the child as an individual who may
have additional problems. The group labelled "hearing
impaired" is a diverse group.

As if to further compound the confusion, Dr. Kevin
Murphy spoke of the three "D's" of disability: detection,
diagnosis, and dealing with. He said there is a continued
need to recognize that there is a real difference between
acuity and function and between impairment and handicap. He
also suggested that, for multiply disabled children, the
shock to parents is usually greater than for a single handicap. By the same token, the parents are more often likely to
become involved in the diagnostic/therapeutic process. Then,
forging full-speed ahead into the methodology controversy,
Doctor Murphy suggested that multiply handicapped children
need as many receptors as possible, and that the key sensory
modality for the multiply handicapped hearing-impaired child
is tactile. It encourages mobility and through a system of
cross modal transfer, it aids in improving auditory function.
I might add here that we did not have representation at the
meeting from the Guberina Verbo-Tonal Method developed in
Yugoslavia. It would have been interesting to have heard
their opinions on all of this.

Mrs. Tell from Jerusalem reported on the long-term
follow-up of children diagnosed as hearing-impaired as babies
in the famous Jerusalem study of 1967 through 1972. She
stressed the role of parent co-operation as being the most
decisive factor in the habilitation program, with approximately 2/3 of the children being able to succeed in integrated
regular schools, regardless of the application of oral or
total communication methods.

Doctor Bentzen told us that the European Economic
Community has studied the problems of the deaf and hearing
impaired in Europe. One of the most significant findings of
their report was that the ability of children with a hearing
loss of 90 dB or greater in the better ear to speak intelligibly differs rather dramatically from country to country.
Noted was the fact that the degree of integration with normal
hearing and speaking children was very important to speech
and language development, as was the earliest possible provision of hearing aids.

Dr. Martha Rubin agreed that hearing aids are only a
part of the total rehabilitation program, but still an important part. To quote her, "the fitting of a hearing aid is
the first tangible sign to the family that the child is
handicapped," and, therefore, it is an extremely critical
phase in the habilitative program. She suggested that it
seems prudent to start with monaural amplification until the
parents accept the aid, and then to move to a binaural fitting.
That is certainly an interesting interpretation, as the majority of the time our decision on a monaural or binaural fitting
is based on the child's response to the hearing aid. She
also suggested the selection of the hearing aid depends on
ergonomic characteristics, electro-acoustic parameters, and
repair capabilities; and that post-auricular aids for babies
can be a reality when preceeded by proper counselling and
fitting, and when parental support is complete.

Mrs. Downs, in her second presentation, agreed with
Doctor Rubin on the question of factors influencing hearing
aid choice. She said that because babies cannot tell us what
they hear, hearing aid selection for them cannot be made on
the basis of the same objective criteria as for adults. Thus,
guidelines for the upper and lower limits and frequency
response characteristics of hearing aids become really critical. Discussion focused on the need to limit saturation output because of the deliterious effects of not doing so.

Mrs. Downs also suggested that use of split frequency band fittings in a fairly standard pattern might be an appropriate methodology for babies. Jacobson, et al, considered the use of ABR not only as a technique for determining the audiogram, but also as a method for evaluating the effectiveness of amplification in very young babies. Jerry Northern proposed a model for using impedance measurements in determining hearing aid fitting.

Mrs. Downs raised the question of how mild a hearing loss can, or should be fitted with a hearing aid, with the opinion offered that losses as low as 15 dB can be successfully aided. That will certainly provide discussion and should be a very controversial issue. All in all, amplification procedures, limitations, and approaches should be a key area for discussion and recommendations.

Finally, Dr. Linda Nober discussed the effects of current legislation in the United States on parent and child rights, facilities, and programming for the hearing impaired.

This has been a long, tiring, interesting, fascinating, confusing, thought provoking and, I hope, exciting conference. The future promises to be more of the same. I hope we have stimulated your ideas and titillated your minds. I hope you can think about what you have read here, and apply at least some of it in your everyday work situation.

You have heard "The way we are." Our recommendations are "The way we ought to be." We hope they, too, will be helpful, meaningful, and most important, useful.

Doctor Shea concluded with that beautiful quote from Dr. Burton Jaffe, one of the participants in the Saskatoon Conference: "Deafness never, of itself, killed anyone; but who can count the lives it has wasted." Let us hope that the results of this conference can significantly reduce that number!!

AUTHOR INDEX